MANAGERIAL
EPIDEMIOLOGY

SECOND EDITION

MANAGERIAL EPIDEMIOLOGY

SECOND EDITION

STEVEN T. FLEMING, PhD

Health Administration Press, Chicago
Asscociation of University Programs in Health Administration, VA

AUPHA

Library of Congress Cataloging-in-Publication Data

Fleming, Steven T., 1950–
   Managerial epidemiology : concepts and cases / by Steven Fleming. — 2nd ed.
      p. ; cm.
   Includes bibliographical references and index.
   ISBN-13: 978-1-56793-292-8 (alk. paper)
   ISBN-10: 1-56793-292-4 (alk. paper)
 1. Health services administration. 2. Epidemiology—Methodology. I. Title.
   [DNLM: 1. Epidemiologic Methods. 2. Health Services Administration. WA 950 F598m 2008]
   RA971.F54 2008
   614.4—dc22

                              2007046084

Project manager: Eduard Avis; Acquisitions editor: Janet Davis; Cover design: Chris Underdown

Health Administration Press   Association of University Programs
A division of the Foundation   in Health Administration
   of the American College of   2000 14th Street North
   Healthcare Executives   Suite 780
One North Franklin Street   Arlington, VA 22201
Suite 1700   (703) 894-0940
Chicago, IL 60606-3529
(312) 424-2800

Printer: Cushing-Malloy
Typeface: Galliard

To my loving wife Alayne, my very best friend of 35 years, confidante, and consultant extraordinaire. Thank you for sharing my life with me.

To a great mentor and brilliant theorist, Avedis Donabedian.

BRIEF CONTENTS

DETAILED CONTENTS

FOREWORD

James W. Holsinger, Jr.

Late one night when I was a young surgery resident, several other residents and I were recuperating with a midnight snack when one of our group asked the intern among us why he was so old. The intern told us that he had not entered college immediately following high school but had worked in his family's ranching and crop-dusting business. He was asked if he knew how to fly, and his response was a classic: "I've been flying as a crop duster since I was 16. I am the third-best crop duster in the state of Florida, but the two best are dead. You see, I don't get the 5 percent in the corners." His answer was a paradigm for life, since "squaring the corners," getting the one and a quarter percent in each corner, is what kills crop dusters—just as struggling to get that last 5 percent for a perfect healthcare management decision is what keeps many good decisions from being made.

For many years in my career as a physician executive, I struggled with making management decisions at a 95 percent confidence level. Only late in my career did I realize the importance of epidemiology in making those decisions. In retrospect, a managerial epidemiology course early in my career would have been a major benefit in reaching sound healthcare decisions.

Managerial epidemiology is as critical to managing healthcare organizations as managerial accounting. However, healthcare leaders often relegate epidemiology to the realm of infection control or public health. Understanding the health of populations and communities is essential for the careful planning and execution of good healthcare decisions.

The usefulness of managerial epidemiology was proven time and again while I served as Kentucky's Secretary of Health and Family Services. For example, epidemiology played a major role in the revitalization of the state's Medicaid program, and it helped create a financially sound program for the University of Kentucky's self-insured health plan. To succeed, managers must bring a keen understanding of managerial epidemiology to the decision-making process. To do less results in an inadequate process, often ending in suboptimal decisions.

This second edition of *Managerial Epidemiology: Concepts and Cases*, authored by my colleague Steve Fleming, provides the prospective healthcare manager with the tools needed to use epidemiology in healthcare decision making. Healthcare managers who use these skills can make decisions at a 95 percent confidence level. *Managerial Epidemiology* is clearly the product of an excellent course syllabus, as it flows from theory to practice to application. It shows students how epidemiology applies to finance and evidence-based management. The final section of this book demonstrates the usefulness of epidemiology applied to specific chronic diseases: cardio-vascular disease, AIDS, and Alzheimer's disease.

The many cases, a hallmark of this textbook, have been crafted with great care to provide the student with real-life examples that clarify the text and provide practical direction. Questions posed for each case help the student grasp the issues presented. Feedback is immediate, since suggested answers are provided for each question. The cases are an integral part of the teaching methodology, not simply an end-of-chapter exercise.

Healthcare managers often try to square the corners on their decisions without using epidemiology. That's unfortunate, because without the tools provided by epidemiology, healthcare management practitioners will be unable to meet the challenges of twenty-first-century healthcare. With the tools provided by *Managerial Epidemiology*, they will succeed admirably.

James W. Holsinger Jr., M.D., Ph.D.
Charles T. Wethington Endowed Chair in the Health Sciences,
College of Public Health, and
Chancellor-Emeritus,
Chandler Medical Center,
University of Kentucky

PREFACE

This book is a comprehensive introduction to the concepts and principles of epidemiology and an examination of how those principles are applied to healthcare management. The book could be a stand-alone text for (1) a course that introduces students to the field of epidemiology and provides applications to management, (2) a course that seeks to apply epidemiologic principles to management, and (3) a basic "introduction to epidemiology" course.

This second edition of *Managerial Epidemiology: Concepts and Cases* represents a significant departure from the first edition in that it removes the paradigm that was used in the first edition. In the first edition, managerial epidemiology was discussed as the application of epidemiologic principles organized around the functions of a manager. In this new edition, the book is structured more along the lines of basic principles first, then specific applications to management.

A second major change with this second edition is the expansion of the descriptive epidemiology chapter (Chapter 2 in the first edition) into four chapters.

A third major change with this edition is the use of more and longer case studies. These 41 case studies are integrated into the text (though highlighted by shaded boxes) and include detailed answers or solutions. The case studies in this book are not optional exercises at the end of each chapter, but rather important aspects of the teaching methodology.

A fourth change with this second edition is the organization of the methods chapters into Part III: "Evidence-Based Management and Medicine." These chapters include the statistics chapter, the three study design chapters, and the clinical epidemiology chapter.

A final major change with this edition is the addition of three specific application chapters. The purpose of these chapters is to focus on specific kinds of patients (those with cardiovascular disease, HIV, and dementia), discuss the epidemiology associated with each group of patients, and give case studies that refer back to many of the basic concepts that were discussed in earlier chapters.

Many of us have reviewed or adopted textbooks and asked ourselves, "Why did the authors arrange the chapters in this order?" We designed the syllabus and arranged chapters in what we thought was a logical order. The "pioneer" students of the course on which this book is based complained of too much theory and not enough application. In an effort to face their honest and reasonable criticism, I have integrated numerous case study applications throughout the text. Beyond that, however, the chapters are arranged in a more integrated order: morbidity; then two application chapters; then mortality and descriptive epidemiology across time, place, and person.

In an effort to encourage the instructor to embrace the case-study approach to teaching, Health Administration Press maintains online Instructor Resources for this textbook. On this website, there are numerous case studies. Some of the cases on this website are cases from the text with changed parameters. Other cases include some written by students in my managerial epidemiology courses. Instructors are encouraged to visit the website and use the case studies either in class, as didactic exercises, or as assigned homework for the students. Also available to instructors who use this book are PowerPoint slides. For access information to the Instructor Resources, write to hap1@ache.org.

I have numerous people to thank for their contributions of time, energy, and enthusiasm. Thank you to Alayne for listening to me babble epidemiology-speak far too often, I'm sure. To my colleagues and friends Tom Tucker and Doug Scutchfield, who coauthored the first edition of this text, thank you for getting me into this business of managerial epidemiology. To my talented contributors, dear colleagues and seasoned experts, thank you for adding depth, breadth, and luster to the text. The staff of Health Administration Press is to be commended for their encouragement and support, particularly Janet Davis, acquisitions editor, with whom I must have exchanged hundreds of e-mails. Eduard Avis, the project manager, provided an unbelievable amount of critical review, not just of spelling and grammar, but also epidemiologic theory and technique. My two student assistants, Tim Crawford and Rachel Hall, edited the text and provided helpful comments from a distinctly student perspective. And finally, as a man of faith, I acknowledge my limitations, confess to errors of commission or omission in the text, and attribute the occasional insight or brilliance to someone other than me.

Steven T. Fleming
February 2008

CONCEPTS, PRINCIPLES, AND APPLICATIONS

Epidemiology is the study of the distribution and determinants of disease in human populations. Thus, the study of epidemiology can be broadly divided into two main areas: descriptive epidemiology (distribution of disease) and analytical epidemiology (determinants of disease). Managerial epidemiology is the study of the application of epidemiologic concepts and principles to the practice of management. This first part focuses primarily on descriptive epidemiology, with selected applications to two critically important tasks of healthcare managers: planning and quality control.

Chapter 1 presents an overview of the entire text, as well as a case study of a fictitious managed care organization. The case study shows how valuable epidemiologic information is to healthcare decision making. Chapter 2 reviews infectious disease epidemiology, or how diseases are transmitted, particularly in healthcare settings. The third chapter is a study of morbidity—the nature, definition, and natural history of disease, including the sources and measurement of such conditions. Chapters 4 and 5 are application chapters where epidemiologic principles are applied to healthcare planning and quality control. Chapter 6 is a study of mortality, with a focus on the use of risk-adjusted mortality rates as measures of quality of care. Chapter 7 summarizes how descriptive epidemiology is typically oriented along three dimensions time, place, and person. A particular focus of this chapter is describing patterns of disease across geographic regions with the aid of Geographic Information Systems (GIS).

AN INTRODUCTION TO MANAGERIAL EPIDEMIOLOGY

Steven T. Fleming, Thomas Tucker, and
F. Douglas Scutchfield

Epidemiology is the study of the distribution and determinants of disease in human populations. Epidemiology has developed the tools by which we (1) measure the burden of disease in specific populations, (2) determine differences in the burden of disease between populations, (3) explore the origins or causes of differences in disease burdens, and (4) determine the effect of treatments and interventions on reducing the burden of disease. In other words, we can think of epidemiology as the tools we use to determine everything we know about interventions, treatments, and healthcare services.

This text examines ways to apply the principles and tools of epidemiology to the management of health services. Much like managerial accounting applies the principles of accounting to various management functions, this book applies the principles of epidemiology to the management of health services.

Health services management can be described many ways. One common way is to list the functions that managers perform, describe them one by one, elaborate on the descriptions, and form connections. Rakich, Longest, and Darr (1992) list the functions as planning, staffing, organizing, directing, and controlling. With each of these functions, health services managers must make decisions. For example, in the planning function, they decide which services they will provide and which they will not. As part of the staffing function, managers determine the skills required to provide specified services and decide on the type and number of staff needed to provide them. The organizing function requires managers to decide how various parts of the organization will relate to each other in order to maximize positive impact on health outcomes. As part of the directing function, managers provide vision and leadership to focus the organization on important goals. With the controlling function, managers determine if the organization is effective in producing the desired results. Each of these managerial functions requires decisions, and the decisions made in one functional domain almost always have consequences in other functional areas.

Managerial epidemiology uses the principles and tools of epidemiology to help managers make better-informed decisions in each of these functional domains; that is, *managerial epidemiology* is the application of the principles and tools of epidemiology to the decision-making process. The first edition of this text was organized specifically around the functions of a manager. The second edition is not organized that way. The first edition devoted only one chapter to descriptive epidemiology (Chapter 2). The second edition expands this coverage to four chapters (chapters 2, 3, 6, and 7). The first edition included short case studies (without answers) at the end of each chapter. The second edition integrates longer case studies (with answers) into the context of each chapter, and as such, the case studies become part of the formal didactic process, not an "optional" homework assignment at the end of each chapter. The second edition also includes three integrative "capstone" chapters at the end of the text on three modern-day "plagues"—cardiovascular disease, AIDS, and Alzheimer's disease.

This text is organized into four main parts. Descriptive epidemiology is covered in Part I (chapters 2 through 7), with specific applications to healthcare planning and quality of care. The application of epidemiology to financial management is discussed in Part II (chapters 8 and 9). Part III, on evidenced-based decision making, comprises chapters 10 through 14. Finally, Part IV provides a three-chapter capstone conclusion to the text by describing in epidemiological terms three critical important diseases to modern society.

Chapter 2 provides an overview of disease transmission and control, with a specific focus on infectious diseases. This includes the relationship between agent, host, and environment; concepts of disease transmission, incidence, and prevalence rates; the various kinds of epidemics; and methods to prevent and control disease. The two case studies in this chapter are about a food poisoning outbreak at the fictitious Bluegrass Hospital and an outbreak of influenza in a New York nursing home.

Chapter 3 deals with the measurement and interpretation of morbidity data. This includes the nature, definition, and "natural history" of disease, and sources of morbidity data. This chapter focuses on describing the important characteristics of diagnostic and screening tests. The three case studies in this chapter deal with product lines for a managed care organization, comparing the performance of digital and film mammography screening, and evaluating the performance of two different methods of prostate cancer screening executed in sequence.

Chapters 4 and 5 show how descriptive epidemiology applies to two important functions of a manager: planning and quality measurement and control. The application of epidemiology to planning is the topic of Chapter 4. Here the authors differentiate between community and institutional planning, discuss human resources planning and healthcare marketing, and summarize the basic principles of needs assessment. Three case studies are integrated into the text, one dealing with community health planning for a managed care organization in eastern Kentucky, one focused on determining bed demand for cardiac care in a new hospital construction project, and one dealing with a needs assessment for stroke services in Ontario, Canada. Chapter 5 applies epidemiologic principles to quality of care issues. The chapter discusses the various ways quality can be assessed using epidemiologic measures, and explores the concepts of rates, surveillance, risk adjustment, and quality measurement using various quality indicators. Ambulatory care-sensitive conditions and avoidable hospitalization rates are discussed as measures of quality within the context of managed care. Finally, the chapter explores ways epidemiology can play a fundamental role in total quality management. The three case studies woven into this chapter include one dealing with methicillin-resistant *Staphylococcus aureus* surveillance at a university hospital, another focused on complication rates in a small rural hospital, and a third discussing inpatient quality of care indicators at Bluegrass Hospital.

Chapter 6 concentrates on mortality, and discusses the sources and measurement of mortality data, methods for standardizing mortality rates by age, and the process of risk-adjusting mortality rates. Four case studies are included in this chapter: one that compares breast cancer mortality rates among immigrants and emigrants to/from Australia and Canada, one dealing with standardizing mortality rates for both age and gender, a third dealing with risk-adjusted mortality using contingency tables in Pennsylvania, and a fourth focused on risk-adjusted mortality using the multivariate approach of New York State.

Chapter 7 focuses on descriptive epidemiology in terms of measuring morbidity and mortality burden across time, place, and person, and includes discussion of spot maps, clusters, and geographic information systems (GIS). Case studies in this chapter include one dealing with infant mortality disparities by race, and a second dealing with using GIS to decide where to locate an HIV clinic in Kentucky.

Chapter 8 reviews the principles of epidemiology as they relate to financial management. Here the authors thoroughly expostulate the concept of risk, differentiate between the kinds of risk (or exposure) facing the patient, and describe the capitation environment. In addition to a discussion on the basics of capitation and risk adjustment, the chapter suggests possible ways of using morbidity and risk factors to adjust capitation rates. Case studies in this chapter include one dealing with incorporating risks into capitation rates, and one dealing with how a managed care organization could adjust for smoking and obesity in its capitation rates.

Cost-effectiveness analysis (CEA) is described in Chapter 9. The discussions include the process of program specification, how to measure costs and effectiveness (including quality-adjusted life years), how to control for biased estimates and uncertainty, and how to choose among programs using cost-effectiveness ratios. Case studies in this chapter include the Oregon

Medicaid Prioritization of Health Services Program, a CEA of treatment options for acute otitis media (earache), the cost-effectiveness of health insurance, and a CEA for targeted or universal prostate cancer screening.

Chapter 10 presents the basic statistical tools used in epidemiology and distinguishes between descriptive and inferential epidemiology, within the context of decision making for the healthcare manager. The chapter discusses the difference between continuous and categorical variables with measures of central tendency and variability for each type, and it describes various types of sampling methods. For inferential statistics, the authors discuss hypothesis testing, the concept of a p-value, and the distinction between type I (a) and type II (b) errors.

Chapters 11, 12, and 13 relate to various types of epidemiologic study designs. Chapter 11 explores the case control design by describing selection of cases and controls; the concepts of exposure, relative risk, and confounding variables; attributable fraction; and various kinds of bias, with a focus on misclassification bias. Prospective and retrospective cohort studies are compared in Chapter 12. The authors discuss selection, exposure, and relative risk within the context of a cohort study, and the difference between attributable fraction and attributable risk, as well as the methods by which incidence is measured over time. Randomized clinical trials are the subject of Chapter 13, which includes the concepts of protocols, randomization, historical controls, crossover designs, and treatment effects. The authors also describe the importance of blinding, ethics, and integrity within the randomization process. The chapter summarizes the concept of a hospital firm, the technique of meta-analysis, and the research design referred to as a community trial. Case studies in these chapters include those dealing with coffee and pancreatic cancer, smoking and low birth-weight newborns, smoking and prostate cancer, the Rand Health Insurance Experiment, and inpatient staffing at Henry Ford Hospital, among others.

Clinical epidemiology is the focus of Chapter 14. This acquaints the reader with how physicians can use epidemiology to make clinical decisions. It is useful and pragmatic for healthcare managers to be at least somewhat familiar with how physicians think. In this chapter, the authors distinguish between tradition-based and evidence-based medical practice, where epidemiologic studies can inform the latter. The chapter describes the clinical encounter in terms of diagnosis, treatment, and prevention, and discusses how epidemiology should provide the evidence necessary for rational decisions. Case studies in this chapter include making a diagnosis for a patient presenting with chest pain; treatment options for a patient diagnosed with gastroesophageal reflux disease; prevention and control strategies; family history and numbers-needed-to-treat; and the use of clinical decision-making tools.

Chapters 15, 16, and 17 focus on the application of epidemiologic principles to three major diseases that incur a substantial burden on society, in terms of both human suffering and financial resources. Two of the diseases, cardiovascular disease and Alzheimer's, are classified as chronic diseases. The third disease, HIV/AIDS, is relatively new and has elements of both an infectious and a chronic disease. The purpose of these three chapters is to present a capstone experience for the reader with a focus on these three diseases. Case studies in these chapters include screening for coronary artery calcium using electron beam computed tomography, testing for HIV with the ELISA test, cost-effectiveness of HIV testing, and study designs for Alzheimer's disease, among others.

Below is a detailed, multifaceted case study (with solution) involving a fictitious managed care organization in the Boston area. The purpose of this case study is to convince the reader that managers need to embrace the methods of epidemiology. Step into Mr. Jones's shoes as he wrestles with the issues.

Case Study 1.1. Group Health East

Group Health East (GHE) is a 100,000-member managed care organization (MCO) located in southern New England. GHE is a mixed-model MCO affiliated with two large multispecialty groups—Physicians Associates (PA) and Bayside Multispecialty Group (BMS)—in addition to 500 individual physicians in the community. PA provides in-house services in the north clinic; BMS provides services in the south. GHE is affiliated with two major metropolitan hospitals in the Boston area. The chief executive officer (CEO), Mr. Jones, is a 55-year-old hospital executive who crossed over into the managed care sector three years ago. GHE is going through a time of transition attributable to increased market competition, and it faces a number of important decisions that will affect its future. These decisions relate to organizational structure, staffing, incentives and performance appraisals, surveillance of adverse outcomes, strategic planning, and rate setting.

Each large GHE clinic maintains a functional organizational design with two main divisions—Support Services and Clinical Services—and separate departments in each division based on specific functions, such as housekeeping in Support Services and medicine in Clinical Services. An organization-wide medical staff, as well as separate medical staff organizations, practice at each of the two clinics. Based on his experience in large academic medical centers in the acute care sector, and on the recommendation of the system's governing board, Mr. Jones is considering moving to a matrix model organizational design, with separate product lines that affiliate with, and draw services from, the functional departments (e.g., nursing).

Mr. Jones is wrestling with a number of critical and fundamental questions at this juncture:

- What are the advantages and disadvantages of a matrix model for GHE in terms of direct and indirect costs, as well as benefits such as improved coordination?
- How many product lines should the organization identify?

• How should the organization determine which product lines ought to maintain separate identities as part of the matrix design?

In the past, Mr. Jones has distanced himself from clinical issues, and he is unfamiliar with the disease burden of the enrolled population served by the MCO. However, he wants to make better use of the experts within the organization to provide him with the epidemiological input that he needs. What kinds of data are needed to make him better informed?

The move to a matrix model is expected to affect staffing in a number of significant ways. Although the new model is expected to improve efficiency with regard to coordination of services, the effect of the new organizational structure is unclear in terms of the number of employees needed, both professional and otherwise, by the organization. More specifically, Mr. Jones is worried that the new structure will increase the total number of required physician generalists and specialists. His concern is founded, at least in part, on the uncertainty associated with the new structure and physician productivity. The focus on product lines may also break the market into segments in ways that would increase the demand for services. In addition to these staffing concerns, the nurse practitioners in two of the five satellite clinics have voiced concerns about workload and the amount of time they can spend with each patient.

Mr. Jones is dealing with a number of critical staff questions at this point:

• How can he estimate the number of affiliated physicians that will be needed to support the north and south clinics when the matrix model of organization is in place?
• Will the new structure increase or decrease physician productivity?
• What kinds of data are necessary to determine staffing needs with regard to nurse practitioners at the satellite clinics?

A recommendation of the board has also moved GHE to consider restructuring the incentive and performance appraisal system, specifically for physicians. Based on the experience of U.S. Healthcare, GHE would like to link capitation payments to outcomes. Currently, GHE negotiates separate capitation contracts with both PA and BMS, wherein the two groups are paid monthly per-member-per-month payments based on the total number of enrolled members for which each group is responsible. Separate capitation contracts are negotiated with other affiliated physicians in the community. Currently, GHE withholds 20 percent of capitation payments until the end of the fiscal year and returns all or part of that amount based on expenses in three categories: hospitalization, emergency room use, and out-of-plan specialty services. GHE would like to provide incentives for physicians to deliver good quality care by linking capitation payments to patient outcomes. Although Mr. Jones has resisted this idea, the board has insisted that he develop a plan based on performance appraisal. Since Mr. Jones has eschewed contact with the medical staff in the past, he approaches this challenge with some degree of trepidation. His questions are many at this point:

- What aspects of performance, or quality of care, should be considered?
- Is it necessary to measure different outcomes for each type of physician specialist, or are there generic outcomes that can be assessed?
- How will the outcome measures incorporate risk?
- To what degree should capitation payments depend on performance appraisal?
- Will performance appraisal be the responsibility of GHE or the group practices or both?
- How will performance be assessed for the 500 individual physicians in the community?

For the last three years, GHE has retained most of the withhold payments because of substantial hospitalization expenses. This has increased friction between GHE and the two physician groups. The director for hospital services has presented Mr. Jones with a case-mix breakdown by diagnosis-related group (DRG). The concern seems to be that many of the hospital episodes are potentially avoidable. GHE does not currently have a surveillance program that would flag these specific episodes, nor does it have a system to identify conditions that could result in hospital care if ambulatory care is deficient. The chief financial officer (CFO) calculates the potentially avoidable cost to be $18.8 million. Dr. Practice, medical director for BMS, urges Mr. Jones to reduce these episodes by developing a more sophisticated system for targeting ambulatory care-sensitive conditions that are at risk for costly hospitalization.

Mr. Jones faces a number of decisions at this point:

- Which ambulatory care-sensitive conditions need to be included in the surveillance system?
- How will these conditions be identified among the enrolled population?
- How will avoidable hospital episodes be monitored over time?
- How will GHE measure progress in this area?

GHE has contracts with several of the largest employers in the Boston area and with 50 mid-size businesses. Each employer contract is negotiated separately with past utilization primarily determining the capitation rates, although within companies the employees are assessed the same premium (i.e., they are community rated). The GHE board has urged Mr. Jones to become more proactive in setting capitation rates. More specifically, it has encouraged him to include not just the estimated disease burden of the enrolled population, based on past experience, but also the burden of risk factors to which enrollees are exposed (e.g., obesity, smoking, and alcoholism).

Mr. Jones is puzzling over finding answers to a number of sensitive, but imperative, questions:

- How can the present and future disease burden of the enrollees be accurately measured or estimated?
- What are the significant risk factors of disease that can be measured?
- To what extent do they predict future morbidity?
- How should these risk factors be included in setting capitation rates?
- How feasible would such a rate-setting system be?
- To what extent would such a system affect profitability and market share?

In addition to all of these decisions, Mr. Jones is laboring over a five-year strategic plan. GHE has been well-positioned in the market and is having difficulty meeting the demand for services at both the north and south clinics, and GHE enrollment has grown by 30 percent in the last five years. Moreover, the GHE plan has evolved to include a substantial number of elderly and poor members as the result of a decision made five years ago to accept Medicare and Medicaid risk contracts. Mr. Jones is concerned that the membership profile has changed over the last several years, and he does not know the effect this will have on the kinds of services promised to enrollees. The planning director, Mr. Thompson, has been a strong advocate of building a new clinic on the western side of Boston, where several large employers have been the source of thousands of new members in the last few years.

Mr. Jones has a number of questions at this point:

- What kinds of needs assessment approaches should be used at this juncture?
- What measures of morbidity can be used to predict the demand for clinic services?
- How should risk factors of disease enter into the needs assessment?

As part of the strategic plan, Mr. Jones is considering a major effort to reduce the proportion of members who are overweight or obese. Part of this initiative involves including such risk factors as obesity in capitation rates. The other part is a proactive, multi-program, coordinated effort at weight reduction with financial incentives. Mr. Jones is curious about the extent to which obesity plays a role in various kinds of diseases.

He has a number of questions at this point:

- What different kinds of studies support the relationship between obesity and disease?
- How can one tell the difference between a good study and a bad one?
- To what degree does obesity increase the risk of various kinds of disease?
- What proportion of various kinds of diseases can be attributed to obesity?
- Is it possible to calculate how much disease could be avoided if the obesity risk factor were reduced?

GHE faces substantial, probably painful, changes outside and within the organization. The CEO has lost the respect of his senior staff, he has frustrated mid-level managers, and he has alienated the medical staff. He is being urged by others, including the governing board and affiliated medical groups, to make critical and significant decisions within the organization. Mr. Jones will make more efficient and effective decisions if he gathers the relevant epidemiologic measures and evaluates these data from an epidemiologic perspective.

ANSWER

Many believe that enrolled members of a managed care organization form an excellent denominator for epidemiology purposes. They represent a delineated "at risk" population, from which one could establish morbidity and mortality rates (chapters 3 and 6) using the total number of members, or covered lives, as the denominator. This also suggests that managed care organizations, properly run, can not only influence the acute care of the members for which they are responsible, but also assume responsibility for the health of the enrolled population. Using epidemiology tools with this group can improve the decision-making process, particularly if enlightened leadership is focused on improving population health and not exclusively on the bottom line. This paradigm shift— from a reactive medical care system that treats illness, to a proactive one that is concerned with maintaining health—is discussed in Chapter 8.

Mr. Jones needs to make some decisions regarding the move to a matrix model organization for GHE. With a matrix model organization, the product lines are on one axis, and functional departments on the other. The first set of decisions involves choosing which product lines should be arrayed along one axis of the matrix organization. Clearly, the disease burden of the subscribers is one area that could be used to make that decision. A review of DRGs would provide insight into the morbidity burden associated with hospital episodes. The frequency of diagnoses and/or procedures could be evaluated in the ambulatory setting with the commonly used physician coding scheme Current Procedural Terminology (CPT). Mr. Jones could develop rates of hospitalization by specific condition, or rates of ambulatory care encounters by CPT code. Conditions with the highest rates in either setting or both settings could be evaluated as candidates for separate product lines.

Since Mr. Jones is an epidemiologically informed manager, he is concerned about the health of the entire population at risk, which in this case would be the enrolled members of GHE. Because of this concern, Mr. Jones should collect and evaluate risk factor data (e.g., smoking, obesity) on his subscribers to identify potential areas of improvement. Risk factor intervention programs could improve the financial health of GHE as well. GHE may want to complete a behavioral risk factor study on subscribers to determine which programs need to be developed. The target should be risk factors that are modifiable through changes in behavior. These behavioral modification programs (e.g., smoking cessation) may be separate product lines, or part of another product line. For example, smoking cessation could be a "stand-alone" product line, or part of a chronic obstructive pulmonary disease and emphysema line.

Mr. Jones may also want to decide about product lines based on the cost of care for various kinds of morbidity, and the extent to which the enrolled population has, or is at risk of developing, those conditions (Chapter 8). With a focus on the high-cost conditions, Mr. Jones would need to know the prevalence of disease and the prevalence of risk factors that may lead to disease. The DRGs and CPT codes could be used to develop rates. It may be more difficult to associate a specific cost with each code, especially in a managed care environment, but Mr. Jones could borrow the Medicare "prices" assigned to DRGs and CPT codes and assume a fee-for-service environment for the sake of prioritizing product lines.

Finally, Mr. Jones may want to know the time, place, and person descriptors of the enrolled population with regard to morbidity. Some product lines may be age-specific, such as juvenile diabetes and Alzheimer's disease. Others may be affected by specific settings or places in which the enrolled population lives or works. For example, lead screening and abatement might be important in older neighborhoods or among certain groups, such as employees of a battery factory.

There are also a number of staffing issues. These include the uncertainty about how the new matrix model would affect GHE staffing patterns, particularly with regard to the generalist/specialist mix, and the concerns of the nurse practitioners in the satellite clinics. Mr. Jones uses the morbidity data (Chapter 3) from the product line analysis to project the number of enrolled members that can be expected in each product line. He assumes an optimistic and pessimistic scenario with regard to demand increases from market segmentation. Further, he uses industry benchmarks to predict the number of generalists and specialists needed to treat each product line, assuming productivity remains constant. For the satellite clinics, he collects weekly workload statistics by clinic for each practitioner, and analyzes these data to determine if there is a statistically significant increase in patient load. He compares each quarter to the previous quarter, and each week to the same week one year ago. A statistically significant increase in workload that persists over time would argue for increased staffing in this area.

Having made some progress in organizational design and staffing, Mr. Jones moves ahead to directing issues. As you recollect, the board had charged Mr. Jones with looking at an incentive system that would reward outcomes. He begins to review the literature on outcomes and is amazed at some of the material he finds, such as the work in New York and Pennsylvania on coronary artery bypass surgery. Using risk adjustment and other epidemiologic tools, they have provided information to consumers, providers, and plans on expected and actual mortality associated with that procedure (Chapter 6).

Futhermore, the board has been encouraging Mr. Jones to consider applying for accreditation by the National Committee on Quality Assurance (NCQA). Mr. Jones looks into that process and realizes that a couple of outcome measures might be in order. Specifically, the NCQA expects health plans to examine quality by reporting results on the Healthcare Effectiveness Data and Information Set (HEDIS). As Mr. Jones examines the measures that compose HEDIS, he realizes that they are good outcome indicators, and that many are drawn from a planning document he has seen before, *Healthy People 2010*. He recalls the previous problem, that of product lines in a matrix organization, and realizes that a behavioral risk factor survey of enrolled members might also provide information about baseline levels of several of the key HEDIS measures for his population.

Mr. Jones realizes that there are other outcome and baseline variables that he needs to know about the population. Two commonly used outcome measures, for example, are the 36-item short form survey (SF-36) and patient satisfaction measures. SF-36 was developed as the result of the Rand Medical Outcomes Study. This allows for individuals to classify their health status on general, mental, and physical scales.

After careful consideration, he decides to take several interim steps. First, he decides to incorporate a quality indicator in the decision about how much (if any) of the 20 percent withholding to return to each physician. Further, he determines that the quality indicator should be tied to the HEDIS measures and patient satisfaction. With that in mind, he proposes to conduct a patient satisfaction survey and undertake a behavioral risk factor survey of his enrollees. He also is persuaded of the need to know the health status of his plan members, and does a random sample survey using the SF-36.

Mr. Jones is convinced that the withholding incentive system will work better with quality indicator(s), but is appropriately concerned about hospitalization costs consuming most of the withholding cache in recent years. This has caused considerable discord among physician providers who feel they are being penalized for provided high-quality care, albeit in a hospital setting. Fortunately, Jones is aware of a promising solution to the problem. The CFO has acquired hospital case-mix information on GHE enrollees for the past several years. Several of the diagnoses that have prompted admissions are for ambulatory care-sensitive conditions (ASCs), such as asthma, diabetes, and congestive heart failure. These conditions typically should not result in hospitalization if effective primary care is provided. Thus any hospital episode related to these conditions is considered a "preventable" or "avoidable" hospitalization.

Ambulatory sensitive conditions (Chapter 5) can be categorized into one of three areas. Some conditions are totally preventable, such as hospitalization for an immunizable disease, such as measles. Other conditions should not typically require hospitalization if primary care is sought early enough, for example, cellulitis or community acquired pneumonia. The third group includes chronic diseases, which, if tightly controlled, should not require hospitalization. These diseases include asthma, diabetes, and congestive heart failure. Mr. Jones needs to ponder the burden of diseases like these in the enrolled population, and the financial cost to GHE for these conditions. While epidemiology is not critical to the consideration of the latter, it certainly is to the former.

Mr. Jones decides to implement a surveillance system (Chapter 5) for several high-cost and high-frequency ACSs. This monitoring system will identify potential targets for intervention to decrease hospital costs. The surveillance system will describe ACSs and preventable hospitalizations in terms of the epidemiologic concepts of time, place, and person. The problem of preventable hospitalization may occur during a particular time of year, within certain neighborhoods of the city, or among specific population groups. This problem may be caused by a lack of access to care, cultural barriers, or other factors, only some of which may be corrected by an organization intervention, such as an outreach program.

The strategic plan is ambitious and difficult since GHE has undergone so much growth in recent years. Chapter 4 outlines the various kinds of needs assessment approaches that could be undertaken, such as those involving the use of surveys, (e.g., the National Health Interview Survey), risk factor data (e.g., the Behavioral Risk Factor Surveillance System, or insurance claims. GHE could estimate future morbidity based on past utilization, hospital DRGs, or clinic records, or try to estimate future morbidity based on risk factors in the population (see Case Study 4.2, page 76, for example). The increase in proportion of members who are poor and elderly makes future planning even more difficult, because past utilization may not necessarily predict future utilization. Medicare claims would be a good source of data to predict future physician and hospital utililization among the elderly population. Medicaid claims may be available to predict physician and hospital utilization among the Medicaid population.

With regard to Mr. Jones's weight reduction program(s), different kinds of studies support the link between obesity and diseases. Chapters 11–13 discuss these studies. In general, case-control studies and cohort studies can be used to measure the degree to which a particular risk factor, such as obesity, increases the risk of disease. Randomized clinical trials are more often used to evaluate the efficacy of a particular intervention, such as a new weight loss medication. There are various characteristics, or features, of each study that reflect its "quality," such as the strength of the relationship between the risk factor and the outcome, and whether there is a "dose-response" relationship between the risk factor and outcome. These features are discussed in Chapter 14. Different studies in the literature report on the "relative risk" of obesity and a given disease, such as heart disease (Chapter 15). Relative risk refers to the number of times more likely a person who is obese is to develop a disease compared with a person who is not obese. Mr. Jones could calculate the proportion of various kinds of diseases that can be attributed to obesity in the GHE-enrolled population by obtaining the relative risks associated with obesity and each disease, and determining the prevalence of obesity in the GHE-enrolled population. This is referred to as the *attributable fraction*. To estimate how much disease could be avoided, Mr. Jones would also need to go to the literature to determine the relative success of various weight loss programs.

Finally, Mr. Jones turns to the issue of setting capitation rates (Chapter 8). He is pleased with the previous decisions that he has made with regard to product line and quality of care. These decisions have put in place a mechanism to collect the data needed to determine capitation rates. Specifically, the SF-36 should give him information about the health of his population, and how he might go about determining whether his enrollees are sicker than the normal population. If he could convince employers that GHE members are sicker, on average, than other insured people in the area, he might be able to argue for higher capitation rates. Mr. Jones realizes that the behavioral risk factor data could also be an important part of that discussion, particularly if the members of his plan have worse risk factor prevalence than others across the state.

He decides to examine the attributable morbidity associated with several major risk factors, to evaluate the extent to which such morbidity is responsible for a major portion of the per-member-per-month fee. He realizes that if he can bring these risk factors under control, through education, outreach, or other programmatic improvements, there is the potential to increase profitability, particularly if he can use the data that he has gathered in rate negotiations.

Mr. Jones has, as the result of learning more about epidemiological reasoning, begun to improve his ability to make decisions and solve problems. This case study illustrates a principle that we suggested at the beginning of this chapter, that epidemiology can be a useful tool in all of the managerial functions. Moreover, as is apparent, epidemiology tools can frequently be used simultaneously in several managerial functions. The epidemiology perspective influences a manager's practice style in positive ways, and epidemiology can function as an integrative approach to management decision making. The use of the epidemiologic method and the epidemiology perspective can improve management, and, more important, can help the manager reach the goal of improving population health.

Resources

Austin, C. 1974. "What Is Health Administration?" *Hospital Administration* 19 (27): 27–34.

Hodgetts, R., and D. Cascio. 1983. *Modern Healthcare Administration*. New York: Academic Press.

Lilienfeld, D., and P. Stolley. 1994. *Foundations of Epidemiology*, 3rd ed. New York: Oxford University Press.

Neumann, B., J. Suver, and W. N. Zelman. 1988. *Financial*

Management: Concepts and Applications for Healthcare Providers,
2nd ed. Owings Mills, MD: National Publishing/AUPHA Press.
Rakich, J., B. Longest, and K. Darr. 1992. *Managing Health Services
Organizations,* 3rd ed. Baltimore, MD: Health Professions Press.

INFECTIOUS DISEASE EPIDEMIOLOGY

Glyn G. Caldwell and Steven T. Fleming

"Louis Pasteur's theory of germs is ridiculous fiction." Pierre Pachet,
professor of physiology at the University of Toulouse, 1872

Disease, that is, any impairment of physiological function of the body, is an adverse health condition arising from one of four causes: trauma, degenerative changes, metabolic abnormalities, or infection or parasitism by another living agent (*International Webster New Encyclopedic Dictionary* 1975; Last 2000). In this chapter we will discuss diseases that result from infection by predominantly microbial agents, especially those that are communicable from person to person.

Infectious diseases have probably been in existence as long as plants, animals, and humans have inhabited the planet. Data from ancient ice, permafrost, and imprints in rock indicate that microorganisms have a long and varied history, but of the millions of known species, the majority are not pathogenic to either animals or humans (Castello and Rogers 2005).

Studies of the bones of prehistoric animals have revealed evidence of injury and diseases affecting bone, but because most organs have decayed, virtually nothing is known about diseases affecting soft tissues. Early humans were afflicted with a variety of ailments, as demonstrated from Egyptian mummies and pre-Columbian bones. The diseases that left their mark on prehistoric bones or bony tissues are fractures, osteomyelitis, osteitis, periosteitis, arthritis (cave gout), dental abscesses, pyorrhea, and caries (Lyons and Petrucelli 1978).

Infectious diseases, because they frequently affect and damage only soft tissues, have only been recorded since the onset of cave drawings and writing, approximately 4000 B.C. (Lyons and Petrucelli 1978). Because early humans were primarily hunters and gatherers living in small nomadic family or tribal units, they had limited contact with other humans, and most of their infections were likely caused by trauma and secondary infection or their diet. Populations were small and crowding was minimal. However, as animals were domesticated and a more agrarian society developed, there were more opportunities for contact with infectious agents from livestock and other humans. Early cultures experienced dysentery, fevers, gonorrhea, leprosy, malaria, parasitic infections, plague, pneumonia, smallpox, tuberculosis, and urinary tract infections—all clearly observed and documented in biblical texts (Anonymous 1957) and the writings of the early Greeks (Lyons and Petrucelli 1978; Conrad et al. 1995).

As populations grew and people traveled from their home areas, there was an increased opportunity for contact with other people, other environments, and a variety of different animals, increasing the possibility of contact with new diseases (Lyons and Petrucelli 1978; Conrad et al. 1995). As populations grew, so did epidemics. Bubonic plague, or the Black Death, devastated large parts of the Mediterranean world and Europe, killing roughly 30 percent of the population. Entire towns and villages ceased to exist (Kelly 2005; Platt 1996; Ziegler 1996). In 1347, the plague arrived in Caffa, a Genoese city on the Black Sea, with the Mongol invasion led by Khan Janiberg. Bodies of plague victims were hurled by catapult into the city during the siege to cause plague in the defenders and force the surrender of the city (Kelly 2005).

The plagues of the sixth, fourteenth, sixteenth, seventeenth, and eighteenth centuries devastated the population repeatedly, and disrupted industry, agriculture, and commerce. This damaged the economy of many countries (Platt 1996). In England, during the mid-1300s, mortality was generally between 40 and 50 percent, but in some places mortality was much lower (in Market Roding it was 25.6 percent) or disastrously higher (Bibury 76 percent and Aston 80 percent) (Platt 1996). Not until the influenza pandemic in 1918 would the world suffer similar mortality rates (Barry 2005).

The enormity of past plagues and their effects on industry, commerce, transportation, agriculture, and especially the healthcare systems is a major reason managers and administrators need to know sufficient infectious disease epidemiology to cope with the necessary planning, preparedness, and response that future epidemics and pandemics may engender.

Agent, Host, and Environment

The agent, host, and environment are the primary factors to be considered when investigating disease cases and potential epidemics. These are displayed as a triad or triangle (Figure 2.1) (Centers for Disease Control and Prevention 1992a). It is the intersection of these factors that leads to disease. This can be represented as intersecting circles, a Venn or Boolean logic diagram (Figure 2.2).

Managers and administrators of health facilities of every kind, but especially hospitals, nursing homes, free-standing clinics, and ancillary healthcare facilities, are likely to face an infectious disease concern. They may see infectious diseases as individual cases or an outbreak, and they must understand the relationship of the agent, host, and environment. Each contributes to the cause of the disease in its own unique way, with a specific group of people, during some specific period.

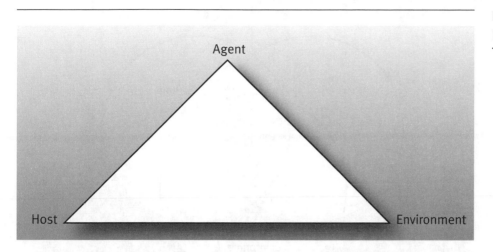

FIGURE 2.1
Epidemiologic
Triad

The agent, host, and environmental determinants of disease are shown in the box on page 20. The manager is primarily concerned with the environment, especially the facility (the place) under his or her control, and how it contributes to the risk, maintenance, and transmission of disease among his customers, patients, and staff (Siegel et al. 2007; Tietjen, Bossemeyer, and McIntosh 2003). Many of the environmental determinants affect specific facilities, but may affect different facilities in different ways. However, not all factors apply to all facilities. All are controlled to some extent by the facility operators, management, and staff.

For example, excessive humidity and moisture enhance mold growth in airshafts, walls, or carpeting where either plumbing or roofing leaks have occurred (Arundel et al. 1986; Ehrlich, Miller, and Walker 1970; Lester 1948). *Legionella pneumophila*, a species of bacteria, populates air conditioning units, and depending on circumstances related to air intake and distribution systems, may affect all or only parts of a facility (Fraser et al. 1977 Fraser 1980). In addition, this same organism has been transmitted through hospital water distribution systems (Naphaetian et al. 1991; Stout, Yu, and Best 1985). Although the determinant "neighborhood" may appear to be more applicable to homes or schools, the location of a hospital or clinic near construction sites has been linked to infections from fungal spores aerosolized by earth-moving equipment operation. One only has to think of Hurricane Katrina to understand the effect of a natural disaster on homes, neighborhoods, hospitals, and evacuation centers and to realize how many of these environmental determinants play a role in infectious disease.

Although there are many agents that cause disease—including chemicals, physical agents such as ionizing radiation, and nutritional deficiencies—this chapter focuses on the role of biological agents.

Infectious agents play a role in nosocomial (hospital-acquired) illness and epidemics in hospitals, other healthcare facilities, and non-health-related

FIGURE 2.2
Epidemiologic
Triad as a
Venn
Diagram

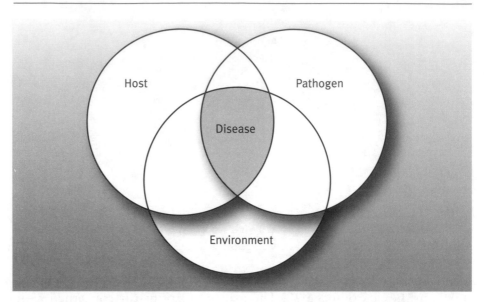

AGENT, HOST, AND ENVIRONMENT FACTORS

Infectious Agents	Environmental Determinants	Host Factors
Metazoa	Temperature	Age
Protozoa	Humidity	Sex
Fungi	Altitude	Race
Bacteria	Crowding	Ethnicity
Rickettsia	Housing	Religion
Viruses	Neighborhood	Occupation
Prions	Water	Heredity/genetics/family background
	Milk	
	Food	Marital status
	Radiation	Previous illnesses
	Pollution	Comorbidities
	Sewage management	Immune status
	Noise	Lifestyle (behavioral factors)
	Animal contacts	Physiological state
	Disruptions (wars, disasters)	Trauma (including surgery)
	Emergencies	Medical procedures used
		Vaccination status
		Susceptibility/resistance

institutions. The biological agents listed in the box on page 20 are those that could, under a variety of circumstances, cause disease in institutions. The majority of institutional infectious diseases are the result of bacterial or viral infections. Fungi, rickettsia, prions, and metazoa (insects, parasitic worms, mites, and ticks) are less likely to be problems in healthcare facilities (though obviously some patients are admitted to hospitals or treated in clinics for diseases caused by those pathogens).

Most infectious organisms have specific requirements for moisture, temperature, and nutrients. When those requirements are met, the organisms survive, live, reproduce, and thrive, though sometimes only within a specific host (Dunklin and Puck 1948; Farrell and Rose 1967; Price and Tom 1992). For example, the infectious agents of tetanus (*Clostridium tetani*) and anthrax (*Bacillus anthracis*) produce spores that can survive for years and move from one generation of hosts to another, while the organisms of syphilis (*Treponema pallidum*) and gonorrhea (*Neisseria gonorrhea*) are so delicate that they require constant moisture and cannot survive in a dry environment for more than a few minutes (Burrows 1959; Holmes et al. 1999). A far larger group of microbial agents (*Staphylococcus aureus*, *Escherichia coli*, *Vibrio cholera*, and *Mycobacterium tuberculosis*) can survive for varying periods in the environment, especially in water, food, and sewage; on hands and fomites (toys, eating utensils, catheters, or medical devices); or on surfaces (floors, bedrails, or tables), depending on humidity (Cox 1976; Makison and Swan 2006; Stine et al. 2005).

Each agent has determinants that characterize its ability to colonize, infect, damage tissues, and produce disease (Nelson and Masters Williams 2007). Agents that cause disease are said to be *pathogenic*, and the severity of the resulting disease is a property of the agent termed *virulence*. Although all microbial agents that produce disease are termed *infectious*, not all are communicable. Only those transmissible from animals or other persons are considered communicable; agents such as *C. tetani* or *B. anthracis*, which are acquired directly from the environment, are called infectious, not communicable (Heymann 2004). Similarly, infectious agents that can survive only within a specific host species may be infectious and/or communicable within that species, but not communicable to humans. An example is the virus of hoof and mouth disease.

Management must spend considerable time and effort maintaining a clean and sanitary facility, which minimizes transmission of bacterial and viral disease and avoids the development of hospital strains of disease with high levels of antibiotic resistance. This involves careful planning and attention to detail in food preparation and distribution, cleaning and sanitizing rooms following patient occupancy, and training staff to prevent transmission of disease agents.

Similarly, the health status of the host (patient, inmate, or customer) plays an important role in the development of a disease or outbreak within a facility's walls. Although the majority of the host determinants, listed in the box on page 20, are important factors related to the possible acquisition of a microbial agent and subsequent development of disease, they are not generally controllable by the facility operators or staff. The caregivers are responsible for preventing infection in highly susceptible patients, especially those who have had invasive diagnostic or therapeutic interventions. Post-surgery patients and patients with burns or severe trauma have a heightened likelihood of infection.

Transmission

Infectious diseases come from outside the host. There must be a pathway for the infectious agent to reach each new host, and the agent must be transmitted from infected host or reservoir to a susceptible host. Transmission can be described as direct or indirect, and each has specific modes of transmission within those two categories (see below) (Nelson and Masters Williams 2007; Timmreck 2002).

Carriers are a special example of transmission. A *carrier* is a person who spreads an infectious disease to other susceptible persons. A carrier may be a healthy person—not ill—who is nevertheless colonized with an infectious agent. A carrier can transmit the agent continuously or intermittently. Similarly, individuals who have been infected and are incubating the disease (incubatory carrier) may transmit the agent before they develop the disease. Likewise, individuals who are recovering from an infectious disease can transmit that disease during recovery. These people are called *convalescent carriers* (Nelson and Masters Williams 2007).

In most circumstances, the management of facilities or institutions is more concerned with agents that can be transmitted within the institution. It is management's responsibility to develop and implement infection control policies and procedures to ensure the protection of patients, staff,

MODES OF TRANSMISSION

Direct
    Contact-kissing, sexual activity, in utero, via breast milk
    Airborne droplet or droplet nuclei

Indirect
    Animate—from a human carrier, mechanically transmitted on
        hands, etc.
    Animate—by an insect or other animal vector
    Inanimate—from free-living organisms in the environment, from water,
        sewage, dust, fomites, etc.

FIGURE 2.3
Chain of
Infection

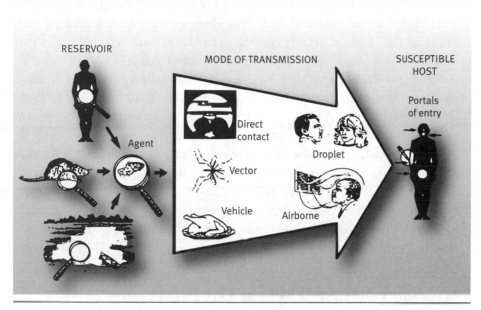

SOURCE: Centers for Disease Control and Prevention (1992a, 45).

and visitors from infectious agents present in the hospital environment and patients undergoing treatment. The likely pathways for transmission are (Beggs 2003; Buccheri et al. 2007; Dennesen, Bonten, and Weinstein 1998; Gikas et al. 2006; Nguyen 2007; Tipple et al. 2004):

- airborne from infected staff or visitors;
- from the environment as a result of contamination from patients;
- improper cleaning;
- on caregivers' hands or clothing;
- from ingestion of food or water.

Outbreaks have occurred in hospitals and nursing homes as a result of these pathways (Figure 2.3) (Centers for Disease Control and Prevention 1992a).

Portals of entry and exit into and from the host body are necessary for transmission of disease (see box on page 24). A pathway through air, water, food, contact, etc. from an infected host to a susceptible host is also needed (Nelson and Masters Williams 2007; Timmreck 2002). If the infectious agent cannot gain entry, it cannot multiply and cause disease. Similarly, if there is no way for the infectious agent to leave the body and attack another susceptible host, it cannot survive.

Once an infectious disease agent gains entry into a susceptible host, it must evade the host defenses and find an appropriate cell to invade and begin multiplication. The time from the first entry of the disease agent until disease becomes evident is called the *incubation period*. This period is variable, and depends on the particular infecting agent, the infecting dose (number of organisms in the exposure), and the immunological condition and relative resistance or susceptibility of the host. Most acute bacterial and viral illnesses have incubation periods from 24 to 72 hours. However, the incubation period may be as short as a few hours (*Staphylococcal enterotoxin*) or as long as 30 days (Hepatitis A virus), 60 days (Hepatitis B virus), or occasionally up to a year (human immunodeficiency virus) (Nelson and Masters Williams 2007). Table 2.1 lists some typical incubation periods, and Figure 2.4 shows examples of incubation periods for foodborne illnesses.

Each disease has specific stages of infection and illness. Exposure to an organism via any pathway or route of transmission may lead to illness. The incubation period begins when infection occurs. In the early period of infection, before signs and symptoms generally appear, the carrier doesn't look ill. The next stage is the "prodrome," the latter part of the incubation period. Sometimes signs or symptoms occur during

INFECTIOUS DISEASE ENTRY AND EXIT POINTS

Entry	Exit
Conjunctiva	Respiratory tract
Gastrointestinal tract	Gastrointestinal tract
Genito-urinary tract	Genito-urinary tract
Percutaneous (trauma, injection)	Percutaneous (trauma, injection)
Transplacental	
Organ transplantation	

TABLE 2.1
Incubation
Periods

Disease	Incubation Period
Botulism	8–36 hours
Common cold	12–72 hours (usually 24)
Conjunctivitis	1–3 days
Influenza	1–3 days
Bacterial/viral pneumonia	1–3 days
Gonorrhea	2–5 days
Meningitis	2–10 days
Herpes simplex virus	up to 2 weeks
Measles	12–26 days
Dysentery	2–4 weeks
Epstein-Barr (Mononucleosis)	4–7 weeks
Infectious hepatitis	15–50 days
Serum hepatitis	45–160 days

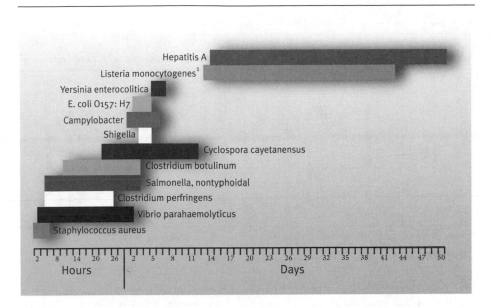

FIGURE 2.4
Usual Incubation Period Ranges for Select Foodborne Diseases

[1]Invasive form; incubation period for diarrheal disease unkown.

SOURCE: Data on the "usual" incubation period obtained from Centers for Disease Control and Prevention (1996).

prodrome, but they are generally nonspecific and usually attributed to the person being tired. The acute phase of illness begins when signs and symptoms become obvious, at the end of the prodrome period. The acute phase may last for a few days (the common cold) or years (tuberculosis, leprosy, or HIV/AIDS). Whether the patient survives depends on the response of the host immunological defenses or treatment. When the patient begins to improve, it is called the *resolution phase*. For most illnesses this will be a few days, although some may require treatment for months to a year (tuberculosis) or for life (HIV/AIDS). Finally, the surviving patient enters into the convalescent period, during which all the signs and symptoms disappear and the patient feels well again (Nelson and Masters Williams 2007).

Prevention

For the individual, general wellness, immune status, and acquired immunity from previous illnesses and immunizations minimize the likelihood of colonization, infection, or reinfection (Nelson and Masters Williams 2007). However, if any of these parameters diminish due to illness or age, recrudescent disease may occur. Prevention of disease may be primary, secondary, or tertiary (Timmreck 2002).

FIGURE 2.5
How Herd
Immunity
Prevents an
Epidemic

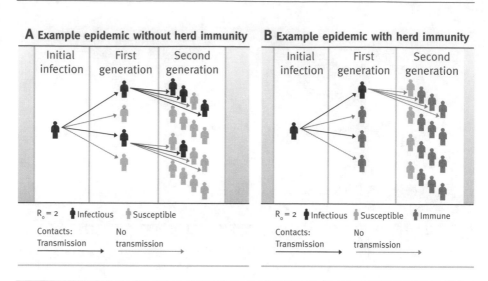

A Example epidemic without herd immunity

Initial infection	First generation	Second generation

$R_o = 2$ Infectious   Susceptible

Contacts:
Transmission   No transmission

B Example epidemic with herd immunity

Initial infection	First generation	Second generation

$R_o = 2$ Infectious   Susceptible   Immune

Contacts:
Transmission   No transmission

Effect of herd immunity on the spread of an infection in a homogeneous population. A. Schematic illustration of two generations of spread of infection with a basic reproductive number (R_o) of 2, when no individuals in the population have immunity. B. Spread of the same infection, with $R_o = 2$, in a population with the same number of contacts but with 75 percent of the population immune.

SOURCE: Garnett, G. P. 2005. "Role of Herd Immunity in Determining the Effect of Vaccines Against Sexually Transmitted Disease." *Journal of Infectious Diseases* 191 (Suppl. 1): S97–S106. Copyright © 2005, Infectious Diseases Society of North America. Used with permission.

The goal of primary prevention is to avoid illness altogether, generally by preventing disease development even if exposed, through the use of immunization (measles, tetanus, smallpox, etc.), or in some circumstance by prescribing specific prophylactic drugs (*Neisseria meningitidis*) or post exposure vaccines (rabies). Sanitation and environmental management of the water supply, sewage disposal, air purification, and general cleaning of living spaces may also contribute to prevention of transmission and thus be primary prevention methodologies (Duffy 1992). These efforts also reduce the overall incidence of disease in a population.

Immunization also contributes to the prevention of transmission by reducing the number of susceptible persons in the population. Figure 2.5 illustrates how "herd immunity" can prevent the spread of a communicable disease in a population (Nelson and Masters Williams 2007; Garnett 2005). The basic reproductive number (R_o) is the "average number of new infections caused by one infected individual in an *entirely susceptible population*" (Garnett 2005, S98). In Figure 2.5, that number is two. If the average number of contacts is four, 50 percent of those contacts will become infected. Notice that only 50 percent of both first- and second-generation contacts in panel A become infected. With a herd immunity of 75 percent (panel B), only 25 percent of the population is susceptible, thus only one individual in the first generation is susceptible. Of the two contacts with infectious hosts (one in the first generation and one in the second), only one of these contacts becomes infectious (50 percent). The epidemic is propagated geometrically with no herd immunity (panel A), but fizzles out with a herd immunity of 75 percent (panel B).

Secondary prevention is aimed at reducing illness onset, duration, or further transmission once infection has occurred, or in the case of cancer, a tumor has developed. For example, someone exposed to *Mycobacterium tuberculosis* may have no apparent signs or symptoms, even though she was infected for a few days to several weeks. The only change may be the development of a positive response to a tuberculin skin test. In this event, preventive (or prophylactic) treatment will prevent development of active disease and the further transmission of disease. This contributes to reducing both the incidence and prevalence of disease in the community. More typically, secondary prevention is associated with screening, the purpose of which would be to discover the disease at an early, curable stage. An example is mammography screening for breast cancer.

Tertiary prevention strives to cure the illness once obvious symptoms have appeared. It also seeks to reduce complications, suffering, and long-term impairments and disabilities (for example, mastectomy for breast cancer). Tertiary prevention may have no effect on the incidence or prevalence of disease in the community.

Management of a healthcare facility must ensure that the facility's staff is appropriately immunized to protect the staff, patients, and visitors from vaccine-preventable diseases (Bolyard et al. 1998; Centers for Disease Control and Prevention 1997; Krause et al. 1994; Ziegler 1996). In addition, an outbreak of a vaccine-preventable disease can temporarily diminish, or in rare cases destroy, the ability of a healthcare facility to function because of illness in critical staff (Izurieta et al. 2002; Hanna et al. 2000; Krause et al. 1994; Sepkowitz 1996; Terada et al. 2001).

Even when employees are properly immunized, there are other ways disease can spread. Transmission may occur via the facility itself, the water supply, other patients, or contaminated food (Bezanson, Khakhria, and Bollegraaf 1983; Helms et al. 1983).

Management must constantly ensure that the facility is adequately sanitized to prevent the transmission of microbes from badly cleaned and disinfected beds, rooms, and equipment, especially considering the number of ill and elderly people occupying the facility. Management must ensure the availability of an adequate and well-trained cleaning staff, who know the proper methods for cleaning and disinfecting rooms following patient discharge, especially rooms occupied by patients with an infectious disease. Appropriate infection control requires that all spills of blood, body fluids, or other organic materials be removed to avoid the possibility of causing a subsequent patient to be colonized or infected by the previous occupant's microbes. In addition, special attention must be given to rooms where invasive procedures will be carried out. Operating rooms, intensive care units, and burn units require meticulous cleaning and disinfecting between procedures and patients to minimize the possibility of transmission from either the room itself or from multiple-use equipment that is not disposable (Sehulster and Chinn 2003; Zerr et al. 2005).

Professional and lay staff must also be aware of the policies and procedures for infection control, including personal hygiene (Boyce and Pittet 2002). Outbreaks have occurred when staff failed to be meticulous in infection control, particularly by inadequately implementing isolation procedures when visiting patients with an infectious disease. Critical to infection control, in this situation, is the use of personal protective equipment (gown, glove, and mask) and careful hand washing between patients. Studies have shown that hand washing decreases nosocomial infection rates in hospitals, and standardized hand-hygiene protocols reduce the level of bacterial hand contamination (Colombo et al. 2002; Lucet et al. 2002; Gastmeier et al. 2002). Unfortunately, breaks in infection control result in nosocomial infections in approximately 2 million people per year, or 5 percent of all acute care admissions, with attendant costs of $30.5 billion and approximately 100,000 deaths annually (Nibley 2007; Nguyen 2007; Zerr et al. 2005).

Although management is mostly concerned with the risk from infection by airborne or hand contact, water (Doebbeling and Wenzel 1987; Squier, Yu, and Stout 2000; WHO 2003) and foodborne illnesses can occur in hospitals, although somewhat less frequently than in community settings (Bezanson, Khakhria, and Bollegraaf 1983; Sabetta et al. 1991; Gikas et al. 2006).

Diarrheal illness, especially, is frequent in hospitals, child care, and nursing facilities. Foodborne and diarrheal illnesses are frequently caused by staff who are poorly trained. When staff fail to safely prepare and store raw foods, or risk cross-contamination of cooked with unprocessed foods, disease can spread. When there is an infection-control failure in the kitchen, a common-source epidemic may occur, resulting in large numbers of affected persons. Such outbreaks are expensive; prevention always costs less (Tietjen, Bossemeyer, and McIntosh 2003). Case Study 2.1 illustrates such an outbreak at the fictitious Bluegrass Hospital.

Case Study 2.1. Food Poisoning Outbreak at Bluegrass Hospital

An outbreak of food poisoning occurred among the 300 staff and patients at Bluegrass Hospital a few hours after eating dinner. Among the 50 people who became ill, the symptoms were mainly nausea, vomiting, and diarrhea. The infection-control nurse investigated the outbreak and reported results in Table 2.2 below.

Table 2.2. Foodborne Outbreak at Bluegrass Hospital

Type of Food	Consumed Food		Did Not Consume Food	
	No. People	No. Ill	No. People	No. Ill
Apple juice	50	10	250	40
Cantaloupe	30	6	270	44
Taco salad	100	30	200	20
Hot dogs	80	20	220	30
Chipped beef with sauce	80	45	220	5
Egg salad	90	20	210	30
Apple pie	120	20	180	30
Layer cake	125	25	175	25

QUESTIONS

1. What is the "crude" attack rate?
2. What are the food-specific attack rates for those who consumed, and did not consume, each food item?
3. How many times more likely are people who consumed specific food items to get sick compared to those who did not consume each item?
4. Which food item is the most likely cause of this "common source" outbreak?
5. What are the incubation period and most likely cause of the outbreak?

ANSWERS

1. The crude attack rate is (50/300) × 100 = 16.7%.
2. These rates are reported in Table 2.3 below.
3. The ratio of food-specific attack rates (consumed/not consumed) provides these "relative risks." Those who consumed apple juice or cantaloupe are 1.25 and 1.2 times as likely, respectively, to get sick as those who did not consume these items. Those who consumed taco salad or hot dogs are 3.0

Table 2.3. Food-Specific Attack Rates (per 100) for Bluegrass Hospital

Type of Food	Consumed Food	Did Not Consume Food
Apple juice	20	16
Cantaloupe	20	17
Taco salad	30	10
Hot dogs	25	14
Chipped beef with sauce	56	2
Egg salad	22	14
Apple pie	17	17
Layer cake	20	14

and 1.8 times as likely, respectively, to get sick as those who did not consumer these items. Chipped beef or egg salad consumers are 28 and 1.6 times as likely, respectively, to get sick, while apple pie and layer cake consumers are 1.0 times and 1.4 times as likely to get sick.

4. Chipped beef had an extremely high relative risk and is the most likely cause of the outbreak.

5. The incubation period is about three hours. The most likely cause of this outbreak would be *Staphylococcus aureus*.

Epidemic Investigation

All communities and facilities are at risk for an outbreak or epidemic. Managers must ensure that adequate infection control policies are in place, with sufficient monitoring by staff to detect any change in the frequency of disease. This means that management must know how to ascertain that an increased frequency of disease above that usually seen (the endemic level) in the facility has occurred. Generally, management will have some data or records of the diseases that have occurred in the hospital's patients or residents, either from informal monitoring and tracking of disease frequency or by some specific dedicated surveillance system of data collection, compilation, analysis, and interpretation. Additionally, management could use disease data from the state or Centers for Disease Control and Prevention (CDC). Such data are recorded and disseminated in state reports, or the *Morbidity and Mortality Weekly Report* and its annual summaries (www.cdc.gov/mmwr/).

If an outbreak is suspected, management must report their suspicions to the local health departments. Following the report they will be required to respond with an investigation to determine the cause of the outbreak, how to control the epidemic, and what changes need to be made to policies, procedures, and operations to prevent a recurrence.

Observations of specific communicable disease cases and unusual increases in other infectious disease are required by law to be reported to the local and state health departments for evaluation and investigation if necessary. All states statutorily require specific diseases to be reported, within specific time frames using that state's reporting form.

Once an epidemic is suspected and supported by local data, a systematic investigation should be planned and implemented rapidly. The activities that should be considered are listed in the box below. Although all the steps are considered in sequence, some may occur simultaneously.

STEPS IN THE INVESTIGATION OF AN OUTBREAK

1. Establish the existence of an outbreak (epidemic).
2. Verify the reported diagnosis.
3. Prepare a case definition and count cases.
4. Prepare for fieldwork.
5. Compile descriptive epidemiology.
6. Develop hypotheses.
7. Evaluate hypotheses.
8. Reconsider and refine hypotheses.
9. Plan and implement additional necessary studies (clinical, environmental, epidemiological, laboratory).
10. Implement control and prevention actions.
11. Communicate findings.

The first step is to ascertain that an outbreak exists, by comparing the known local data about disease frequency to those observed or reported. Does the number of cases exceed that usually seen in this facility or community? For example, the state health department will generally keep a running tally and rate of specific diseases for some period of years, as part of its reportable disease surveillance system. And if the number of persons at risk, in either the facility or community, is known or can be estimated, a rate may be calculated from these data.

FIGURE 2.6
Outbreak
from a
Common
Source of
Infection

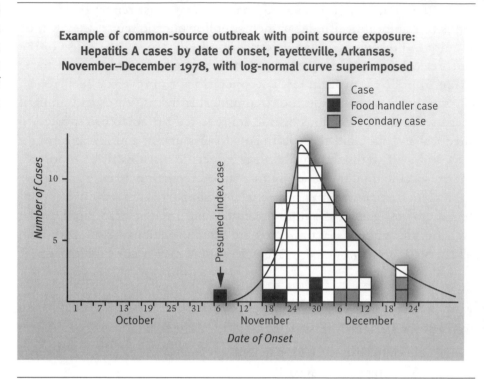

Example of common-source outbreak with point source exposure: Hepatitis A cases by date of onset, Fayetteville, Arkansas, November–December 1978, with log-normal curve superimposed

SOURCE: Centers for Disease Control and Prevention (1979).

At the same time, the facility and local health department must confirm that the cases of disease suspected to be in excess of normal expectancy are in fact the same disease. Officials may do this by reviewing clinical records, microbiology laboratory data, pathology reports, or other pertinent data. If the cases appear to be the same disease, and the number is increased, then a more formal and systematic investigation is warranted.

If it is determined that the cases are indeed the same disease and that the disease frequency exceeds that usually seen in the population, preparation for fieldwork may occur. The persons assigned to the investigation need to have the knowledge, equipment, and support for the mission. This planning requires administrative assistance from the facility to allow access to the records and patients; help from the investigator's organization to facilitate travel and logistics; and, in some situations, consultations with experts in the field. Once the decision has been made to investigate, the resources are amassed and prepared for transit to the epidemic location.

The case definition should be clear, be concise, and present a uniform set of criteria to include or exclude a particular case. For example, in a recent outbreak of diarrheal disease in day care centers in a Kentucky county, a case was defined as "a child with diarrhea enrolled in a day care center during May through August, 2004 with a microbiological culture of Shigella sonnei." Other examples abound in the literature.

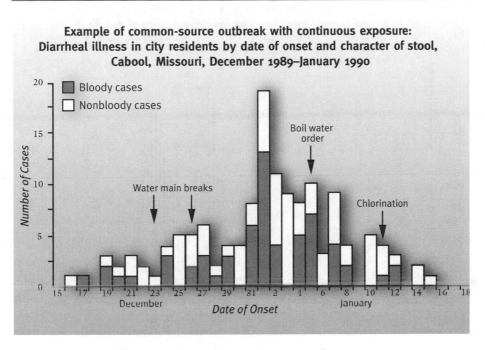

Example of common-source outbreak with continuous exposure: Diarrheal illness in city residents by date of onset and character of stool, Cabool, Missouri, December 1989–January 1990

SOURCE: Centers for Disease Control and Prevention (1992a, 57)

FIGURE 2.7
Outbreak with Common–Source of Infection and Continuous Exposure

Now cases need to be counted, and additional cases need to be sought. It is possible that an epidemic is suspected in one facility, when in fact cases are occurring in other facilities as well. Such information will help the investigator determine if only one facility is affected, or if the epidemic is a community-wide outbreak. If the investigator determines two or more facilities are affected, then he tries to learn if there was movement of persons from one facility to another, possibly spreading the disease.

Early in the process, the investigator will develop an attack curve or epidemic curve. This may show if the epidemic is likely resulting from a common source of infection, such as a contaminated food item (Figure 2.6), or a continuous common source, such as a contaminated water supply (Figure 2.7). The curve could also show if the epidemic was propagating sequential waves of infection (Figure 2.8), or show a mixed pattern. The development of the attack curve is also likely to provide some information about the incubation period (Figure 2.9) (Centers for Disease Control and Prevention 1992a).

Early in the investigation, a simple listing (Figure 2.10) of cases and noncases needs to be compiled using available data to determine what other information is needed (Centers for Disease Control and Prevention 1992a). The listing should include identifying data, demographic data, clinical data, and risk factor data. This listing, along with the attack curve, will assist in the development of the preliminary hypotheses.

FIGURE 2.8
Propagated
Epidemic

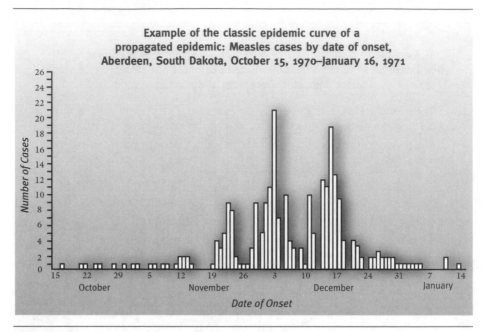

Example of the classic epidemic curve of a
propagated epidemic: Measles cases by date of onset,
Aberdeen, South Dakota, October 15, 1970–January 16, 1971

SOURCE: Centers for Disease Control and Prevention (1992a, 58).

FIGURE 2.9
Attack
Curves and
Incubation
Periods

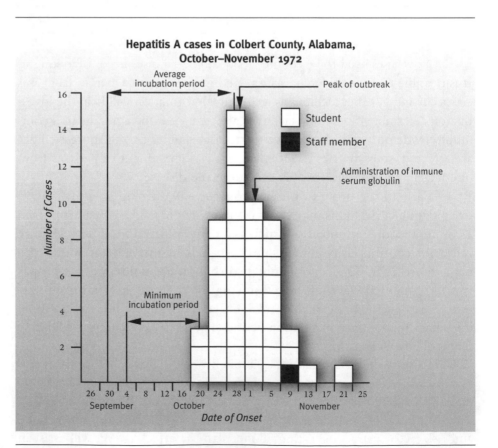

Hepatitis A cases in Colbert County, Alabama,
October–November 1972

SOURCE: Centers for Disease Control and Prevention (1992a, 58).

The risk factor data need to be tailored to the specific disease or circumstance at hand. For example, if the disease is hepatitis, risk factors related to food and water sources need to be considered. If the attack curve shows an abrupt rapid increase in cases compatible with a common-source outbreak, then information about where the cases ate and the foods they ate could be critical data.

The preliminary analysis of these data constitutes the descriptive epidemiology of the outbreak. The attack curve helps determine if there is a common source; the clinical and laboratory data provide information about the diagnosis; and the line listing describing the persons involved, the timing of the outbreak, and its location helps determine the further direction of the investigation.

It is at this point, with the majority of the data in hand, that a hypothesis can be developed. As the data have been collected, compiled, organized, and analyzed, however, preliminary hypotheses have probably been considered, discarded, and modified, as the facts of the outbreak were accumulated. When a more complete analysis is presented with virtually all of the data complete, the hypothesis can spell out more precisely what happened, and possibly why it happened. With further evaluation of the data and hypotheses, the investigator can determine if further epidemiologic studies are needed to confirm, or more accurately identify, the risk factors.

FIGURE 2.10
Listing of Cases and Noncases for Hepatitis A

Case #	Initials	Date of Report	Date of Onset	MD Dx	N	V	A	F	DU	J	HA IgM	Other	Age	Sex
					Diagnostic — Signs and Symptoms						Lab			
1	JG	10/12	10/6	Hep A	+	+	+	+	+	+	+	SGOT↑	37	M
2	BC	10/12	10/5	Hep A	+	−	+	+	+	+	+	ALT↑	62	F
3	HP	10/13	10/4	Hep A	±	−	+	+	+	S*	+	SGOT↑	30	F
4	MC	10/15	10/4	Hep A	−	−	+	+	?	−	+	HBs Ag-	17	F
5	NG	10/15	10/9	NA	−	−	+	−	+	+	NA	NA	32	F
6	RD	10/15	10/8	Hep A	+	+	+	+	+	+	+		38	M
7	KR	10/16	10/13	Hep A	±	−	+	+	+	+	+	SGOT = 240	43	M
8	DM	10/16	10/13	Hep A	−	−	+	+	+	−	+		57	M
9	PA	10/18	10/7	Hep A	±	−	+	±	+	+	+		52	F
10	SS	10/18	10/11	r/o Hep	+	+	+		+		pending		24	

S* = scleral
N = nausea
V = vomiting
A = anorexia
F = fever
DU = dark urine
J = jaundice
HA IgM = Hepatitis A IgM antibody test

SOURCE: Centers for Disease Control and Prevention (1992a).

The analytical study designs available for further work will probably include either a case control study or cohort studies. At this point the basic epidemic investigation is nearly complete.

Although control and prevention are far down the list in the "Steps in the Investigation" box, they should always be uppermost in the minds of the investigators, community leadership, or facility management. With the results of the studies at hand, control should be possible.

If the problem was a foodborne outbreak of nausea, vomiting, and diarrhea, the determination of how the food became contaminated, and which conditions allowed the organism to multiply and be served, will be critical. With appropriate treatment of the cases, the immediate crisis may end. However, a review of policies and procedures may lead to modifications in food handling, processing, or serving that would prevent future outbreaks.

If this is an outbreak in a healthcare facility that resulted from transmission by staff from patient to patient, the policies and procedures related to environment cleaning, and the implementation of universal precautions—including hand washing—should be reviewed. The review may indicate the need for facility modification, staff education and retraining, or further study. For example, if the results of the epidemic investigation revealed that transmission from patient to patient occurred, then management may want to implement surveillance procedures to audit the use of appropriate hand washing and infection-control practices by staff. In addition, microbiological surveillance of staff and the environment, while expensive and time consuming, may also be necessary to identify problems with cleaning and sanitation of the patient rooms and other parts of the facility.

Prevention, through constant review and monitoring of the facility, operations, and professional and lay staff, will always be the responsibility of management, along with a rapid response to investigate and resolve outbreaks. Case Study 2.2 describes an outbreak of influenza in a New York nursing home despite a high rate of vaccination.

Case Study 2.2. Outbreak of Influenza in a New York Nursing Home

An outbreak of influenza A occurred among 337 residents of a New York nursing home during December 1991 and January 1992, despite the vaccination of 295 of them between mid-October and mid-November of 1991. The residents, 76 percent of whom were female, had a mean age of 83 years and shared common recreational and dining areas (CDC 1992b). Widespread activity and substantial mortality characterized the 1991–92 influenza season.

QUESTIONS

1. If 65 of the residents developed influenza-like illness (ILI), what proportion of the residents became sick?
2. Of those with ILI, 34 developed pneumonia, 19 required hospitalization, and 2 died. What proportion of those with ILI developed pneumonia? What percentage of those with ILI and pneumonia were hospitalized? What proportion of those with ILI died?
3. Of the 295 residents who were vaccinated, 52 developed ILI. Of the 42 residents who were not vaccinated, 13 developed ILI. What percentage of vaccinated residents developed ILI? What percentage of unvaccinated residents developed ILI? How many times higher is the rate of ILI among those who were unvaccinated compared to those who were vaccinated?
4. Of the 295 vaccinated residents, 27 developed pneumonia following ILI compared to 7 residents among the 42 who were not vaccinated. What percentage of vaccinated residents developed pneumonia following ILI? What percentage of unvaccinated residents developed pneumonia following ILI? How many times higher is the pneumonia rate following ILI among those who were unvaccinated compared to those who were vaccinated?
5. Supposedly, how high was the herd immunity in this population of nursing home residents? What was the vaccine efficacy for preventing ILI and pneumonia?

ANSWERS

1. The incidence rate (Chapter 3) of ILI is $(65/337) \times 100 = 19.3\%$.
2. The incidence rate of pneumonia among those with ILI is $(34/65) \times 100 = 52.3\%$. The hospitalization rate among those with ILI and pneumonia is $(19/34) \times 100 = 55.9\%$. Of those with ILI, the proportion who died (case-fatality rate, Chapter 6) is $(2/65) \times 100 = 3.1\%$.
3. Of those who were vaccinated, $(52/295) \times 100 = 17.6\%$ developed ILI. Of those who were not vaccinated, $(13/42) \times 100 = 31.0\%$ developed ILI. The ratio of the two rates, $31.0/17.6 = 1.76$, is called a relative risk (Chapter 12) and indicates that the unvaccinated group was 1.76 times as likely to develop ILI as the vaccinated group.
4. Of those who were vaccinated, $(27/295) \times 100 = 9.2\%$ developed pneumonia following ILI. Of those who were not vaccinated, $(7/42) \times 100 = 16.7\%$ developed pneumonia following ILI. The ratio of the two rates, $16.7/9.2 = 1.82$, indicates that the unvaccinated group was 1.82 times as likely to develop pneumonia following ILI as the vaccinated group.
5. For herd immunity, $295/337 \times 100 = 87.5\%$ of the nursing home population was immunized. However, according to Last (2000), the resistance to infection of a population of people, such as nursing home residents, depends on the number of susceptible hosts (presumably those not

immunized) as well as the chance that a susceptible host will come in contact with a carrier of disease. The fact that 52 of the immunized residents contracted influenza suggests that the vaccine was not entirely protective. Thus, this was an outbreak of influenza among a population with relatively high herd immunity. The vaccine efficacy is calculated as the difference in illness rates (unvaccinated – vaccinated) divided by the unvaccinated rate. In this case, that would be $(0.31 - 0.176)/0.31 = 0.432$ (43.2%) for vaccine efficacy in preventing ILI, and $(0.167 - 0.092)/0.167 = 0.449$ (44.9%) for vaccine efficacy in preventing pneumonia.

Summary

Louis Pasteur's germ theory of disease was proven to be much more than "ridiculous fiction," ushering in a paradigm shift in our understanding of the cause of disease. Healthcare managers certainly should be aware of the fundamental principles of infectious disease epidemiology: the agent/host/environment triangle, the process and types of disease transmission, and how diseases can be prevented or controlled. They must recognize the potential for an outbreak in their institution and the need and timing for the initiation of an epidemic investigation. Such understanding should not be entirely delegated to the infection control division. Managers may be involved in future decisions such as isolation procedures (such as in an outbreak of sudden acute respiratory disease syndrome in the local hospital), routine testing (e.g., active surveillance for methicillin-resistant *Staphylococcus aureus*) (Case Study 5.1), or outbreaks of disease (e.g., Case Study 2.2 discussed earlier). Infectious disease epidemiology has become even more relevant in the last several decades with the emergence of new or "renewed" diseases such as HIV/AIDS, Legionnaires' disease, Lyme disease, West Nile virus, and antibiotic resistance among older diseases such as tuberculosis. Chapter 17 of this text focuses in on just one of these new emergent infectious diseases, HIV/AIDS.

References

Anonymous. 1957. Lev. 13, 15; 1 Sam. 6. *New Catholic Edition of the Holy Bible*. Totowa, NJ: Catholic Book Publishing Corp.

Arundel, A., E. Sterling, J. Biggin, and T. Sterling. 1986. "Indirect Health Effects of Relative Humidity in Indoor Environments." *Environmental Health Perspectives* 65: 351–61.

Barry, J. 2005. *The Great Influenza*. London: Penguin.

Beggs, C. B. 2003. "The Airborne Transmission of Infection in Hospital Buildings: Fact or Fiction?" *Indoor and Built Environment* 12: 1–2, 9–18.

Bezanson, G., R. Khakhria, and E. Bollegraaf. 1983. "Nosocomial Outbreak Caused by Antibiotic-Resistant Strain of Salmonella Typhimurium Acquired from Dairy Cattle." *Canadian Medical Association Journal* 128: 426–27.

Bolyard, E., O. Tablan, W. Williams, M. Pearson, C. Shapiro, S. Deitchman, and the Hospital Infection Control Practices Advisory Committee. 1998. "Guideline for Infection Control in Healthcare Personnel." *American Journal of Infection Control* 26: 289–354.

Boyce, J., and D. Pittet. 2002. "Guideline for Hand Hygiene in Health-Care Settings. Recommendations of the Healthcare Infection Control Practices Advisory Committee and the HICPAC/SHEA/APIC/IDSA Hygiene Task Force." *Morbidity and Mortality Weekly Report* 51 (RR-16): 1–44.

Buccheri, C., A. Casuccio, S. Giammanco, M. Giammanco, M. La Guardia, and C. Mammina. 2007. "Food Safety in Hospital: Knowledge, Attitudes, and Practices of Nursing Staff of Two Hospitals in Sicily, Italy." *BMC Health Services Research* 7: 45–58.

Burrows, W. 1959. *Textbook of Microbiology.* Philadelphia: W. B. Saunders.

Castello, J., and S. Rogers, eds. 2005. *Life in Ancient Ice.* Princeton, NJ: Princeton University Press.

Centers for Disease Control and Prevention (CDC). 1979. Unpublished data. Atlanta, GA: Centers for Disease Control and Prevention.

———. 1992a. "Self Study Course 3030-G." *Principles of Epidemiology*, 2nd ed. Atlanta, GA: U.S. Department of Health and Human Services, Public Health Service, Centers for Disease Control and Prevention, Epidemiology Program Office, Public Health Practice Program Office.

———. 1992b. "Outbreak of Influenza A in a Nursing Home—New York, December 1991–January 1992." *Morbidity and Mortality Weekly* 41 (8): 129–31.

———. 1996. "Surveillance for Foodborne Disease Outbreaks–United States, 1988-1992." *Morbidity and Mortality Weekly Report* 45, (SS-5): 58-66.

———. 1997. "Immunization of Health-Care Workers: Recommendations of the Advisory Committee on Immunizations Practices (ACIP) and the Hospital Infection Control Practices Advisory Committee (HIC-PAC)." *Morbidity and Mortality Weekly Report* 46 (RR-18): 1–42.

Colombo, C., H. Giger, J. Grote, C. Deplazes, W. Pletscher, R. Luthi, and C. Ruef. 2002. "Impact of Teaching Interventions on Nurse Compliance with Hand Disinfection." *Journal of Hospital Infection* 51: 69–72.

Conrad, L., M. Neve, V. Nutton, R. Porter, and A. Wear. 1995. *The Western Medical Tradition 800 BC to AD 1800.* Cambridge, UK: Cambridge University Press.

Cox, C. 1976. "Inactivation Kinetics of Some Microorganisms Subjected to a Variety of Stresses." *Applied and Environmental Microbiology* 31: 836–46.

Dennesen, P., M. Bonten, and R. Weinstein. 1998. "Multiresistant Bacteria as a Hospital Epidemic Problem." *Annals of Medicine* 30: 176–85.

Doebbeling, B., and R. Wenzel. 1987. "The Epidemiology of Legionella Pneumophila Infections." *Seminars in Respiratory Infections* 2: 206–21.

Duffy, J. 1992. *The Sanatarians: A History of American Public Health.* Urbana, IL: University of Illinois Press.

Dunklin, E., and T. Puck. 1948. "The Lethal Effect of Relative Humidity on Airborne Bacteria." *Journal of Experimental Medicine* 87: 87–101.

Ehrlich, R., S. Miller, and R. Walker. 1970. "Relationship Between Atmospheric Temperature and Survival of Airborne Bacteria." *Applied Microbiology* 19: 245–49.

Farrell, J., and A. Rose. 1967. "Temperature Effects on Microorganisms." *Annual Review of Microbiology* 21: 101–20.

Fraser, D. 1980. "Legionellosis: Evidence of Airborne Transmission." *Annals of the New York Academy of Sciences* 353: 61–66.

Fraser, D., T. Tsai, W. Orenstein, W. Parkin, H. Beecham, R. Sharrar, J. Harris, G. Mallison, S. Martin, J. McDade, C. Shepard, and P. Brachman. 1977. "Legionnaires Disease: Description of an Epidemic of Pneumonia." *New England Journal of Medicine* 297: 1186–96.

Garnett, G. P. 2005. "Role of Herd Immunity in Determining the Effect of Vaccines Against Sexually Transmitted Disease." *Journal of Infectious Diseases* 191 (Suppl. 1): S97–S106.

Gastmeier, P., H. Brauer, D. Forster, E. Dietz, F. Daschner, and H. Ruden. 2002. "A Quality Management Project in 8 Selected Hospitals to Reduce Nosocomial Infections: A Prospective, Controlled Study." *Infection Control and Hospital Epidemiology* 23: 91–97.

Gikas, A., S. Maraki, E. Kritsotakis, D. Babalis, M. Roumbelaki, E. Scoulica, C. Panoulis, E. Saloustros, E. Kontopodis, G. Samonis, and Y. Tselentis. 2006. "Food-borne Nosocomial Outbreak of Salmonella Enteritica Serotype Enteritidis in a Teaching Hospital in Greece." Abstract presented to the 16th European Congress of Clinical Microbiology and Infectious Diseases, April.

Hanna, J., A. Richards, D. Young, S. Hills, and J. Humphreys. 2000. "Measles in Healthcare Facilities: Some Salutary Lessons." *Tropical Public Health Unit CDC Newsletter* 32: 2–3.

Helms, C. M., R. M. Massanari, R. Zeitler, S. Streed, M. J. Gilchrist, N. Hall, W. J. Hansler, Jr., J. Sywassink, W. Johnson, L. Wintermeyer, and W. Hierholzer. 1983. "Legionnaires' Disease Associated with a Hospital Water System: A Cluster of 24 Nosocomial Cases." *Annals of Internal Medicine* 99: 172–78.

Heymann, D. 2004. *Control of Communicable Diseases Manual*, 18th ed. Washington, DC: American Public Health Association.

Holmes, K., P. Sparling, P. Mardh, S. Lemon, W. Stamm, P. Piot, and J. Wasserheit. 1999. *Sexually Transmitted Diseases*, 3rd ed. New York: McGraw-Hill.

International Webster New Encyclopedic Dictionary. 1975. Chicago: English Language Institute of America.

Izurieta, H., M. Brana, P. Carrasco, V. Dietz, G. Tambini, C. de Quadros, N. Lopez, D. Rivera, L. Lopez, M. Vargas, E. Maita, C. Garcia, D. Pastor, C. Castro, J. Boshell, O. Castillo, G. Rey, F. de la Hoz, D. Caceres, M. Velandia, W. Bellini, J. Rota, P. Rota, F. Levano, and C. Lee. 2002. "Outbreak of Measles—Venezuela and Colombia, 2001–2002." *Morbidity and Mortality Weekly Report* 51: 757–60.

Kelly, J. 2005. *The Great Mortality: An Intimate History of the Black Death: The Most Devastating Plague of All Time.* New York: HarperCollins.

Krause, P., P. Gross, T. Barrett, E. Dellinger, W. Martone, J. McGowan, Jr., R. Sweet, and R. Wenzel. 1994. "Quality Standard for Assurance of Measles Immunity Among Healthcare Workers." *Clinical Infectious Diseases* 18: 431–36.

Last, J. 2000. *A Dictionary of Epidemiology,* 4th ed. New York: Oxford University Press.

Lester, W., Jr. 1948. "The Influence of Relative Humidity on the Infectivity of Air-Borne Influenza Virus (PR8 Strain)." *Journal of Experimental Medicine* 88: 361–68.

Lucet, J., M. Rigaud, F. Mentre, N. Kassis, C. Deblangy, A. Andremont, and E. Bouvet. 2002. "Hand Contamination Before and After Different Hand Hygiene Techniques: A Randomized Clinical Trial." *Journal of Hospital Infection* 50: 276–80.

Lyons, A., and R. Petrucelli. 1978. *Medicine: An Illustrated History.* New York: Abradale.

Makison, C., and J. Swan. 2006. "The Effect of Humidity on the Survival of MRSA on Hard Surfaces." *Indoor and Built Environment* 15: 85–91.

Naphaetian, K., O. Challemel, D. Beurtin, S. Dubrou, P. Gounon, and R. Squinazi. 1991. "The Intracellular Multiplication of Legionella Pneumophila in Protozoa from Hospital Plumbing Systems." *Research in Microbiology* 142: 677–86.

Nelson, K., and C. Masters Williams. 2007. *Infectious Disease Epidemiology, Theory and Practice,* 2nd ed. Boston: Jones and Bartlett.

Nguyen, Q. 2007. "Hospital-Acquired Infections." [Online article; retrieved 7/8/07.] www.emedicine.com/ped/topic1619.htm.

Nibley, M. 2007. "Hospital Infection Control Saves Lives, Cuts Costs." *Medical News Today,* May 11.

Platt, C. 1996. *King Death: The Black Death and Its Aftermath in Late-Medieval England.* Toronto: University of Toronto Press.

Price, R., and P. Tom. 1992. "Environmental Conditions for Pathogenic Bacterial Growth." [Online information; retrieved 7/18/07.] www.seafood.ucdavis.edu/Pubs/pathogen.htm.

Sabetta, J., S. Hyman, J. Smardin, M. Carter, J. Hadler, and Enteric Diseases Branch, Centers for Disease Control and Prevention. 1991. "Foodborne Nosocomial Outbreak of Salmonella Reading—Connecticut." *Morbidity and Mortality Weekly Report* 40: 804–5.

Sehulster, L., and R. Chinn. 2003. "Guidelines for Environmental Infection Control in Health-Care Facilities, Recommendations of CDC and the Healthcare Infection Control Practices Advisory Committee (HIC-PAC)." *Morbidity and Mortality Weekly Report* 52 (RR-10): 1–42.

Sepkowitz, K. 1996. "Occupationally Acquired Infections in Healthcare Workers: Part I." *Annals of Internal Medicine* 125: 826–34.

Siegel, J., E. Rhinehart, M. Jackson, L. Chiarello, and the Healthcare Infections Control Practices Advisory Committee. 2007. *2007 Guideline for Isolation Precautions: Preventing Transmission of Infectious Agents in Healthcare Settings.* [Online report; retrieved 7/10/07.] www.cdc.gov/ncidod/dhqp/pdf/isolation2007.pdf.

Squier, C., V. Yu, and J. Stout. 2000. "Waterborne Nosocomial Infections." *Current Infectious Disease Reports* 2: 490–96.

Stine, S., I. Song, C. Choi, and C. Gerba. 2005. "Effect of Relative Humidity on Preharvest of Bacterial and Viral Pathogens on the Surface of Cantaloupe, Lettuce, and Bell Peppers." *Journal of Food Protection* 68: 1352–58.

Stout, J., V. Yu, and M. Best. 1985. "Ecology of Legionella Pneumophila Within Water Distribution Systems." *Applied Environmental Microbiology* 49: 221–28.

Terada, K., T. Niizuma, S. Ogita, N. Kataoka, and Y. Niki. 2001. "Outbreak of Measles in a Hospital and Measures Taken Against Hospital Infection—Evidence of Cost and Benefits." [English abstract.] *Kansenshogaku Zasshi* 75: 480–84.

Tietjen, L., D. Bossemeyer, and N. McIntosh. 2003. *Infection Prevention: Guidelines for Healthcare Facilities with Limited Resources.* Baltimore, MD: JHPIEGO.

Timmreck, T. 2002. *An Introduction to Epidemiology*, 3rd ed. Boston: Jones and Bartlett.

Tipple, M., W. Heirendt, B. Metchock, K. Ijaz, P. McElroy, and the Division of TB Elimination, Centers for Disease Control and Prevention. 2004. "Tuberculosis Outbreak in a Community Hospital—District of Columbia, 2002." *Morbidity and Mortality Weekly Report* 53: 214–16.

World Health Organization (WHO). 2003. "Hospital Infection Control Guidance for Severe Respiratory Syndrome (SARS)." [Online information; retrieved 7/8/07.] www.who.int/csr/sars/infectioncontrol/en/print.html.

Zerr, D., M. Garrison, A. Allpress, J. Heath, and D. Christakis. 2005. "Infection Control Policies and Hospital-Associated Infections Among Surgical Patients: Variability and Associations in a Multicenter Pediatric Setting." *Pediatrics* 115: 387–92.

Ziegler, P. 1996. *The Black Death*. London: HarperCollins.

MEASURING AND INTERPRETING MORBIDITY

Steven T. Fleming and F. Douglas Scutchfield

> *"It is time to close the book on infectious diseases, declare the war against pestilence won, and shift national resources to such chronic problems as cancer and heart disease."* U.S. Surgeon General William H. Stewart, 1967

The current surgeon general would certainly disagree with this statement, made over 40 years ago. Despite the massive shift in cause of death from infectious to chronic diseases over the last century, the "war against pestilence" has not been won. Enemies such as HIV/AIDS (Chapter 16), methicillin-resistant *Staphylococcus aureus* (Case Study 5.1), and influenza, among others, are still formidable foes.

This chapter focuses on the measurement and interpretation of disease statistics. We describe the nature, definition, and classification of disease, while making a distinction between disease and illness. We discuss the natural history of disease, or quite simply, how the disease "plays out" over time; the various sources of morbidity data; and how morbidity can be measured with incidence and prevalence statistics. Finally, we focus on screening and diagnostic tests; review their characteristics, such as sensitivity and specificity; and present three case studies regarding product lines and breast and prostate cancer screening to illustrate these points.

The Nature and Definition of Disease

Disease can be defined in a number of ways. Timmreck (2002, 28) defines *disease* as "any disruption in the function and structure of the body...an abnormal state in which the body is not capable of responding to or carrying on its normally required functions." Koepsell and Weiss (2003, 18) define disease simply as "almost any departure from perfect health." Susser (1973) distinguishes between *disease* and *illness*, the former being "physiological or psychological dysfunction" and the latter a "subjective" state where a person does not feel well. The single term *morbidity* is defined by Last (2001) as "any departure subjective or objective, from a state of physiological or psychological well-being," a definition that includes disease and illness. Timmreck (2002) expands this definition to include "injuries" as well.

Many different types of diseases affect human beings, thus posing a challenge to classify these diseases in a meaningful and efficient way. One could classify diseases by their means of transmission—for example, those that are airborne (such as influenza), vector-borne (such as malaria), or transmitted through intestinal discharge (such as cholera). One could also classify diseases by their source, such as those caused by microorganisms (such as plague) or inanimate sources (such as radiation or noise). The most comprehensive and widely used method of disease classification is the International Classification of Diseases (ICD), now in its tenth edition, which classifies diseases into more than 65,000 categories. The diseases are categorized primarily by body system—there are separate chapters for the nervous, circulatory, respiratory, and digestive systems, with codes of up to seven digits. For example, with diabetes, the first three digits denote the type of diabetes (e.g., E10, insulin-dependent diabetes). The fourth digit classifies the type of complications (e.g., E102, renal), and a fifth digit denotes specific complications (e.g., E1023, diabetes mellitus with diabetic renal failure). A sixth digit can further refine complications. A seventh digit is used in a number of situations, such as to distinguish between initial and subsequent encounters (in the case of injuries), to indicate which fetus is involved in the complication (in the case of pregnancies), or to indicate the severity of a coma. Although the tenth edition represents a substantial refinement over the earlier ICD-9-CM (for example, four times as many codes for diabetes alone), the changes in classification and expansion in number of codes pose problems for monitoring changes in morbidity over time.

Natural History of Disease

The natural history of disease refers to the course of disease over time from onset to resolution, or more simply, how the disease unfolds over time.

Valanis (1999) illustrates the natural history of disease as consisting of a number of distinct phases (Figure 3.1). Exposure to the agent occurs during the pre-pathogenesis phase (before the disease process begins). The susceptibility phase denotes the period during which the host may be particularly susceptible to the agent, because of low resistance, poor nutrition, and so on. If the host is successful in resisting disease, this would occur during the adaptation phase. The pathogenesis phase consists of the development of disease, with the early pathogenesis phase being before symptoms occur. One can distinguish the early from the late clinical phase, with the former being the period during which diagnosis occurs. The period between exposure and onset of symptoms is referred to as the *incubation period* for infectious agents, and *induction period* or *latency period* for noninfectious agents.

FIGURE 3.1
Natural
History of
Disease

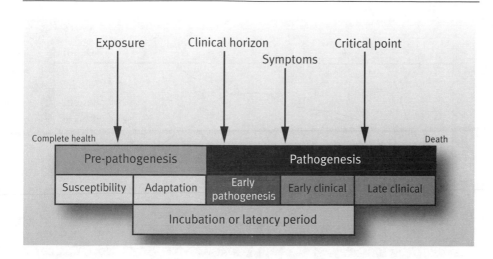

SOURCE: Adapted from Valanis, Barbara. *Epidemiology in Health Care*, 3rd Edition, © 1999, p. 22. Adapted by permission of Pearson Education, Inc., Upper Saddle River, NJ.

Valanis also defines terms that are useful for assessing whether a screening program would be effective. The *clinical horizon* is the "imaginary line dividing the point where there are detectable signs and symptoms from that where there are not" (Valanis 1999, 23). The *critical point* is "a theoretical time in the natural history that is crucial in determining whether there are major or severe consequences of the disease" (Valanis 1999, 274). For the latter, one might envision serious disabilities, coma, or, in the case of cancer, spread of the cancer throughout the body.

For a screening program to be effective, the clinical horizon must occur before the critical point. In other words, we must be able to detect disease at a point in its natural history before major consequences occur. If the critical point occurs before the clinical horizon, as is the case with some cancers (e.g., pancreatic cancer), serious consequences occur before the disease can be detected, so screening is ineffective. In such cases, it is the challenge of medical technology to move the clinical horizon to an earlier point in the natural history of the disease.

Each disease has a characteristic natural history, though some diseases may share similar manisfestations over time. Acute diseases are relatively severe, treatable diseases of short duration, with an outcome of either recovery or death. Chronic diseases are typically less severe and of longer duration, and often do not conclude with complete recovery but progressive disability. Subacute diseases are intermediate in both severity and duration.

With this in mind, another way to conceptualize natural history is to graph the progress of disease over time in terms of severity of disease or departure from wellness or health, as postulated by Donabedian (1973, 73) 35 years ago. Figure 3.2 illustrates the wide range of natural histories. Line

FIGURE 3.2
Hypothetical
Time–
Intensity
Relationships
in Disease

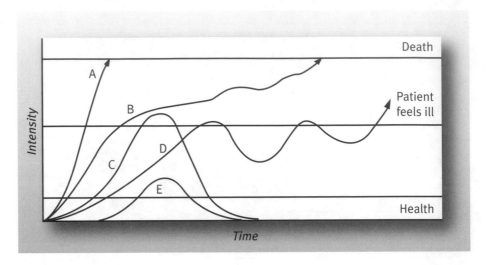

SOURCE: Reprinted by permission of the publisher from ASPECTS OF MEDICAL CARE ADMINISTRA-
TION: SPECIFYING REQUIREMENTS FOR HEALTH CARE by Avedis Donabedian, p. 72, Cambridge,
MA: Harvard University Press, Copyright © 1973 by the President and Fellows of Harvard College and the
Commonwealth Fund.

A represents an acute disease leading to death. B is a chronic disease leading to progressive disability. C is an acute, self-limited disease that normally
concludes with the patient at complete health. D is a chronic disease with
relapsing episodes (e.g., multiple sclerosis). E is an acute asymptomatic disease (i.e., a disease that infects a person but produces no symptoms).

Sources of Morbidity Data

Morbidity data can be obtained from a number of different sources in the
United States and elsewhere. In this country, physicians and laboratories
submit data to the public health departments, who in turn submit these
data to the Centers for Disease Control and Prevention (CDC).

Specific "notifiable" diseases must be reported within certain time
frames depending on the degree to which each is a threat to public health.
For example, botulism (a deadly foodborne illness that causes paralysis)
must be reported by telephone immediately; hepatitus A, malaria, and
measles must be reported within one day; AIDS, mumps, and Lyme disease must be reported within a week. CDC publishes regular reports of
these diseases and others through the weekly publication *Mortality and
Morbidity Weekly Report* (www.cdc.gov/mmwr).

Clinical records from physicians and hospitals are another source of
morbidity data. Medical records in both settings are a rich repository of morbidity data, though the recent Health Insurance Portability and Accountability

Act regulations protect the confidentiality of such data, making it more difficult to access. Some would argue that medical records represent a biased source of morbidity statistics, since people who are treated in healthcare settings may not be representative of the community at large. Some people are sick but do not seek medical attention for various reasons, such as problems accessing care or a lack of insurance.

Financial "claims" derived from patient encounters are a related source of morbidity data, inasmuch as each claim is tagged with one or more diagnoses. Claims are tied to reimbursement by third-party providers such as Medicare and Medicaid, and as such are driven by financial incentives. The diagnoses associated with each claim may be those that maximize reimbursement, rather than those that are most clinically relevant.

Morbidity registries are a third source of morbidity data. Perhaps the most mature registry system in this country is the network of registries coordinated by the North American Association of Central Cancer Registries. The National Cancer Institute administers the Surveillance Epidemiology and End Results program, which collects registry data from states and cities representing about 25 percent of the U.S. population.

A fourth source of morbidity data is the periodic surveys that are undertaken by various federal, state, and local agencies. The National Center for Health Statistics (www.cdc.gov/nchs/) compiles morbidity information through its numerous surveys. These include the National Health Interview Survey, the Health and Nutrition Survey, the National Hospital Discharge Survey, the National Nursing Home Survey, and the National Ambulatory Medical Survey, among others. Much of this information is available to the public and can be downloaded from the center's website.

Measuring Morbidity

The burden of illness in a population can be expressed by two different kinds of rates: prevalence and incidence.

Prevalence comes in two varieties: point prevalence and period prevalence. *Point prevalence* is the number of events occurring in a population at a point in time. For example, the number of individuals with asthma in Kentucky on July 1, 2007, was 250 per 100,000. *Period prevalence* is the number of people who had the condition during a specific period, such as a month or year. Prevalence rates are often used for the purpose of healthcare planning, where the knowledge of the number of people with a certain condition or disease is particularly helpful in estimating future resource needs.

The incidence rate, on the other hand, measures how many new cases of a given disease occur in a defined population over a certain period. Incidence is important in the examination of disease etiology. Although it is useful in health planning, frequently it is less useful than prevalence rates. However, because of the proximity of the development of the disease to the causes of that disease, the research epidemiologist often prefers to use incidence rates, since those rates are more likely to reflect causation.

Consider the example of HIV/AIDS. In 2005, newly diagnosed cases numbered 37,331, but an estimated 475,220 people were living with HIV/AIDS (CDC 2007). The first figure is used to calculate the incidence rate and the latter the prevalence rate. So with these numbers, the incidence rate for 2005 was 19.8 per 100,000 and the prevalence rate was 252.5 per 100,000:

37,331/188,222,674 (est. U.S. pop. 33 states) × 100,000 = 19.8/100,000
475,220/188,222,674 (est. U.S. pop. 33 states) × 100,000 = 252.5/100,000

Clearly, incidence and prevalence are related. Figure 3.3 illustrates this relationship. The faucet dripping into the bowl represents the incidence. That is how the addition of new cases is accumulated in the prevalence rate. The volume in the bowl represents the prevalence. The faucet representing the outflow from the bowl reflects the fact that people with the illness either die or get well and no longer are in the prevalence bowl. Thus, prevalence and incidence are related by duration. The relationship is measured as Prevalence = Incidence × Duration.

This illustrates that an increase in prevalence may be the result of increases in incidence, duration, or both. If you know two terms of the equation, it is possible to solve for the third term.

FIGURE 3.3
Relationship
Between
Incidence
and
Prevalence

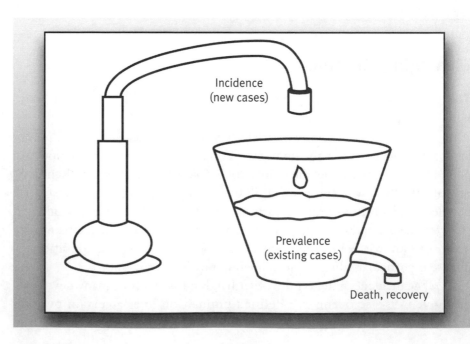

When collecting morbidity statistics, the epidemiologist must decide what to do with recurrent cases of disease, that is, disease that occurs more than once in the same person. Both the nature of disease and the period between episodes are important. If the nature of the disease lends itself to recurrences (e.g., gonorrhea), then recurrent cases are usually counted as new cases, as long as the period between disease episodes is long enough to treat the recurrent case as a "new case" rather than a "relapse" of an earlier illness.

To illustrate these points, consider Figure 3.4, which summarizes the occurrence of a particular disease (say, gonorrhea) among 1,000 college students. Gonorrhea often recurs, so we can specify the time window between episodes (say, one month). The incidence rate is calculated as the number of new cases over a specified period (say, one year) divided by the population at risk (in this case, 1,000 students). In Figure 3.4, we see that the new cases for 2007 include cases 2, 3, 4, 5, 7 (recurrence), 8, 10, and 11. (Student F suffered a recurrence [case 7], because the second episode occurred outside the specified time window. This would count as a new incident case. Student H suffered an "episode" within the time window. We presume this to be the same case [case 9], rather than a new case.) Thus, there are eight new cases, divided by an at-risk population of 1,000, for an incidence rate of 8 per 1,000.

The period prevalence rate is the number of existing cases during a specified period. Since reoccurring cases that occur within the specified time window count, this would include all 11 cases, for a period prevalence

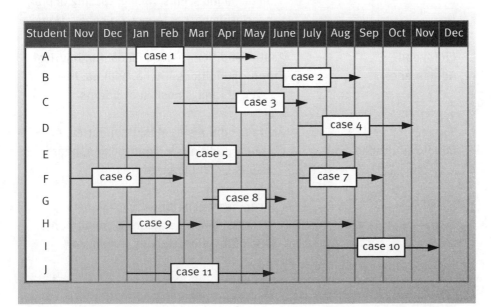

FIGURE 3.4
Prevalence and Incidence Rates Among 1,000 College Students, Nov. 2006–Dec. 2007

rate of 11 per 1,000. The point prevalence rate is evaluated at a particular point in time, say July, 15, 2007. At that point in time, there were five existing cases, for a point prevalence rate of 5 per 1,000.

Incidence and prevalence rates can be used to characterize patterns of disease by age group. Table 3.1 summarizes the work of Valanis (1999), in which she describes the kinds of disease and related issues and problems by age groups including (1) infancy/pregnancy, (2) childhood and adolescence, (3) young to middle adulthood, and (4) the elderly.

For example, among infants, respiratory distress, congenital malformations, sudden infant death syndrome (SIDS), and low birth weight (LBW) are the critical morbidities. For pregnant women, AIDS, toxemia (pregnancy-induced high blood pressure), ectopic pregnancies, and hemorrhage are the critical morbidities. Related issues include declining fertility, pregnancy among older women and adolescents, and the timing and spacing of pregnancies. Acute conditions such as head colds, influenza, and injuries are replaced by chronic

TABLE 3.1 Patterns of Morbidity by Age Group	

Age Group	Morbidity
Infancy/Pregnancy	Infants: respiratory distress, congenital malformations, SIDS, LBW newborns Pregnancy: prenatal care, AIDS, toxemia, ectopic pregancies, hemorrhage, adequate nutrition and weight gain, fertility declining, pregnancy among older women, pregnancy among adolescents, timing/spacing of pregnancies, impact of tobacco, alcohol, drugs
Childhood/ Adolescence	Acute conditions—head colds, flu, injuries Chronic conditions—acne, asthma, hay fever, chronic sinusitis, accidents
Young/ Middle adulthood	Acute conditions—colds, flu, injuries, AIDS Chronic conditions—hypertension, heart disease, diabetes, arthritis
Elderly	Cancer, heart conditions, hypertension, arthritis, diabetes, hearing impairments, loss of function, nursing home use

SOURCE: Valanis (1999).

conditions such as hypertension, heart disease, cancer, and diabetes as a person gets older. Case Study 3.1 illustrates how morbidity data could inform the decision of Group Health East to develop a product line for asthma care.

Case Study 3.1. Product Lines for Group Health East

Group Health East (GHE), a fictitious 100,000-member managed care organization, is interested in moving away from a functional or divisional structure to a matrix model. The challenge is to identify and develop relevant product lines or programs.

Initially this involves a "needs assessment" (Chapter 4) both in terms of an internal assessment of capacity (i.e., current products and current physical and human resources) and an external assessment of the environment (markets, competitors, needs of the population, and so forth). The latter is characterized by epidemiological measures, such as the incidence/prevalence of acute and chronic disease.

Within the hospital, GHE must examine case-mix patterns over a period of years, say, ten. Diagnosis-related groups (DRGs) represent specific hospital products for the Medicare population, whose data have been available since 1983. It would be useful to examine changes in DRG mix over time, and across competitors in the hospital service area, to describe the need for specific "hospital" products in the service area.

Since GHE is a managed care organization, it may also want to get measures of ambulatory care need, if available, such as a breakdown of visits to physicians by diagnosis. It will also be worthwhile to collect data on the enrolled population, in terms of various risk factors that lead to disease, such as obesity, smoking, and hazardous workplaces. This information would be key to forecasting future product lines.

QUESTIONS

1. Along which dimensions could one characterize the enrolled population in this managed care organization; how might one measure these dimensions; and how could this information be used to develop product lines?
2. GHE is considering the care for asthma as a possible product line since the incidence of asthma in the United States and throughout the world has increased dramatically over the past several decades (Pearce 1998; Chadwick and Cardew 1997). Suppose GHE reported 250 hospitalizations for asthma in 2007 (a rate of 2.5 per 1,000 enrolled members), based on an evaluation of DRGs. At least some of these inpatient episodes were potentially avoidable. To what state or national statistics could GHE compare this rate?
3. The ambulatory visit profile for GHE showed 3,500 physician visits for

asthma, for a rate of 3.5 per 100 enrolled members, somewhat lower than the state average. To what sources of data could GHE compare this rate to national statistics?

4. What actions might GHE take with regard to the care for asthma patients? Consider that 35 percent of the enrolled population of GHE are considered regular smokers, a suspected risk factor for pediatric asthma.

ANSWERS

1. The enrolled population could be characterized on three dimensions: acute care, ambulatory care, and risk factors. For acute care, the prevalence of disease/disability could be measured by case mix and described over a five-year period by DRG. Some DRGs could be clustered together into larger hospital products, or labeled as "potentially avoidable" (Chapter 5). In terms of ambulatory visits, members could be grouped into classes based on diagnosis. For risk factors, members could be assessed on the basis of smoking, obesity, substance abuse, and employment in a hazardous workplace. The three dimensions could then be integrated into potential product lines or programs.

2. The Massachusetts Division of Health Care Finance and Policy collects statewide hospital discharge data. GHE could use this information to compare the asthma hospitalization rate. Nationally, there are two sources of hospital discharge data. The National Hospital Discharge Survey, sponsored by the National Center for Health Statistics, contains about 270,000 inpatient records from a national sample of about 500 hospitals. The Nationwide Inpatient Sample, sponsored by the Agency for Healthcare Research and Quality, is a large, all-payer database of about 8 million records from 1,004 hospitals in 37 states. Either of these databases would provide excellent national statistics on the asthma hospitalization rate nationwide.

3. For national data, GHE could access the National Ambulatory Medical Care Survey, which provides reliable information on the utilization of ambulatory medical care services in the United States. Each physician in the survey is randomly assigned to a one-week period, over which data are collected on a random sample of patient visits.

4. Smoking cessation programs would be critical here, but many asthma patients also lack access to healthcare or education regarding the disease process and proper use of inhaler treatments. GHE could adopt a more proactive posture on the monitoring of asthma patients, so as to reduce the incidence of avoidable hospitalizations.

Screening

Secondary prevention typically involves the use of screening tests to identify individuals with a particular disease in the hope of finding the disease at an early and treatable stage. *Screening* is the "identification of unrecognized disease or defect by the application of tests, examinations, or other procedures that can be applied rapidly and inexpensively to populations" (Valanis 1999).

Screening and diagnostic tests differ in a number of ways. Screening tests are typically done before, rather than after, symptoms occur. These tests do not need to be ordered by a physician, as is the case with diagnostic tests, and may be obtained in nonmedical settings, such as health fairs. Diagnostic tests typically require expensive, specialized equipment; are more time consuming; and may incur pain, discomfort, or risk. Screening tests are usually simpler, quicker, and painless. Screening tests are applied to healthy populations to identify disease before symptoms occur, so it can be treated early. Diagnostic tests are applied to patients with symptoms to determine an accurate diagnosis.

Two measures of the quality of a test are validity and reliability. *Validity* refers to the accuracy with which a measure, such as a screening test, represents a particular phenomenon. For example, suppose a five-question screening test was developed for clinical depression; the test would have validity to the extent that the questions accurately characterized this mental disorder. As another example, the prostate-specific antigen (PSA) screening test for prostate cancer has validity if a measurement of PSA accurately portrays prostate cancer.

Reliability is a measure of consistency. Reliable screening tests yield the same results regardless of the number of times they are repeated. *Interrater reliability* measures the degree to which different reviewers get the same results with single or multiple applications of a test. *Intrarater reliability* refers to the consistency of test results found by the same reviewer. For example, one could assess the interrater reliability of a blood pressure screening test by determining the consistency of results with multiple tests by different nurses. The intrarater reliability of mammography could be assessed by measuring the consistency of test results when a single radiologist interprets a number of films on multiple occasions.

Ideally, the screening test should distinguish individuals who have the disease (the true positives) from those who do not (the true negatives). The test should minimize the number of individuals who do not have the disease but test positive (the false positives) and those who have the disease but test negative (the false negatives).

The logic of the screening test involves the choice of a particular level (e.g., blood pressure level or level of prostate-specific antigen) as

FIGURE 3.5
Screening for
Disease

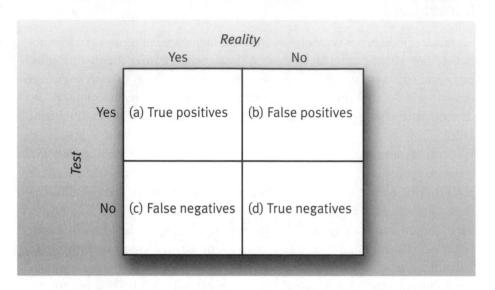

the critical juncture between the positive and false negative test result, in an effort to minimize false positives and negatives. Unfortunately, this represents a trade-off. If one wants to be sure that the test identifies all true positives, then one must accept a higher level of false positives. By the same token, to ensure that those who test positive for the disease do in fact really have the disease, one must accept more false negatives. These concepts are called sensitivity and specificity.

Sensitivity measures the proportion of those who are diseased and test positive, whereas *specificity* measures the proportion of those who are not diseased and test negative. Thus, sensitivity is the ability of the test to identify those who are truly sick, whereas specificity is the ability of the test to correctly identify those who are well.

This relationship is illustrated mathematically in the two-by-two table of Figure 3.5. The columns represent those with and without the disease, labeled "reality." The rows represent those who test positive and negative. Cell a represents the true positives, b represents false positives, c is the false negatives, and d is the true negatives.

Assume that 2,000 people are tested, 1,000 with the disease and 1,000 without. Figure 3.6 is an example of what might be found when the test is done. The sensitivity is calculated by dividing a by a + c, and the specificity is calculated by dividing d by b + d. In our hypothetical case, the sensitivity is 80 percent and the specificity is 90 percent. This represents a less-than-ideal test, but one consistent with several commonly used laboratory tests. One can also calculate a false positive ratio as b divided by b + d and the false negative ratio as c divided by a + c. With a sensitivity of 80 percent and a specificity of 90 percent, the false positive

FIGURE 3.6
Sensitivity,
Specificity,
PPV, NPV by
Disease
Prevalence

		Disease (50%)		Disease (10%)		Disease (1%)	
		Yes	No	Yes	No	Yes	No
Test	Yes	800	100	160	180	16	198
	No	200	900	40	1,620	4	1,782
Totals		1,000	1,000	200	1,800	20	1,980

Sensitivity = 80%	Sensitivity = 80%	Sensitivity = 80%
Specificity = 90%	Specificity = 90%	Specificity = 90%
PPV = .89	PPV = .47	PPV = .07
NPV = .82	NPV = .98	NPV = .998

and false negative ratios are 0.10 (10 percent) and 0.20 (20 percent), respectively.

The number of false positives and false negatives will vary with the prevalence of the disease, even though the sensitivity and specificity of the test will remain the same. The hypothetical example just presented assumed a prevalence of 50 percent, that is, of the 2,000 people tested, half had the disease.

Figure 3.6 also illustrates the case with the same specificity and sensitivity in a group of 2,000 individuals where the prevalence is 10 percent. With a 50 percent prevalence, 100 people are incorrectly labeled as positive. With a 10 percent prevalence, the number rises to 180 of the 2,000 population. As you can see, the number of false positives increases as the prevalence rate decreases. If the prevalence rate were 1 percent, 198 people would be mislabeled as false positives.

The measure that examines the ability of a test to predict disease is called the *predictive value*. One can measure both the positive and the negative predictive value of a test. The positive predictive value (PPV) is the proportion of those who test positive and who actually have the disease. The negative predictive value (NPV) is the proportion of those who test negative and who actually do not have the disease. Returning to the two-by-two table of Figure 3.5, the positive predictive value is a divided by a + b and the negative predictive value is d divided by c + d. Note the positive and negative predictive value in the circumstance where the prevalence of the disease is 50 percent, 10 percent, and 1 percent (Figure 3.6). The positive predictive value falls to less than 10 percent in the situation where the prevalence is 1 percent. Case Study 3.2 illustrates some of these concepts with digital and film mammography for breast cancer.

Case Study 3.2. Breast Cancer Screening

Pisano and colleagues (2005) compare the performance of digital to film mammography for breast cancer screening with sensitivities and specificities in Table 3.2 below.

TABLE 3.2. SENSITIVITY AND SPECIFICITY OF DIGITAL AND FILM MAMMOGRAPHY BY PATIENT GROUP, 42,760 WOMEN

	Digital		Film	
	Sensitivity	Specificity	Sensitivity	Specificity
Women < 50 years old	0.78	0.90	0.51	0.90
Premenopausal and perimenopausal women	0.72	0.90	0.51	0.90
Women with dense breasts	0.70	0.91	0.55	0.90
All women	0.70	0.92	0.66	0.92

SOURCE: Pisano et al. (2005).

Assume that 0.04 percent of women below age 50 will have breast cancer. Moreover, assume that women with dense breasts are three times as likely to get breast cancer and that the prevalence of breast cancer among symptomatic women is about 10 percent.

QUESTIONS

1. How successful is film mammography in identifying women with breast cancer?
2. How successful is film mammography in correctly ruling out the disease in women without breast cancer?
3. Of all those without breast cancer, what percentage will incorrectly test positive (false positives)?
4. Suppose that you screened a population of 100,000 women under age 50 using both the digital and film mammograms. How confident would a women who tests positive or negative be that she has breast cancer?

5. Suppose that you screened 1,000 *symptomatic* women under the age of 50 using digital mammography. How confident could these women be in a positive or negative test result?

ANSWERS

1. According to this study, only 66 percent of all women and 51 percent of women under age 50 who have breast cancer will be identified by this screening test.
2. The test correctly identifies 90 percent of women under age 50 without breast cancer.
3. With a specificity of 90 percent, 10 percent of all those without breast cancer will be false positives.
4. From the information, one can derive the following 2 × 2 table (Table 3.3) for digital and film mammography.

TABLE 3.3. DIGITAL AND FILM MAMMOGRAPHY, 2 × 2 TABLES

	Digital Mammography			Film Mammography		
	Cancer	No Cancer	Total	Cancer	No Cancer	Total
Test positive	31	9,996	10,027	20	9,996	10,016
Test negative	9	89,964	89,973	20	89,964	89,984
Total	40	99,960	100,000	40	99,960	100,000

Step 1: If there are 100,000 women who are screening and the prevalence of breast cancer is 0.04 percent, then $0.0004 \times 100,000 = 40$ of them actually have breast cancer.

Step 2: Of the 40 women who actually have cancer, 31 of them will test positive with a digital mammography (sensitivity $0.78 \times 40 = 31$) and 20 of then will test positive with a film mammography ($0.51 \times 40 = 20$).

Step 3: Of the 99,960 women without breast cancer, 89,964 of them will test negative with both mammograms if the specificity is 0.90 ($0.90 \times 99,960 = 89,964$).

The positive predictive value for digital mammography is $31/(31 + 9,996) = 0.0031$. The positive predictive value for film mammography is $20/(9,996 + 20) = 0.0020$. Thus, less than 1 percent of women who are under 50 years old who test positive (with either of these tests) actually have breast cancer.

TABLE 3.4. DIGITAL MAMMOGRAPHY, 2 × 2 TABLE

	Cancer	No Cancer	Total
Test positive	78	90	168
Test negative	22	810	832
Total	100	900	1,000

SOURCE: Pisano et al. (2005).

5. From the information, one can derive the above 2 × 2 table (Table 3.4) for digital mammography.

Step 1: If there are 1,000 symptomatic women who are screened and the prevalence of breast cancer for symptomatic women is 10 percent, then 0.10 × 1,000 = 100 of them actually have breast cancer.

Step 2: Of the 100 women who actually have cancer, 78 of them will test positive with a digital mammography (sensitivity 0.78 × 100 = 78).

Step 3: Of the 900 women without breast cancer, 810 of them will test negative if the specificity is 0.90 (0.90 × 900 = 810).

The positive predictive value for digital mammography is 78/168 = 0.46. Thus, a symptomatic woman can be 46 percent confident that she has breast cancer if she tests positive with digital mammography.

The difference between sensitivity and positive predictive value, on the one hand, and specificity and negative predictive value, on the other, is not entirely intuitive. Sensitivity and specificity are intrinsic characteristics of the test itself and of the ability of that test to make a distinction—on the basis of some measureable characteristic, such as blood sugar or blood pressure levels—between those who are diseased and those who are not. Positive and negative predictive values are derived not only from characteristics of the test, but also from the prevalence of the disease in the population. As shown earlier, it can be demonstrated empirically that positive predictive value increases as disease prevalence does. The test itself has not changed, but one can place more trust in a positive test result from a screening test applied to a population wherein the disease is highly prevalent. On the other hand, negative predictive value falls as disease prevalence rises. One can trust a negative test result more with rare diseases than with common diseases.

In assessing the usefulness of a screening test, it is necessary to ensure that it is both sensitive and specific; however, it is also important to examine the predictive value of a test, as discussed earlier. A classic example of this issue is HIV testing. When the causative agent for AIDS was identified and a test was developed to screen for HIV, a great deal of pressure came into play to test various groups, frequently not of high risk. The obvious downside to testing a low-prevalence population for HIV is that many individuals would falsely test positive. This would result in incorrectly labeling many as having the virus. It would also result in substantial time and energy to evaluate the extent to which the positive test was correct for a specific individual, and would create a great deal of unnecessary anxiety in those who tested positive but did not have the virus. The better strategy was to use the test in high-risk populations, where the prevalence would be high enough to ensure a better positive predictive value. The current HIV-1 enzyme immunoassay test has such high sensitivity and specificity (99.9 percent and 99.85 percent, respectively) that the positive predictive value is high enough, even in a low-risk population, if a repeat test is administered. See Case Study 16.1.

A good screening program is one that is relatively simple to implement and relatively inexpensive. It employs a test with high enough specificity and sensitivity to detect a disease of sufficient importance (in terms of prevalence or severity) at an early enough stage that prompt and available treatment significantly improves outcomes. The test is relatively safe and "acceptable" to patients.

For example, let us compare the mammography and colonoscopy screening for breast and colorectal cancer, respectively. The former is moderately simple and inexpensive, and relatively safe and acceptable to patients, though there is some discomfort. The test has moderately high sensitivity and specificity. It detects the most prevalent cancer among women, and early detection can improve survival. The colonoscopy is an invasive, relatively expensive, surgical procedure carrying a small, but significant, risk of complications. Patient acceptability is a major problem due to the one- or two-day unpleasant "preparation" that is required. Early detection for this leading cause of cancer among both men and women can significantly improve outcomes. Case Study 3.3 illustrates the technique of sequencing two screening tests to improve positive predictive value.

Case Study 3.3. Prostate Cancer Screening

Prostate cancer is the most frequently diagnosed cancer among men in the United States. It can be detected early with a digital rectal examination or a prostate-specific antigen (PSA) blood test. The latter has been the subject of much controversy given the relatively poor characteristics of this test. The enzyme measured by this test increases with age, and is also elevated by benign prostate hypertrophy. As a result, some have suggested an enzyme cut-off level (to distinguish between those who test positive and negative) that is age-specific. Others have suggested measuring the proportion of "free-PSA," or the "PSA velocity," which measures the change in PSA over time. Sun and colleagues (2007) report the sensitivity and specificity of PSA and PSA velocity (PSAV) by enzyme level for men under and over age 50 in Table 3.5.

TABLE 3.5. SENSITIVITY AND SPECIFICITY OF PSA AND PSAV BY AGE GROUP AND LEVEL

| | < 50 | | ≥ 50 | |
PSA Level (ng/mL)	Sensitivity (%)	Specificity (%)	Sensitivity (%)	Specificity (%)
1.0	85.0	73.6	89.3	39.8
2.0	75.0	92.2	83.4	65.5
2.5	73.8	94.1	81.0	72.7
3.0	68.8	95.9	78.3	77.8
4.0	61.3	97.7	71.3	85.2
PSAV (ng/mL/year)	Sensitivity (%)	Specificity (%)	Sensitivity (%)	Specificity (%)
0.10	95.2	41.0	95.0	26.1
0.20	85.7	62.1	91.2	44.1
0.30	71.4	73.2	88.6	54.8
0.40	71.4	78.8	86.2	62.0
0.50	71.4	81.7	82.4	67.7
0.60	71.4	83.7	78.6	71.6
0.70	66.7	85.6	74.6	75.6
0.75	66.7	86.3	73.4	77.1

SOURCE: Reprinted with permission from Sun et al. (2007).

QUESTIONS

1. What is the relationship between sensitivity and specificity for both tests?
2. Which test has the highest sensitivity?
3. In an effort to improve the performance of screening tests, either a repeat test is done on those who screen positive, or a different test is done on the same group. One strategy would be to screen initially with a high-sensitivity

test, and follow up on those who screen positive with a high-specificity test. Suppose that you were to run the PSA test using a cutoff level of 1.0 ng/mL on a group of 1,000 men over age 50, and then run the test again on those who test positive using a 4.0 ng/dL cutoff level. For the sake of argument, let us assume that 25 percent of these men have prostate cancer. What is the final sensitivity and specificity of this two-test sequence? Calculate a PPV for the two-test sequence to show the level of confidence in a positive test result. How does this level of confidence compare to the PSA test with a 1.0 ng/dL cutoff only? Create a separate 2 × 2 table for the PSA test with a 4.0 ng/dL cutoff only, and compare the confidence in a positive test result for the two-test sequence and the 4.0 ng/dL cutoff.

4. Suppose you were to run the test with the highest sensitivity (PSAV test at a 0.1 ng/dL/year cutoff) and then the test with the highest specificity (PSA test with 4.0 ng/dL cutoff) on those who test positive. What is the positive predictive value of each test and the final sequence? What is the sensitivity and specificity of both tests?

5. How could you determine which strategy would be best to maximize sensitivity? Specificity? PPV? Combination of these three measures?

ANSWERS

1. For both tests, as sensitivity increases, specificity decreases.
2. The PSAV test (at 0.1 ng/mL/year) has the highest sensitivity for both age groups but is associated with very low specificity.
3. From the information, one can derive the following 2 × 2 table (Table 3.6) for this PSA–PSA sequence.

Table 3.6. PSA–PSA Test Sequence, Men Age 50 and Above

	PSA Test (1.0 ng/dL Cutoff)			PSA Test (4.0 ng/dL Cutoff)		
	Cancer	No Cancer	Total	Cancer	No Cancer	Total
Test positive	223	452	675	159	67	226
Test negative	27	298	325	64	385	449
Total	250	750	1,000	223	452	675

Step 1: If there are 1,000 men who are screened and the prevalence of prostate cancer is 25 percent, then 250 of them will actually have prostate cancer (0.25 × 1,000 = 250).

Step 2: Of the 250 men who actually have cancer, 223 of them will test positive with the PSA and a cutoff of 1.0 ng/dL (sensitivity 0.893 × 250 = 223).

Step 3: Of the 750 men without prostate cancer, 298 of them will test negative if the specificity is 39.8% (0.398 × 750 = 298).

Step 4: The 675 men who test positive with a 1.0 ng/dL cutoff will be tested again using a higher cutoff of 4.0 ng/dL. Notice that the "total" row of the second test is derived from those who test positive on the first test.

Step 5: Of the 223 men with prostate cancer, 159 will test positive (0.731 sensitivity × 223 = 159). Of the 452 men without prostate cancer, 385 will test negative (452 × 0.852 specificity = 385).

The final sensitivity of this sequence is 159/250 or 63.6%. The final specificity is (385 + 298)/750 or 91%. The positive predictive value is 223/675 = 33%, from the first test only, and 159/226 = 70.3% with both tests. The PPV using a 4.0 ng/dL cutoff would be only 61.6%. Thus the two-test sequence shows an improvement in PPV over either test alone.

4. From the information, one can derive the following 2 × 2 table (Table 3.7) for this PSAV–PSA sequence.

TABLE 3.7. PSAV–PSA TEST SEQUENCE, MEN AGE 50 AND ABOVE

	PSAV Test (0.1 ng/dL/year Cutoff)			PSA Test (4.0 ng/dL Cutoff)		
	Cancer	No Cancer	Total	Cancer	No Cancer	Total
Test positive	238	554	792	170	82	252
Test negative	12	196	208	68	472	540
Total	250	750	1,000	238	554	792

Step 1: If there are 1,000 men who are screened and the prevalence of prostate cancer is 25 percent, then 250 of them will actually have prostate cancer (0.25 × 1000 = 250).

Step 2: Of the 250 men who actually have cancer, 238 of them will test positive with the PSAV and a cutoff of 0.1 ng/dL/year (sensitivity 0.95 × 250 = 238).

Step 3: Of the 750 men without prostate cancer, 196 of them will test negative if the specificity is 26.1 percent (0.261 × 750 = 196).

Step 4: The 792 men who test positive with the PSAV test and a 0.1 ng/dL/year cutoff are tested again using the PSA test and a cutoff of 4.0

ng/dL. Notice that the "total" row of the second test is derived from those who test positive on the first test.

Step 5: Of the 238 men with prostate cancer, 170 will test positive (0.771 sensitivity × 238). Of the 554 men without prostate cancer, 472 will test negative (0.852 specificity × 554).

The final sensitivity of this sequence is 170/250, or 68%. The final specificity is (472 + 196)/750, or 89%. The positive predictive value is 238/792 = 30%, from the first test only, and 170/252 = 67.5% with both tests. The PPV using a PSA with a 4.0 ng/dL cutoff would be only 61.6%. Thus the two-test sequence shows an improvement in PPV over either the PSAV or PSA test alone.

5. You could create a simulation using a computer program such as Excel using all possible combinations of these two tests in sequence. When this was done, the following testing strategies maximized each of the measure(s) listed in Table 3.8.

TABLE 3.8. TWO TEST STRATEGIES THAT MAXIMIZE SELECTED MEASURES

Measure(s)	First Test	Second Test
Sensitivity	PSAV (0.10)	PSAV (0.10)
Specificity	PSA (4.0)	PSA (4.0)
PPV	PSA (4.0)	PSA (4.0)
Sensitivity and specificity	PSAV (0.40)	PSAV (0.40)
Sensitivity and PPV	PSA (3.0)	PSA (3.0)
Specificity and PPV	PSA (4.0)	PSA (4.0)
Sensitivity, specificity, and PPV	PSA (3.0)	PSA (4.0)

Summary

Each disease has a characteristic natural history or "course over time" from onset to resolution. This natural history may involve different stages and specific junctures, such as the clinical horizon (when the disease can be detected) and the critical point (the point after which severe consequences occur). We distinguished between screening and diagnostic tests; discussed sensitivity, specificity, and positive and negative predictive value; and outlined the characteristics of a good screening program. Two of the case studies focused on product lines and on screening for the two most common types of cancer among women and men, breast and prostate cancer.

These two case studies illustrate the problems faced by most screening tests—they are imperfect. For both types of cancer, false positives occur when screening tests incorrectly report positive results for those without the disease. This type of error can lead to additional follow-up tests, costs, or complications, such as those associated with prostate biopsies. False negatives occur when patients with cancer are incorrectly given a negative test result, leading to delay in treatment, at the very least.

The prostate cancer case study illustrates the common dilemma associated with choosing the cutoff level in a screening test to distinguish between those who test positive and negative. In such cases, sensitivity and specificity work contrary to one another; as one increases, the other decreases. Thus the challenge of maximizing both is difficult, and one must decide which type of errors—false positives or false negatives—is most malicious. This choice is obviously disease specific, and depends on the risks associated with "chasing down" a false positive with additional tests compared to missing a diagnosis because of a false negative.

References

Centers for Disease Control and Prevention (CDC). 2007. "Cases of HIV Infection and AIDS in the United States and Dependent Areas, 2005." *HIV/AIDS Surveillance Report* Vol. 17, Revised Edition.

Chadwick, D., and G. Cardew. 1997. *The Rising Trends in Asthma*. New York: Wiley.

Donabedian, A. 1973. *Aspects of Medical Care Administration*. Cambridge, MA: Harvard University Press.

Koepsell, T. D., and N. S. Weiss. 2003. *Epidemiologic Methods: Studying the Occurrence of Illness*. New York: Oxford University Press.

Last, J. M. 2001. *Last's Dictionary of Epidemiology*, 3rd ed. New York: Oxford University Press.

Pearce, N. 1998. *Asthma Epidemiology: Principles and Methods*. New York: Oxford University Press.

Pisano, E. D., C. Gatsonis, E. Hendrick, M. Yaffe, J. K. Baum, S. Acharyya, E. F. Conant, L. L. Fajardo, L. Bassett, C. D'Orsi, R. Jong, M. Rebner, and the Digital Mammographic Imaging Screening Trial (DMIST) Investigators Group. 2005. "Diagnostic Performance of Digital Versus Film Mammography for Breast Cancer Screening." *New England Journal of Medicine* 353 (17): 1773–83.

Sun, L., J. W. Moul, J. M. Hotaling, E. Rampersaud, P. Dahm, C. Robertson, N. Fitzsimons, D. Albala, and T. J. Polascik. 2007. "Prostate-Specific Antigen (PSA) and PSA Velocity for Prostate Cancer

Detection in Men Aged <50 Years." *BJU International* 99 (4): 753–57.

Susser, M. W. 1973. *Causal Thinking in the Health Sciences*. New York: Oxford University Press.

Timmreck, T. C. 2002. *An Introduction to Epidemiology*, 3rd ed. Sudbury, MA: Jones and Bartlett.

Valanis, B. 1999. *Epidemiology in Health Care*. Stamford, CT: Appleton & Lange.

HEALTHCARE PLANNING AND NEEDS ASSESSMENT

Steven T. Fleming, F. Douglas Scutchfield, and Joel Lee

"We must ask where we are and whither we are tending."
Abraham Lincoln

Planning is essential to all managerial functions, and is perhaps one of the most important activities of those responsible for a healthcare program. A plan sets a course of action. It describes the direction an organization is following and how it will achieve results. Without a plan, the manager will not know what is to be done, how it is to be accomplished, or when the final results are achieved.

Most planning proceeds from the model of planning, implementation, and evaluation, leading to further planning. Planning involves not only technical aspects—the major focus of this chapter—but also social processes. Planning is rarely done by an individual. In organizations or communities, planning usually is done with individuals and other organizations that have an interest in the work and results of that organization, sometimes called *stakeholders*.

Typically a plan consists of the following five components, although the order may vary: (1) ends—specification of outcomes in goals and objectives; (2) means—selection of policies, programs, procedures, and practices by which objectives and goals are to be pursued; (3) resources—determination of the types and amounts of resources required, how they are to be generated or acquired, and how they are to be allocated to activities; (4) implementation—design of decision-making procedures and a way to organize them so the plan can be carried out; and (5) control—design of a procedure for anticipating or detecting errors in, or failures of, the plan and for preventing or correcting them.

A major characteristic of planning is whether it is being carried out at the institutional level or the community level. Institutional planning is in some ways easier, as the institution has a hierarchical structure and theoretically all stakeholders are looking out for the institution's best interest. On the other hand, community health planning must involve many institutions and organizations, each with its own vested interest and agenda. The major effort in community health planning is to recognize that each organization has its own agenda. The challenge is to harmonize plans so all are accommodated in one final outcome.

Whether health planning is community- or institution-based, there are five significant categories or levels of planning: strategic, operational, tactical, project (or program), and contingency.

Strategic, operational, and tactical planning focus on the organization, defining its direction and implementation.

The first and most general is *strategic planning*, which has a comprehensive scope, has a long-range timeline, and defines the future structure of the organization. This type of planning is most frequently done at the upper levels of the organization's governing body and senior staff, and frequently has a three- to five-year timeline. A strategic plan normally includes the following components: (1) vision (long-run "view" of the organization); (2) mission (purpose of the organization); (3) goals (broad statements on how to achieve objectives); and (4) objectives (measure-able outcomes linked to goals).

Clearly, an organization should incorporate epidemiologic concepts and measurement into the strategic planning process. Suppose the vision of a healthcare organization is to be recognized for excellence in patient care, education, and research. "Excellence" in patient care is an undefined benchmark for which there are some epidemiologic measures, such as case-fatality rates or risk-adjusted mortality measures.

Suppose the vision is to assist "people in taking responsibility for their own health by actively promoting wellness and facilitating healing" (Duncan, Ginter, and Swayne 1995, 1120). Obviously the foundation here is the vast body of epidemiologic literature that identifies risk factors such as diet, smoking, and other wellness-enhancing or disease-promoting behaviors.

Suppose the mission statement claims an interest in health status improvement of people in a defined geographic area. The mission statement presumes that one can measure health status improvement in a geographic region through epidemiologic measures, such as mortality and morbidity rates.

Goals and objectives can be defined specifically in epidemiologic terms, such as reducing neonatal mortality, the rates of nosocomial infection, risk-adjusted surgical mortality rates for cardiovascular disease (Chapter 5), and so on.

A second level of planning is *operational planning*, which has a functional scope. While its time range is shorter and more functional, operational planning continues to address the organization's broadest levels of operation, such as financial planning.

Other levels of planning are more functional. *Tactical planning* is generally carried out throughout the organization and concerns itself with how mission, vision, goals, and objectives can be achieved on a day-to-day basis. It usually has a shorter time horizon than strategic planning and is concerned with the nuts and bolts of running an organization, such as scheduling of staff to accommodate seasonal variations in demand.

Project or *program planning* addresses the design and management of a specific organizational activity, such as construction of a new facility or service. The scope and time frame of this type of planning varies with the activity, and is sometimes managed by an external construction company.

A final category of planning is contingency planning. A *contingency plan* addresses the possible but not certain occurrence of a specific future event such as a disaster, unplanned weather, a union strike, or an epidemic. Scope varies, and the timeline of the event is normally short, but decisions must be made immediately if the event occurs. As a result, contingency plans are developed in advance to ensure preparedness for these events.

A recent problem with healthcare planning is that a turbulent and uncertain environment has made it difficult to plan a number of years into the future, while many operational tasks require a great deal of time to complete. For example, rapid environmental change limits a strategic plan time horizon to a few years, while implementation of an operational plan—such as a marketing strategy—may require just as many years to achieve.

Despite these limitations, planning remains essential, and each level of planning has an individual and specific function in healthcare. These functions are complementary, and the performance of each planning function is required to maximize organizational performance.

Regardless of whether planning is community or institutional, the first step in developing an effective plan at any level is to collect and analyze data regarding the present situation and the future. This data can be quantitative and/or qualitative.

For example, in addressing tuberculosis, quantitative data for planning might include the number of patients in the community who have active tuberculosis, or the population at risk. These data are usually statistical in nature and can be manipulated using epidemiological and biostatistical tools to address trends or conduct comparisons to other areas.

Qualitative data, on the other hand, are not necessarily statistical. For example, the results of a focus group that has considered a question cannot be statistically manipulated. They are, however, useful data that have an important role in planning. Another type of qualitative data is key informant surveys, which are generally open-ended discussions with major community leaders or stakeholders. Again, they are not random samples and do not lend themselves to the usual epidemiological and statistical techniques available to the health planner. That does not diminish their value; it just limits how they may be manipulated.

Community Health Planning Tools and Benchmarks

It is important in any planning process to have benchmarks. One of the most frequently used tools in community health planning is the Healthy People series. In 1979, *Healthy People: The Surgeon General's Report on Health Promotion and Disease Prevention* was released. This monograph did several things. First, it established a series of goals that we, as a nation, should achieve in the year 1990. These goals were related to decreased mortality, by age group, for those up to 65 years of age and morbidity for those over 65. These goals were as follows (HHS 1979):

Life Stage	1990 Target
Infants	35 percent lower death rate (9 deaths per 1,000 live births)
Children	20 percent lower death rate (34 deaths per 100,000)
Adolescents/Young Adults	20 percent lower death rate (93 deaths per 100,000)
Adults	25 percent lower death rate (400 deaths per 100,000)
Older Adults	20 percent fewer days of restricted activity

The monograph also identified 15 priority programs, under the rubrics of health promotion, preventive services, and health protection.

Immediately following the release of this report, the Centers for Disease Control and Prevention (CDC), along with the federal Office of Disease Prevention and Health Promotion, convened a series of working groups. These groups had the charge of creating specific objectives tied to the 15 priority areas that would help track our ability to achieve the life-stage goals. These were published in 1980, titled *Promoting Health/Preventing Disease: Objectives for the Nation*. This report presents materials in the following standard format:

• Nature and extent of the problem
• Prevention and promotion measures
• Specific national objectives for
  • Improved health status
  • Reduced risk factors
  • Improved public/professional awareness
  • Improved services/protection
  • Improved surveillance

• Principal assumptions underlying the objective
• Data necessary for tracking the objective

The process worked quite well, and as 1990 approached, the U.S. Department of Health and Human Services created a working group to establish objectives for the year 2000. In 1991, the next in the series of prevention benchmarks was published, *Healthy People 2000. Healthy People 2000* had three major goals. These were (HHS 1991):

• Increase the span of healthy life for all Americans
• Reduce health disparities among Americans
• Achieve access to preventive services for all Americans

As with the 1990 objectives, the priorities were grouped into a series of three principal areas (health promotion, health protection, and preventive services), each with health status objectives, risk reduction objectives, and service/protection objectives. To illustrate, here are examples from one priority area, tobacco.

Health status objective:	Reduce coronary heart disease deaths to no more than 100 per 100,000 people.
Risk reduction objective:	Reduce cigarette smoking to a prevalence of no more than 15 percent among those age 20 and older.
Service and protection:	Increase to at least 75 percent the proportion of worksite objectives with a formal smoking policy that prohibits or severely restricts smoking in the workplace.

Healthy People 2010 (http://web.health.gov/healthypeople) builds on the foundation of *Healthy People 1990* and *2000* by providing specific health objectives that allow diverse groups to join forces to improve the health of the "community." The two overarching goals are to increase quality and length of life, and to eliminate health disparities. The following ten leading health indicators are being used to measure the health of the nation over a ten-year period:

1. Physical activity
2. Overweight and obesity
3. Tobacco use
4. Substance abuse
5. Responsible sexual behavior
6. Mental health
7. Injury and violence

8. Environmental quality
9. Immunization
10. Access to healthcare

There are 28 focus areas and 467 specific goals. For example, tobacco use, diabetes, and cancer are three of the focus areas.

The leading health indicators are supposed to represent "important determinants of health for the full range of issues in the 28 focus areas," and as such, each focus area is related to more than one health indicator. For example, the diabetes focus area relates to the leading indicators of tobacco use, physical activity, overweight and obesity, immunization, and access to healthcare. A midcourse review was conducted midway through the decade to consider new science and available data, and to make appropriate revisions of the objectives.

Tobacco use is one of the 28 focus areas of *Healthy People 2010*. The goal of this focus area is to reduce illness, disability, and death related to tobacco use and secondhand smoke. The midcourse review of this focus area indicated the extent to which our nation exceeded the target, moved toward the target, or moved away from the target in each of 21 objectives, many with subobjectives as well. For example, with regard to Objective 1 (tobacco use among those 18 and above), there were three subobjectives that could be measured: (1) cigarette smoking, 18+ years, moved 25 percent toward the target; (2) spit tobacco use, moved 10 percent toward the target; and (3) cigar smoking, moved 17 percent toward the target. Objective 7 (smoking cessation attempts among grades 9–12) moved 33 percent away from the target. Objective 10 (exposure to environmental tobacco smoke among nonsmokers) exceeded the target by 36 percent.

In summary, there were successes and failures with regard to tobacco use. Of the 21 objectives, ten moved toward the target, one (smoking cessation among 9–12 grade students) moved away, and nine could not be assessed. Mixed results were observed for tobacco advertising and promotion, with a movement toward the target in magazine/newpaper advertising (+57 percent), but considerably away from the target (−333 percent) for Internet advertising. In some cases, objectives were either deleted or added with the midcourse review.

Data systems must be designed and developed to track the objectives in the various reports. These usually include vital statistics tracking systems. They may include special studies, such as the Behavioral Risk Factor Surveillance System (BRFSS) used by the CDC and the states to track the various risk factors for disease.

Incidence and prevalence are major elements of the data presentations. In addition, traditional descriptive epidemiology is used to define the time, place, and person variables associated with the objectives.

Effective planning is key to organizational success. There must be clear goals and objectives, and in the case of health programs, a knowledge of the major community health problems. The tools of descriptive epidemiology are imperative in identifying major health problems, and using time, place, and person descriptors of these health problems allows for the most effective planning. The ability to set priorities is influenced substantially by the burden of disease and its impact on the community, which are both epidemiology issues. Finally, it is important to remember that planning is part of a plan, implement, and evaluate cycle. Epidemiology is useful in that evaluation effort, as well.

Case Study 4.1 illustrates how a managed care organization in eastern Kentucky could use community health planning tools (specifically the BRFSS) to target specific population groups and recommend interventions.

Case Study 4.1. Eastern Kentucky Health

Eastern Kentucky Health (EKH) is a fictitious managed care organization that serves patients in a number of counties in southeastern Kentucky. EKH has entered into a partnership with several local communities to meet *Healthy People 2010* objectives, but it is struggling with a number of priority areas dealing with tobacco use, obesity, hypertension, and related mortality (refer to Table 4.1).

QUESTIONS

1. What are the kinds and sources of data that need to be collected to make rational planning decisions?
2. How does Kentucky compare with the United States in terms of the prevalence of smoking?
3. How does Kentucky compare with the United States in term of the prevalence of diabetes, obesity, and lack of exercise?
4. What kinds of interventions should EKH consider to address the key priority areas?

ANSWERS

1. National surveys such as the National Health Interview Survey, the National Hospital Discharge Survey, and the National Ambulatory Medical

TABLE 4.1 CHRONIC DISEASE RISK FACTORS, KENTUCKY AND THE UNITED STATES, 2006

Cigarette smoking (%)	Kentucky	U.S.	Obesity (%)	Kentucky	U.S.
Age			Age		
18–24	35.9	26.8	18–24	19.7	15.8
25–34	29.3	24.2	25–34	29.7	24.0
35–44	34.2	21.2	35–44	29.8	27.6
45–54	35.2	22.2	45–54	33.2	29.0
55–64	26.3	16.5	55–64	31.0	31.4
65+	10.7	8.6	65+	21.0	22.0
Gender			Gender		
Male	29.1	22.2	Male	28.2	25.9
Female	28.0	18.4	Female	27.9	24.4
Race			Race		
White	28.5	19.5	White	27.8	24.2
Black	22.3	22.3	Black	38.0	36.8
Income level			Income level		
<$15,000	43.2	31.5	<$15,000	34.5	30.8
$15,000–24,999	39.8	27.8	$15,000–24,999	33.4	29.3
$25,000–34,999	31.6	24.4	$25,000–34,999	28.6	27.0
$35,000–49,999	33.0	21.8	$35,000–49,999	27.6	26.8
>$50,000	18.9	15.0	>$50,000	25.0	23.1

Diabetes (%)	Kentucky	U.S.	No Exercise in Last Month (%)	Kentucky	U.S.
Race			Race		
White	9.7	7.2	White	30.1	20.7
Black	13.1	11.9	Black	34.5	30.3
Age			Age		
18–24	0.6	0.8	18–24	20.2	16.5
25–34	2.4	1.6	25–34	22.1	18.9
35–44	5.3	3.7	35–44	27.6	19.5
45–54	13.1	7.7	45–54	32.5	22.5
55–64	18.2	14.2	55–64	36.1	26.3
65+	19.3	18.1	65+	42.3	32.6
Income level			Income level		
<$15,000	17.9	14.2	<$15,000	53.0	40.1
$15,000–24,999	12.3	10.5	$15,000–24,999	39.9	34.4
$25,000–34,999	7.3	9.0	$25,000–34,999	30.1	27.0
$35,000–49,999	7.2	7.5	$35,000–49,999	26.8	22.3
>$50,000	6.9	5.1	>$50,000	15.7	14.3

NOTE: *Healthy People 2010* targets are as follows: 12 percent for smoking; age-adjusted rate of 2.5 percent for diabetes; age-adjusted rate of 15 percent for obesity; age-adjusted rate of 20 percent no leisure-time activity.

SOURCE: Centers for Disease Control and Prevention (CDC). *Behavioral Risk Factor Surveillance System Survey Data, 1995, 2005.* Atlanta, GA: U.S. Department of Health and Human Services.

Care Survey can be used to obtain estimates of the prevalence of disease. The Behavioral Risk Factor Surveillance System can be used to derive estimates of some risk factors. EKH may also want to contact the Kentucky Hospital Association about accessing hospital discharge data for southeastern Kentucky. Physician and hospital claims for Medicare patients can be obtained from the Centers for Medicare & Medicaid Services.

2. Kentucky has higher rates of smoking than the United States across all age groups. Rates are much higher for females, whites, and 18- to 24-year-olds. Disparities exist across all income strata with the exception of the wealthy (income >$50,000).

3. Rates of diabetes in Kentucky are higher than the United States for both races, and across all age categories. Rates of diabetes are higher than the United States in most income groups, particularly the lowest income category (<$15,000). Rates of obesity are higher in Kentucky across all age groups, races, gender, and income levels, except age groups 55–64 and over 65. Lack of physical activity is much higher among Kentucky whites versus whites in the United States (30.1 percent versus 20.7 percent), and is about 30–50 percent higher in Kentucky compared with the United States in most age categories.

4. Kentucky has much higher rates of smoking compared to the United States, particularly among whites, women, and young adults (age 18–24); higher rates of diabetes and obesity than the United States; and much higher rates of lack of physical exercise. The focus should be on reducing cardiovascular disease, lung cancer, and chronic obstructive pulmonary disease mortality rates through different interventions, including smoking cessation programs, particularly among white women and young adults, and weight loss initiatives, especially those that focus on increasing the level of exercise.

Institutional Planning

In healthcare organizations, planning tends to be done the way it always has been done. This is a consequence of several factors: Employees do what they know and what they have experience doing, and they do what they are told to do, frequently by people who have a similar set of previous work experiences. As a consequence, planning is frequently limited.

Many proponents have advocated "one best way to plan," rather than recognizing that planning is situational.

Issues of planning can be addressed on a positive or a normative basis. *Positive theory* describes what currently exists and makes predictions of the future, while *normative theory* addresses values and questions of what should exist in the future.

There are four basic models of planning theory: rational/comprehensive, incremental, mixed scanning, and radical planning (Berry 1974).

Rational/comprehensive planning considers the most broad view of the environment and its complexity. The basic elements of the method are to identify all opportunities for possible action by decision makers, identify each consequence of each possible action, and select the action that would result in the most preferred set of consequences. This method considers data concerning all resources for technical decisions and works well if the future is stable, clear trends exist, values are implicit, and efficiency is the highest of all goals. Rational/comprehensive planning is relevant to issues such as developing a long-range master plan, or defining specific health services in a particular community.

Incremental planning involves determining the steps that need to be taken to achieve a predetermined goal. Incremental planning is relevant to long-term issues with step-by-step changes, such as a budget. If a financial situation changes six months after the budget is written, an incremental change can be made to address the new reality. The goal of the budget plan doesn't change, just some steps along the way.

A third method is *mixed scanning*. This strategy creates a blend of the first two strategies, using incremental decisions leading to a fundamental issue. Mixed scanning permits a detailed examination of some aspects of a plan, along with limited detail in other areas. It is particularly applicable in a rapidly changing environment, where decision making requires flexibility. Mixed scanning is appropriate for issues such as operation of a complex medical center.

The fourth planning strategy is *radical planning*. This method emphasizes innovation and spontaneity and considers experimentation a component of the learning process. Radical planning may be most applicable to the resolution of an issue such as establishment of a new type of health program. Case Study 4.2 demonstrates the steps involved in determining bed capacity for a new hospital tower scheduled for construction in 2010.

Case Study 4.2. Determining Bed Demand for Cardiac Patients Age 65–84

University Hospital is a 350-bed tertiary care center located in an urban area of Kentucky with about 200,000 people. As vice president of planning, you are responsible for projecting bed size in the new hospital tower that is scheduled for construction in 2010. Determining bed demand is a complex process that involves consideration of: (1) the service area from which the hospital draws, (2) use rates for various kinds of medical and surgical conditions, (3) service lines, and (4) bed utilization. To simplify the analysis, you are concerned only with the 65–84 age group, and only with medical and surgical cardiac care. Obviously the analysis can be extended to all age groups, and to all medical and surgical conditions, and then aggregated to derive a total estimate of bed demand.

Assume that we have a service area of 60,000 "eligible" patients (age 65–84) from which the hospital draws patients. The care can be broken up into primary (75–80 percent of admissions), secondary (10–15 percent of admissions), and tertiary (5–10 percent of admissions) service areas, each with distinct use rates that reflect underlying demographic characteristics. Assume that you use 2007 utilization rates to project bed demand to 2020.

QUESTIONS

1. Assume that 2007 utilization rates in patient days (per 1,000 population, age 65–84) in the primary, secondary, and tertiary service areas are 150, 254, and 242, respectively, for medically treated cardiac patients, and 112, 90, and 118, respectively, for surgically treated cardiac patients. What might explain these differences in use rates?

2. Assume that the overall 2007 use rate (per 1,000) for all areas combined is 190 and 110 for medical and surgically treated cardiac patients, respectively. With a population of 60,000 eligible patients, age 65–84, how many patient days does this represent?

3. Assume that the eligible population (age 65–84) in the service area grows by 50 percent by 2020, and that the use rates remain the same. How many patient days can be anticipated in 2020? A patient day is one patient occupying one bed for one hospital day; so if one patient stayed in the hospital for an entire year, that patient would accrue 365 patient days.

4. Would you expect the age-specific use rates to increase by 2020? Why or why not?

5. How many medical and surgical beds are required for cardiac care patients in 2007 and 2020 assuming 100 percent utilization (each bed is filled all the time)? What about 75 percent utilization? Why are the number of beds needed at 75 percent utilization higher?

6. Assume that age-specific prevalence rates of cardiac disease are projected to increase in 2020 due to the influence of risk factors such as diabetes and obesity. What effect would this have on 2020 use rates and 2020 bed needs?

7. What other factors might affect both use rates and bed needs in 2020?

8. Table 4.2 presents the prevalence of four major risk factors for cardiovascular disease in Kentucky for the 45- to 54-year-old age group, and two years, 1995 and 2005. The table also presents the ten-year risk of coronary heart disease (cumulative incidence rate) for men and women with these risk factors. Calculate the weighted average cumulative incidence rate for men and women for 1995 and 2005. The prevalence of each risk factor (or combination) in Table 4.2 is expressed as a percentage, with a total of 100 percent for all eight categories. A weighted average can be calculated as follows, for males and females.

$$\sum_{j=1}^{8} p^j i^j$$ where p^j is the prevalence of the jth risk factor expressed as a proportion, and i^j is the ten-year incidence of that risk factor.

Assume that the ten-year risk of heart disease based on 1995 risk factors gets directly translated into 2007 use rates, and that the ten-year risk of heart disease based on 2005 risk factors gets directly translated into projected use rates for 2020. Assume that the eligible population still grows by 50 percent in 2020, and that 50 percent of the population are males in all years. How many beds are now needed?

TABLE 4.2. PREVALENCE[1] (%) AND TEN-YEAR CUMULATIVE INCIDENCE RATES[2] (PER 1,000), AGE 45–54, FOR FOUR CARDIOVASCULAR RISK FACTORS IN KENTUCKY

Risk Factor(s)	Prevalence 1995	Prevalence 2005	Ten-Year Incidence Males	Ten-Year Incidence Females
No risk factors	28.0	19.0	50	50
Diabetes only	1.0	4.7	80	100
Smoking only	15.0	15.5	80	70
High cholesterol only	14.7	15.6	80	60

High blood pressure only	6.8	8.2	90	75
Any two risk factors	26.6	26.0	150	100
Any three risk factors	6.9	9.0	250	180
All four risk factors	1.0	2.0	400	250

1. The prevalence of risk factors is estimated using the following two sources (a) Centers for Disease Control and Prevention (CDC). *Behavioral Risk Factor Surveillance System Survey Data*, 1995, 2005. Atlanta, GA: U.S. Department of Health and Human Services; (b) http://www.qualityprofiles.org/leadership_series/cardiovascular_disease/cardiovascular_managingrisk.asp.

2. Cumulative incidence rates are estimated from the work of Wilson et al. (1998).

ANSWERS

1. Higher use rates for medical cardiac care in the secondary and tertiary markets may reflect an increased prevalence of cardiac disease in these areas, or an increased length of stay for these patients due to discharge planning challenges.

2. For medical patients, this represents $(190/1,000) \times 60,000 = 11,400$ patient days. For surgical patients, this represents $(110/1,000) \times 60,000 = 6,600$ patient days.

3. For medical patients, you can anticipate $(190/1,000) \times (60,000 \times 1.50) = 17,100$ patients days. For surgical patients, you can anticipate $(110/1,000) \times (60,000 \times 1.50) = 9,900$ patient days.

4. All other things being equal, you would expect the rates to be the same, unless there are proportionately more older folks in the 65–84-year-old-group (i.e., more people near the top end of that age range), or there is a change in medical practice, treatment, length-of-stay guidelines, and so forth.

5. For medical cardiac patients, you would need $11,400/365 = 31$ beds in 2007, and $17,100/365 = 47$ beds in 2020 at 100 percent utilization. At 75 percent utilization, you would need $31/0.75 = 41$ beds and $47/0.75 = 63$ beds, respectively. For surgically treated cardiac patients, you would need $6,600/365 = 18$ beds in 2007, and $9,900/365 = 27$ beds in 2007, at 100 percent utilization. At 75 percent utilization, you would need $18/0.75 = 24$ beds and $27/0.75 = 36$ beds, respectively. The number of beds required at 75 percent utilization is higher because more beds are needed if the policy is to leave 25 percent of the beds empty.

6. All other things being equal, an increase in age-specific prevalence of cardiac disease in 2020 would increase both use rates and bed needs in 2020.
7. Both medical and surgical innovation could affect use rates. Changes in medical care practice or service options, such as an increased use of cardiac step-down units, could affect both use rates and bed needs in 2020. Other considerations would include new drug therapies, equipment technology, and so on.
8. Calculate average ten-year incidence rates for males and females, in 1995 and 2005, using a weighted average of the prevalence of each risk factor(s) multiplied by the ten-year incidence rate associated with that factor as follows:

Males (1995): $(0.28 \times 50) + (0.01 \times 80) + (0.15 \times 80) + (0.147 \times 80) + (0.068 \times 90)$ $(0.266 \times 150) + (0.069 \times 250) + (0.01 \times 400) = 105.83$ cases per 1,000

Females (1995): $(0.28 \times 50) + (0.01 \times 100) + (0.15 \times 70) + (0.147 \times 60) + (0.068 \times 75)$ $(0.266 \times 100) + (0.069 \times 180) + (0.01 \times 250) = 80.94$ cases per 1,000

Males (2005): $(0.19 \times 50) + (0.047 \times 80) + (0.155 \times 80) + (0.156 \times 80) + (0.082 \times 90)$ $(0.26 \times 150) + (0.09 \times 250) + (0.02 \times 400) = 115.02$ cases per 1,000

Females (2005): $(0.19 \times 50) + (0.047 \times 100) + (0.155 \times 70) + (0.156 \times 60) + (0.082 \times 75)$ $(0.26 \times 100) + (0.09 \times 180) + (0.02 \times 250) = 87.76$ cases per 1,000

Assuming that the population, age 45–54, comprises 50 percent males and 50 percent females, the overall rates would be as follows:

$105.83 \times 0.50 + 80.94 \times 0.50 = 93.38$ (1995)
$115.02 \times 0.50 + 87.76 \times 0.50 = 101.39$ (2005)

Assume that the increase in cumulative incidence rates gets directly translated into use rates. Estimated use rates for medical and surgical cardiovascular patients are calculated as follows:

Medical: $(101.39/93.38) \times 17,100 = 18,567$ patient days, or $18,567/365 = 51$ beds at 100 percent capacity, and 68 beds at 75 percent capacity.

Surgical: $(101.39/93.38) \times 9,900 = 10,749$ patient days, or $10,749/365 = 29$ beds at 100 percent capacity, and 39 beds at 75 percent capacity.

The increase in cardiovascular risk factors in the population as of 2005 is expected to increase the number of medical and surgical cardiac beds at 75 percent capacity needed in 2020 by five beds and three beds, respectively.

A Strategic Planning Model

A strategic plan is a useful and necessary tool in corporate strategy development—but it is not (nor should it be) the end objective. Strategic planning seeks to define the organization and its future with an emphasis on designing and bringing about a desired future, rather than designing and implementing programs to achieve specific objectives.

While there are a variety of approaches to strategic planning, a general concept does exist. Years ago, Keck (1986) and colleagues developed a model of strategic planning that divided the strategic planning process into four sets of activities seeking to answer four specific questions:

1. Where are we now?
2. Where should we be going?
3. How should we get there?
4. Are we getting there?

These questions focus on the activities of planning. For example, to answer the question "where are we now?" requires a situational analysis where participants must collect and assemble data addressing the organization's environment and operations. This leads to an assessment such as a strengths/weaknesses/opportunities/threats (SWOT) analysis, and concludes with the establishment of a set of issues and challenges for the organization.

The question "where should we be going?" can be answered with goal formulation, including exploration of alternative strategies, and development of organizational direction in the form of statements of vision, mission, goals, and objectives.

Strategy formulation answers the question, "how should we get there?" This includes the development of strategies or actions to achieve goals and the assessment of the resources to achieve each strategy, involving both capital and operational budgets.

Following implementation of the chosen strategy, evaluation and control are addressed through the final question, "are we getting there?" Such monitoring requires the collection and analysis of data, followed by the use of this performance feedback to adjust where the organization should be going—and how operations should be managed to achieve those outcomes.

This process is continuous, and is then repeated from the beginning, using evaluation data as input for the next situational analysis and further refinement of the strategic planning process. This model simplifies a complex process of decision making and requires a great deal of time and effort. In developing such a plan, the objective is not to write a plan, but to get something accomplished, and to take action regarding the future direction and profitability of the organization.

Each of these activities is informed by the collection of epidemiologic data. Morbidity profiles (lists of the prevalence of various morbidities), for instance, describe the "where are we now?" question. For a hospital, this might include case-mix measures, or a breakdown of patients by diagnosis-related groups (DRGs). Physician practices could characterize patient mix by Current Procedure Terminology (CPT) code or resource-based relative values, in the case of Medicare patients.

The "where should we be?" question requires the organization to describe the service population (both current and potential) in terms of need. Descriptors of need would include both current morbidity burden (measured by the prevalence of disease) and future morbidity burden. Future need can be estimated on the basis of demographics, as well as the burden of risk factors that can lead to disease, such as the prevalence of smoking, obesity, high blood pressure, and so on.

The "how should we get there?" question may also require epidemiologic input, to the extent that there are alternative patient care or treatment strategies, or that "best care" strategies, practice guidelines, or critical pathways need to be collected and implemented. The "are we getting there?" question requires epidemiologic input described in more detail in Chapter 5, under surveillance and risk-adjusted outcomes. In the healthcare sector, performance must be measured in terms of patient care as well as financial outcomes.

Suppose, for example, a managed care organization is engaged in the strategic planning process. The organization has described where it is in terms of DRG and CPT profiles, and notices a relatively high proportion of cardiovascular disease among the enrolled population. Epidemiologic data are collected on the service area, which confirm a high prevalence of cardiovascular disease, as well as cardiovascular risk factors such as smoking and obesity. The organization decides to address the "where should we be?" question by focusing specifically on cardiovascular disease, among other things.

The question of how to get there is more complex and involves many decisions, such as whether to promote prevention through smoking cessation and weight reduction programs. Epidemiologic studies may provide useful insight into this decision-making process.

Marketing

An organization's most precious asset is its relationship with customers as defined by quality, service, and price. Although many view marketing as advertising, it is a far more complex set of activities. At the most basic level, *marketing* can be defined as an exchange between two parties to satisfy their needs—in the case of healthcare, an exchange of health services for appropriate compensation.

Traditional marketing can be described by the four "Ps" of marketing: product, place, price, and promotion. *Product* or *service* defines the activity of the organization, and can be described as the set of activities focused on a particular diagnosis, such as acute myocardial infarction. Alternatively, product/service can be described as the benefits the service provides to the patient, such as relief from pain or anxiety or longer life.

Place or *location* refers to how the product or service will be delivered to the patient. This marketing concept refers not simply to the location, but to other factors such as operating hours, referral mechanisms, and enablers and barriers to access based on external market segmentation and internal operational factors.

The third measure, *price* or *fee*, addresses not only the charge for the service (which usually is not paid by the patient), but everything that the organization requires the patient to go through to use the service. Price links revenue and consumer satisfaction, controlling a potential conflict of interest between providing the highest quality product and increasing revenue.

Promotion includes activities to acquaint the prospective patient with the organization and the services it offers. Promotion is a matter of communicating information between an organization and the market. Promotion is how the patient becomes aware of the services offered and develops an interest in using one or more of the services.

Strategic concepts in marketing include: product differentiation, price competition, market segmentation by socioeconomic variables, product segmentation for different populations, and mass marketing/advertising. A subcategory of marketing with a direct relationship to healthcare is known as social marketing. *Social marketing* focuses on behavior, such as changing health behaviors related to smoking or diet.

Although planning and marketing are closely related both conceptually and operationally (MacStravic 1977), the former has received more attention in terms of governmental policy. "Planning presents a method for design and management of change, while marketing offers design and management of exchange relations with important publics" (Lee 1989, 173).

Clearly, both planning and marketing are informed by epidemiologic measures. A critical stage of planning is *environmental assessment* (or needs assessment), in which the organization or agency attempts to characterize the needs of the population served. In the case of healthcare, this must involve morbidity profiles, described specifically in terms of the incidence and prevalence rates of acute and chronic disease.

Marketing strategies should also incorporate epidemiologic measures. Product definition, for instance, depends to some degree on descriptions of need. The development of a women's health "product" should be defined on the basis of dimensions of need in this area—much of which is epidemiologically derived—such as the prevalence of breast and ovarian cancer.

Strategies with regard to place include an assessment of barriers to access. These barriers may be recognized, to some degree, on the basis of proxy epidemiologic measures. For example, the high incidence of cervical cancer among women in eastern Kentucky may indicate that those women either lack access to Pap smears or choose not to get them.

Promotional activities may include motivational messages, based in part on epidemiologic studies. Primary prevention, such as cancer screening, can be promoted by encouraging clients to consider the advantages of early- versus late-stage diagnosis in terms of survival studies. Social marketing has clear epidemiologic roots, to the extent that behaviors, such as smoking, diet, and sexual behaviors, have been epidemiologically linked to morbidity.

Needs Assessment

Epidemiologic methods and measurement are critical for estimating the needs in a population for healthcare services, the formal process of which has been referred to as *needs assessment*. This activity can be done at the state or local level, such as to assess the need for a specific public health program, or at the institutional level, to evaluate and justify new programs or building projects. The incidence and prevalence of specific morbidities and risk factors play a key role in the calculus of this type of assessment.

Years ago, Donabedian (1973) defined *need* as "some disturbance in health or well-being" and conceptualized how need is translated into services (or *utilization*) through two parallel sets of activities involving patients and providers. Utilization of medical services is then translated into health outcomes, which presumably represent some "modification" of need, such as the elimination of a particular morbidity, or change in functional status.

Donabedian would agree that need represents the amount of medical services that *should* be consumed, although we could quibble over whether patients or professionals ought to make these judgments.

Unmet and *unrecognized need* represents the need in the population for services that are not currently being provided by the healthcare system, not currently recognized by either the provider or patient, or to which the patient does not have access. It may represent incongruities between what the patient and physician believes is necessary. Services that are provided in excess of what is required could be referred to as an *overmet need*.

Donabedian (1973) discusses six types of unmet or unrecognized need:

1. need that is thought to be required by the physician but not the client or vice versa—for example, colonoscopy may be the preferable screening option for colorectal cancer, but patients find it unacceptable;

2. services desired by the client but not received, such as weight reduction programs;
3. services required by professionals but not received by patients, such as prenatal care for underprivileged teenagers;
4. resources desired by clients but not present or available, such as doctors in physician shortage areas;
5. resources required by professionals but not present—for example imaging technologies in rural areas; and
6. morbidity caused by the failure to use appropriate services—for example, avoidable hospitalization for ambulatory care-sensitive conditions.

The purposes of needs assessment are therefore to assess the level of need in a population, determine the degree to which current resources or existing programs meet that need, and evaluate whether new programs or projects might fill a gap of unmet need.

Needs assessment also can be defined as "the process of measuring ill-health in a population" (Robinson and Elkan 1996). Epidemiologists would embrace this definition since it relies on the collection of morbidity rates for various kinds of diseases. A problem with this definition is that *need* is defined as "ill health," and one could argue that not all health needs should be viewed in this way, since prevention activities are also needs. It is also difficult to factor into this definition many aspects of public health, such as immunizations, since people in need of these services would not be part of morbidity statistics.

An alternative definition is to define needs assessment as measuring the "capacity to benefit from healthcare services" (Stevens and Raftery 1994; Stevens, Raftery, and Mant 2004). An advantage of this definition is that it recognizes that not all health problems are curable. In other words, it forces us to examine outcomes of care, and the degree to which the recipients of healthcare services derive benefit from these activities. It also forces us, however, to decide who makes these kinds of value judgments—clinicians or patients—and what to do with the logical, but ethically problematic, conclusion that people who do not "benefit" from healthcare are not in "need."

A third definition of needs assessment embraces the methods and measures of epidemiology by defining this process as "the epidemiological approach [that] involves describing need related to particular health problems using estimates of the incidence, prevalence, and other surrogates of health impact measured from the local population or elsewhere. This approach can be extended to the consideration, alongside these measures, of the ways in which existing services are delivered and the effectiveness and cost-effectiveness of interventions intended to meet the needs thus described" (Williams and Wright 1998). This approach is similar to the latter approach by combining measures of "ill health" in a population with recognized epidemiologic tools, such as morbidity rates, but also considering "capacity to benefit" with measures of effectiveness and cost-effectiveness.

Spiegel and Hyman (1991) describe five different needs assessment methods: the key information survey, the community survey, the demographic analysis, inferential indicators, and the analysis of programmatic data.

The *key informant survey* is a relatively simple, low-cost, and quick method of obtaining information on the needs of the community. Key informants include knowledgeable people such as clients, clinic directors, and police.

The *community survey* is a more expensive and time-consuming process of collecting information from a sample of the community, or targeted population group, through some survey instrument.

A *demographic analysis* is a relatively inexpensive assessment of population needs using existing data sources, such as the U.S. Census Bureau, the Department of Health and Human Services, or voter registration lists. These data are widely available, typically cover entire populations, and are used to make projections about need using estimates from target populations.

The *inferential indicator* method primarily uses existing data sets to make inferences about need in a population. These include published and unpublished reports; insurance claims collected by Medicare, Medicaid, or private insurance vendors; and other secondary data, such as the periodic surveys conducted by the National Center for Health Statistics.

Finally, one can assess the needs of a population through an *analysis of programmatic data*, which includes healthcare provider files such as medical records, or interviews with the relevant personnel. Case Study 4.3 reviews a comprehensive needs assessment for stroke services in Ontario, Canada.

Case Study 4.3. Needs Assessment for Stroke Services in Ontario, Canada

The Queen's Health Policy Research Unit (QHPRU) estimated the need for stroke services in Ontario, Canada, using measures of prevalence and incidence of (1) modifiable and nonmodifiable risk factors for stroke, (2) acute cases of stroke, and (3) major sequelae of stroke (Hunter et al. 2000; Hunter et al. 2004). They identified the effective health services targeted at each of these three dimensions, and linked these steps to estimate need for health services. QHPRU compared the estimate of need for health services to compiled measures of levels of stroke-related health services in eastern Ontario to see if there was a gap (unmet need) or surplus (overmet need) of these services.

QUESTIONS

1. Risk factors for stroke include heavy alcohol consumption, atrial fibrillation, diabetes, hypercholesterolemia, hypertension, obesity, low physical activity, smoking, ischemic heart disease, and transient ischemic attack. Where might QHPRU get estimates of the incidence of these conditions?

2. For each risk factor, or stroke sequelae, QHPRU listed the kind of intervention that would be effective, and the proportion of people for whom this intervention would be appropriate. According to Table 4.3 (below), which three interventions are appropriate for hypercholesterolemia, and for what proportion of high-risk individuals?

3. The following types of interventions were recommended for acute stroke services: (a) surgical intervention (carotid endarterectomy); (b) thrombolytic therapy; (c) imaging of the brain, either computed tomography (CT) or magnetic resonance imaging (MRI); (d) noninvasive imaging of the vessels (ultrasonography or magnetic resonance angiography); (e) invasive imaging of the vessels (cerebral angiography); and (f) rehabilitation therapy. For what percentage of at-risk individuals are these services recommended?

4. Estimates of people in eastern Ontario with hypercholesterolemia are as follows: age 25–44 (29,500 men and 12,900 women); age 45–64 (33,300 men and 42,400 women); age 65 and above (17,200 men and 41,900 women). How many residents in Ontario will need fasting lipoprotein analysis, dietary intervention, and pharmacologic intervention for hypercholesterolemia?

5. It is estimated that eastern Ontario provides dietary and pharmacologic intervention for hypercholesterolemia to 65,600 and 15,300 patients, respectively. What is the level of unmet need in terms of the number of patients not receiving each of these two recommended interventions? What percentage of need is currently being met in eastern Ontario?

6. The incidence of acute stroke cases was estimated at 3,525 cases, 106 of whom died before reaching the hospital. The prevalence of chronic stroke cases was estimated to be 4,312. Use Table 4.4 (below) to determine the number of acute and chronic stroke cases needing core stroke services and services for chronic stroke and disability.

7. It is estimated that eastern Ontario provides thrombolytic therapy and carotid endarterectomy to 52 and 196 patients, respectively. CT and MRI brain imaging are provided to 1,006 and 145 patients, respectively. Noninvasive and invasive imaging of the vessels are provided to 432 and

168 patients, respectively. Rehabilitation is provided to 1,385 acute stroke survivors, and home care services are provided to 1,435 chronic stroke with disability patients. What is the level of unmet need in terms of the number of patients not receiving each of the recommended services for acute or chronic stroke victims? What percentage of need is currently being met in eastern Ontario?

TABLE 4.3. INTERVENTIONS FOR HYPERCHOLESTEROLEMIA

Type of Intervention	Indications for Intervention	Proportion of At-Risk Individuals with Indications	
		Proportion (%)	In Practice
Nonpharmacologic fasting lipoprotein analysis	All with risk factor	100	All with risk factor
Nonpharmacologic dietary intervention	High LDL cholesterol level and presence of 1 cardiovascular risk factor	70	Indications for dietary intervention
Pharmacologic	All with high LDL levels concomitantly with diet, all with moderate LDL levels where dietary measures alone over 3–6 months fail to lower lipid levels	20	Indications for pharmacologic intervention

SOURCE: Used with permission from Hunter et al. (2000).

ANSWERS

1. QHPRU got estimates for most of these conditions from the Canadian Heart Health Survey (1986–1992) and the Ontario Health Survey (1996/97).
2. Fasting lipoprotein analysis is recommended for 100 percent of at-risk patients, while dietary and pharmacologic interventions are recommended for 70 percent and 20 percent of at-risk individuals, respectively.

TABLE 4.4. INTERVENTIONS FOR ACUTE AND CHRONIC STROKE VICTIMS

Condition	Estimate Eastern Ontario Frequency	Intervention	Percentage of Acute Stroke Cases Needing Intervention
Acute stroke survivors	3,419	**Core stroke services**	
		Not hospitalized	11% (of the 3,525)
		Hospitalized	86% (of the 3,525)
		Restricted stroke services	
		Thrombolytics	11% of hospitalized
		Imaging of brain	
		CT	97% (of the 3,525)
		MRI	10% of surviving cases
		Imaging of vessels	
		Noninvasive	97% (of the 3,525)
		Invasive	8% (of the 3,419)
		Carotid	4% (of the 3,419)
		Endarterectomy	54% surviving acute
Chronic stroke with disability	4,312	*Rehabilitation*	stroke cases
		Assistance in performing activities of daily living	100%

NOTE: 106 (3%) of the 3,525 patients died and did not need core services.

SOURCE: Used with permission from Hunter et al. (2000).

3. Carotid endarterectomy and thrombolytic therapy are recommended for 4 percent and 11 percent, respectively, of at-risk individuals with indications for intervention. Noninvasive imaging of the brain or vessels is recommended for 97 percent of at-risk individuals, whereas MRIs and cerebral angiography are recommended for only 10 percent and 8 percent, respectively, of at-risk individuals. Rehabilitation is recommended for 54 percent of at-risk individuals.

4. There are 177,200 people in eastern Ontario with hypercholesterolemia. Of these, 100 percent (177,200) will require lipoprotein analysis, 70 percent

(124,040) will require dietary intervention, and 20 percent (35,440) will require pharmacologic intervention.

5. The estimated need for dietary and pharmacologic interventions for hypercholesterolemia was 124,040 and 35,440 respectively. Ontario provides 65,600 and 15,300 of these two interventions. Unmet need for dietary intervention is 124,040 − 65,600 = 58,440 patients, or (58,440/124,040) × 100 = 47% unmet need. Unmet need for pharmacologic intervention is 35,440 − 15,300 = 20,140 or (20,140/35,400) × 100 = 57% unmet need.

6. The estimates are that 388 and 3,031 not hospitalized and hospitalized patients, respectively, will need core stroke services such as diagnostic tests, prevention of recurrent stroke, and assessment of disability. Thrombolytic therapy will be required by 333 patients. Imaging of the brain by CT and MRI will be required by 3,419 and 342 patients, respectively; imaging of the vessels by 3,419 and 274 patients; respectively, carotid endarterectomy by 137 patients; and rehabilitation by 1,846 patients. All 4,312 patients with chronic stroke and disability will require assistance with activities of daily living (home care).

7. The estimated need for thrombolytic and carotid endarterectomy services was 333 and 137 patients, respectively. Eastern Ontario provides these services to 52 and 196 patients, respectively. Unmet need for thrombolytic therapy would be 333 − 52 = 281 patients, or (281/333) × 100 = 84% unmet need. Unmet need for carotid endarterectomy would be 137 − 196 = − 59 or − (59/137) × 100 = 43% *overmet* need. The estimated need for CT brain imaging, MRI brain imaging, and noninvasive and invasive imaging of the vessels is 3,419, 342, 3,419, and 274 patients, respectively. Unmet need for CT brain imaging would be (3,419 − 1,006) = 2,413 patients, or 2,413/3,419 x 100 × = 71% unmet need. Unmet need for MRI imaging would be 342 − 145 = 197 patients, or 197/342 × 100 = 58% unmet need. Unmet need for noninvasive imaging would be 3,419 − 432 = 2,987 patients, or (2,987/3,419) × 100 = 87% unmet need. Unmet need for invasive imaging would be 274 − 168 = 106 patients, or (106/274) × 100 = 39% unmet need. The estimated need for rehabilitation (acute stroke) and home care (chronic stroke) is 1,846 and 4,312 patients, respectively. Eastern Ontario provides services to 1,385 and 1,435 acute and chronic stroke victims, respectively. Unmet need for rehabilitation would be 1,846 − 1,385 = 461 patients, or (461/1,846) × 100 = 25% unmet need. Unmet need for home care would be 4,312 − 1,435 = 2,877 patients, or (2,877/4,312) × 100 = 67% unmet need.

Human Resources Planning

Rakich, Longest, and Darr (1992) describe the human resources planning process as consisting of five steps: profiling, estimating, inventorying, forecasting, and planning.

Profiling involves estimating the quantity and mix of employees needed to staff the organization. With the *estimating* step, industry standards, such as staffing ratios, are used to project the number of employees needed. The skills of current employees are assessed in the *inventorying* step. *Forecasting* involves estimating workforce changes such as deaths, retirements, and transfers. In the *planning* stage, the organization articulates a plan based on the assumptions of the previous four steps to meet the anticipated needs of the organization. Epidemiology should play a significant role, particularly in the profiling stage, of human resources planning, inasmuch as the organization must estimate the need for human resources on the basis of expected demand for services.

Some of the theory and techniques that have been developed to estimate the need for physician workforce in the aggregate (i.e., across the United States) could be adapted for organization-wide workforce profiling. For example, the workforce needs in a managed care environment could be estimated by examining the kinds of present and future morbidity expected among enrolled members. This would not work as well in a nonintegrated, fee-for-service environment, in which each level of care (ambulatory, acute, and long-term care) provides separate, not necessarily coordinated, and perhaps even duplicative services.

A simplified version of the Donabedian (1973) model is illustrated in Figure 4.1, in which "need" can be associated with service equivalents, which can then be associated with resource equivalents. This paradigm was anticipated by Lee and Jones (1933), who were probably the first to estimate the need for physician workforce in their classic study. They estimated the number of people in a population who should receive different kinds of services on the basis of prevalence of disease. They also estimated the amount of time and number of services that would be required for each disease. This relates to the "strategy" of care. Finally, they predicted the number of services that could be provided by each professional, obviously a measure of physician productivity. Thus, in this model, need (as measured by the prevalence of disease) could be translated into services (using strategies, guidelines, or standards), which could then be translated into workforce, on the basis of productivity. Clearly, productivity depends on type of practitioner, setting, organization, and even gender.

The major shortcoming of the "needs-based" methods of Lee and Jones and Donabedian, in terms of forecasting workforce, is that they are based entirely on a normative, rather than an actual, measure of what

FIGURE 4.1
"Need" and Its
Equivalents

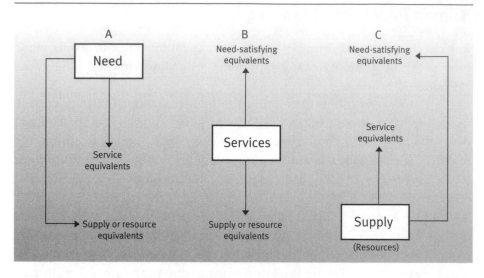

SOURCE: Reprinted by permission of the publisher from ASPECTS OF MEDICAL CARE ADMINISTRA-
TION: SPECIFYING REQUIREMENTS FOR HEALTH CARE by Avedis Donabedian, p. 65, Cambridge,
MA: Harvard University Press, Copyright © 1973 by the President and Fellows of Harvard College and the
Commonwealth Fund.

services are required by each type of morbidity. In other words, with Lee
and Jones, a panel of physicians would prescribe the kinds of services that
"ought" to be provided for each kind of disease. The modern-day approach
would be to use a practice guideline, "clinical trajectory," or critical pathway to predict mix of services.

Regardless of time frame, the point is that normative prescriptions
for service delivery may not directly translate into utilization because of
access barriers, financial or otherwise. Lack of insurance may prevent a
patient from securing medical care regardless of what the practice guideline specifies. Because of this dilemma, some of the more recent models to
predict physician workforce, such as the GMENAC approach (Bureau of
Health Manpower 1978), have attempted to factor market behavior into
the projections. Thus the requirements for workforce are at least in part
based on predicted demand for services.

Even the rather simple needs-based model is encumbered with complexity, and cannot be fully understood or developed without epidemiologic concepts and insight. Clearly, the model is only as good as the measures to assess "need." The measurement of need is doubtless an
epidemiologic concept, expressed formally as the incidence and prevalence
rates discussed in Chapter 3.

The accuracy of the model also depends on the set of standards used
to translate need into service equivalents. The organization trying to predict workforce needs may choose standards that are less than "best practice," for instance, in which case workforce needs may be overestimated.

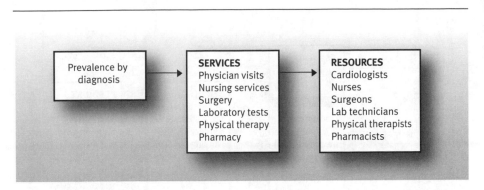

FIGURE 4.2
Need, Services, and Resources for Cardiovascular Disease

Services are translated into workforce through productivity norms, which of course may vary by type of setting or organization, physician office, hospital, clinic, and so on.

Suppose that you are the CEO of a large managed care organization. You are trying to anticipate the future need for staffing, particularly with regard to physicians, nurses, and other allied health workers, such as physical therapists. The simplest approach would be to describe present need in terms of the prevalence of cardiovascular morbidity in the enrolled population, as illustrated in Figure 4.2. You could predict the number of physician visits (generalist and specialist), nursing services, surgical procedures, laboratory tests, and so on, that would be associated with each cardiovascular diagnosis. The number of professional and support personnel that would be required to deliver and support those services could be extrapolated from these data using productivity norms.

A more "upstream" approach to predicting staffing requirements is illustrated in Figure 4.3, where risk factors of disease (such as smoking) are expected to increase the incidence of various kinds of morbidity (such as lung cancer, heart disease, and emphysema). For example, smoking makes you twice as likely to get heart disease and ten times or more as likely to get lung cancer (refer to Chapter 14 on clinical epidemiology). Future incidence of these diseases can be predicted for those with and without a particular risk factor using one or more of the observational and experimental studies described in chapters 11, 12, and 13. The incidence of these diseases can then be associated with services and workforce resources, as was the case in Figure 4.2.

Clearly, the issue is the extent to which medical care organizations care about predicting future staffing on the basis of risk factors in a population, or whether staffing requirements can be developed solely on the basis of current morbidity.

For hospitals and group practices not affiliated with managed care organizations, staffing could be determined on the basis of current patient load as measured by case mix—for example, DRGs for hospitals, CPT codes for physicians. This information would have to be projected into

FIGURE 4.3
Risk Factors,
Need,
Services, and
Resources

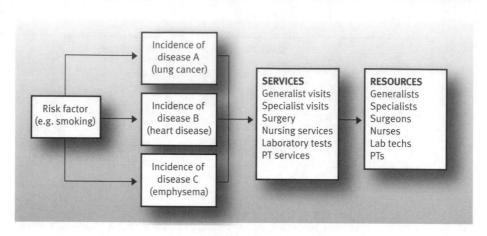

the future, taking into consideration any expected changes in demand for services or market share.

If managed care organizations recognize the promotion of health as a priority, then they should care about how risk factors are ultimately translated into future incidence of disease. It is clear that society has an interest in reducing risk factors. Few managed care organizations have that same interest because of how frequently consumers change insurance plans. The poignant question is whether these organizations will operate within a short rather than long time horizon, expecting that future morbidity will be somebody else's problem.

Summary

Earlier, we described planning as assessing and making provision for the future, or making current choices to influence the future, which may involve guiding the process of change. We have demonstrated how both community and institutional planning should be intimately acquainted with epidemiologic measures. The *Healthy People 2010* initiative, for example, comprises 467 specific goals, many of which point to epidemiologic measures. With institutional planning, questions regarding current and future position or role within a health service market require both internal and external assessment, processes that thrive on valid epidemiologic measures. We have described how needs assessment is the formal process of assessing the healthcare needs in a population for the purposes of program development, and how human resources planning should be based on the underlying model that morbidity translates into services required, which translates into manpower needed to provide those services. Finally, to the extent that planning and marketing are flip sides of the same coin, organizations would benefit from using epidemiology to describe morbidity and risk factor burden of current and potential markets, and using epidemiologic studies to facilitate the promotion of healthcare products to the consumer.

References

Berry, D. E. 1974. "The Transfer of Planning Theories to Health Planning Practice." *Policy Sciences* 5: 343–61.

Bureau of Health Manpower. 1978. "Physician Requirements Forecasting: Need-Based Versus Demand-Based Methodologies." Department of Health, Education, and Welfare Pub. No. (HRA) 78-12. Washington, DC: U.S. Government Printing Office.

Donabedian, A. 1973. *Aspects of Medical Care Administration.* Cambridge, MA: Harvard University Press.

Duncan, W. J., P. M. Ginter, and L. E. Swayne. 1995. *Strategic Management of Health Care Organizations.* Malden, MA: Blackwell.

Hunter, D. J. W., R. A. Spasoff, J. L. Dorland, M. P. H. Purdue, and N. Bains. 2000. *Determining the Need and Provision of Health Services for Stroke in Eastern Ontario: An Epidemiologic Approach to Needs Assessment.* Kingston, ON: Health Information Partnership, Eastern Ontario Region.

Hunter, D. J., H. J. Grant, M. P. Purdue, R. A. Spasoff, J. L. Dorland, and N. Bains. 2004. "An Epidemiologically-Based Needs Assessment for Stroke Services." *Chronic Diseases in Canada* 25 (3/4): 138–46.

Keck, R. K., Jr. 1986. "Strategic Planning in the Health Care Industry: Concentrate on the Basics." *Health Care Issues* (September), reprinted in *Handbook of Business Strategy* 1985–1986 Yearbook. New York: PricewaterhouseCoopers.

Lee, J. M. 1989. "Marketing in Health Services Administration." In *Handbook of Human Services Administration*, edited by J. Rabin and M. Steinhauser. New York: Marcel Decker.

Lee, R. I., and L. W. Jones. 1933. *The Fundamentals of Good Medical Care.* Publication of the Committee on the Costs of Medical Care, No. 22. Chicago: University of Chicago Press.

MacStravic, R. E. 1977. *Marketing Health Care.* Germantown, MD: Aspen Systems.

Rakich, J. S., B. B. Longest, and K. Darr. 1992. *Managing Health Services Organizations.* Baltimore, MD: Health Professions Press.

Robinson, J., and R. Elkan. 1996. *Health Needs Assessment: Theory and Practice.* New York: Churchill Livingstone.

Spiegel, A. D., and H. H. Hyman. 1991. *Strategic Health Planning: Methods and Techniques Applied to Marketing and Management.* Norwood, NJ: Ablex.

Stevens, A., and J. Raftery. 1994. "Introduction." In *Health Care Needs Assessment: The Epidemiologically Based Needs Assessment Reviews,* vol. I, 11–30. Oxford, UK: Radcliffe Medical Press.

Stevens, A., J. Raftery, and J. Mant. 2004. "An Introduction to HCNA: The Epidemiological Approach to Health Care Needs Assessment." [Online article; retrieved 11/5/04.] http://hcna.radcliffe-oxford.com/introframe.htm.

U.S. Department of Health and Human Services. 1979. *Healthy People: The Surgeon General's Report on Health Promotion and Disease Prevention.* Pub. No. (PHS) 79-55071. Washington, DC: U.S. Government Printing Office.

———. 1991. *Healthy People 2000: National Health Promotion and Disease Prevention Objectives.* Pub. No. (PHS) 91-50212. Washington, DC: U.S. Government Printing Office.

Williams, R., and J. Wright. 1998. "Health Needs Assessment. Epidemiological Issues in Health Needs Assessment." *British Medical Journal* 316 (7141): 1379–82.

Wilson, P. W., R. B. D'Agostino, D. Levy, A. M. Belarger, H. Silbershatz, and W. B. Kannel. 1998. "Prediction of Coronary Heart Disease Using Risk Factor Categories." *Circulation* 97 (18) 1837–47.

QUALITY OF CARE MEASUREMENT

Steven T. Fleming

> *"To assess the quality of medical care one must first unravel a mystery: the meaning of quality itself. It remains to be seen whether this can be done by patiently teasing out its several strands or whether one must, in despair, use a sword to cut the Gordian knot."* Avedis Donabedian, The Definition of Quality and Approaches to Its Assessment, 1980

The "control function" of a healthcare manager is perhaps one of the most critical components of the job. The control function, which includes both assessment and intervention activities, includes such tasks as quality of care assurance and management and patient safety.

Control activities link planning with operation. Without planning, there is no direction. Without the control function, there is no assurance that what is planned will ever get accomplished. Most control activities relate to either quality assessment/improvement or financial management. The former includes quality assessment and improvement, risk management, utilization review, and credentialing, and the latter consists of budgeting, case-mix accounting, and ratio or volume analysis (Rakich, Longest, and Darr 1992).

This chapter focuses on quality of care measurement, assurance, and management. The purpose is not to train managers to replace or become hospital epidemiologists, but rather to cultivate a way of thinking that facilitates thoughtful discussion with clinicians and other experts, enriching operational and strategic decisions. The concepts and principles of epidemiology for financial management are discussed thoroughly in Chapter 8.

A generic control system is illustrated in Figure 5.1 (Rakich, Longest, and Darr 1992). Inputs are converted through various processes into outputs, with information generated at each stage. As the information is interpreted (assessment), intervention or change can occur at either the input or process stage. Inputs and processes can be replaced, refined, or reconfigured.

The control function is data driven, which explains the need for information systems to collect and disseminate critical information to key decision makers. The concept of control involves monitoring, assessment, feedback, and regulation, and implies that there are standards, ideals, or objectives to which the organization is compared. If the standards are not met, then intervention through a corrective adjustment is required. Control should be simple, timely, flexible, directed at critical elements, and based on accurate and relevant information (Ginter, Swayne, and Duncan 1998).

FIGURE 5.1
Generic
Control
System

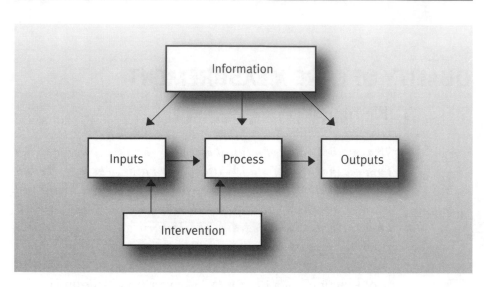

SOURCE: Rakich, Longest, and Darr (1992). Used with permission.

The standards to which the organization is compared can be derived from and focused on inputs, processes, or outputs. *Input standards* refer to the characteristics and configuration of human and physician resources, a concept similar to what Donabedian refers to as "structure."

The credentials of physicians and nurses are a simple example. Their defined relationships and turf are more complicated.

Process standards are based on the machinations of healthcare delivery—the complex web of processes through which inputs are converted to outputs. Clinical guidelines, which describe ideal physician behavior, have been arduously developed and disseminated to the medical community. Critical pathways describe standardized care patterns. Although developed primarily for the hospital setting, these pathways have been expanded to include pre- and post-hospital care. The widespread adoption of a continuous quality improvement (CQI) philosophy signals a sincere interest, on the part of healthcare providers, to examine the processes of care, and to set standards or "benchmarks" to which healthcare organizations can compare.

Output standards refer to the characteristics of the products of healthcare delivery, the most significant of which is the extent to which patients enjoy an improvement in health status or amelioration of symptoms. The outcomes research movement should spawn clinical recommendations and expectations, outcome standards, and "best practices." It should be obvious to the reader that the structure, process, and outcome paradigm of quality assessment espoused by Donabedian captures the essence of the feedback control system illustrated in Figure 5.1.

Ginter, Swayne, and Duncan (1998) distinguish between operational control, which focuses on individual performance or specific processes (e.g., operations and budgeting), from strategic control, which involves determining if an organization's strategy will result in progress toward meeting objectives.

For strategic control, the standards are typically more financial and market oriented, such as market standing, innovative performance, productivity, liquidity and cash flow, and profitability. Perhaps in the future quality will be more widely recognized as a performance standard to which organizations are compared both operationally and strategically. For this to happen, managers would have to develop at least some familiarity with the collection and interpretation of clinical data, and an understanding of the basic concepts and principles of epidemiology.

The purpose of this chapter is to argue that the methods and tools of epidemiology are a critical means of converting the data gathered through the assessment of inputs, process, or outputs into useful information for the purpose of deciding whether intervention is necessary.

Furthermore, a practical understanding of epidemiological principles would assist the manager with strategic control to the extent that performance standards are defined in clinical terms.

Epidemiology and quality are defined and compared in the first section of the chapter. Rates and surveillance are discussed in second section, followed by a case study on methicillin-resistant *Staphylococcus aureus* (MRSA) surveillance. Complication rates are the focus of section three, which includes a case study on risk-adjusted complication rates. Managed care and avoidable hospitalization are the topics of section four. Quality indicators, with a case study on the use of such indicators at the fictional Bluegrass Hospital, compose section five. Finally, the integration of epidemiology and quality improvement is discussed in section six.

Epidemiology and Quality

Quality, at the most fundamental level, is derived from clinicians making judgments about balancing benefit and harm to achieve desirable patient objectives (Donabedian 1980). A more inclusive definition of quality would include such dimensions as access to care and patient satisfaction. Donabedian argues that quality of care also has an "epidemiology" in the sense that one can study the determinants of quality and its distribution among two different populations—providers and clients. Furthermore, one can study quality against the framework of the traditional epidemiological triad—time, place, and person. Studies of this sort are particularly useful for strategic control, where intervention and change of strategy may result in better quality outcomes.

Quality also has a distribution across settings and localities. Within the traditional epidemiology context, disease is investigated in different settings to identify particular agents, vectors, or risk factors. A study of quality within and across different settings (such as hospitals or nursing homes) viewed through the epidemiology prism would be concerned with the determinants of quality in those settings. Within organizations, one should be concerned with how quality is distributed across units or clinics and what characteristics of those divisions are associated with the higher levels of quality. In fact, a healthcare organization may be designed specifically to evaluate alternative interventions and outcomes of care in distinct units (see discussion of hospital firms in Chapter 13). Finally, quality is distributed among the groups of people—providers and clients.

> Knowledge of the distribution of quality among providers of health services...is the product of the more usual studies of quality that throw light on the relation between structure, on the one hand, and either process or outcome on the other...[whereas] the distribution of specified levels of quality among various groupings of the consumers of care is, of course, the ultimate measure of the success or failure in achieving the social objectives of a healthcare system (Donabedian 1985, 282).

The epidemiologist is concerned with identifying causal relationships between agents or risk factors and disease. At least to some extent, the incidence, severity, and progression of disease depend on the characteristics of the agent (e.g., virulence) or risk factor (e.g., strength) and the characteristics of the host or population (e.g., immunity or susceptibility).

Quality is antithetical to disease in the sense that it is desirable and beneficial. Therefore, the emphasis should be on identifying and measuring provider characteristics, such as training, experience, specialization, and age, that engender favorable outcomes of care.

As difficult, perhaps, is the embarrassing task of identifying characteristics (such as race or socioeconomic status) that render patients susceptible to poor quality or inadequate care. For example, the study by Bindman and colleagues (1995), which examines access to care for preventable hospitalizations, suggests a barrier to inpatient care that the uninsured face even if they are very ill.

Donabedian's thesis that quality has an epidemiology validates our argument that the concepts and principles of epidemiology are relevant to the control function of the manager. Moreover, an extension of this thinking provides a useful metaphor through which to understand what quality is and how it can be controlled. Disease and quality are not quite two sides of a coin. Both have a distribution across time, place, and people that can be measured and analyzed. Both are derivative, in the sense that they can be causally related to an exposure—an agent, a risk factor, a provider, a setting, or a process of care. And both can be controlled through intervention, such as elimination or modification of the exposure. This is where continuous quality improvement and risk management come into play.

Beyond the argument that quality of care has an epidemiology is the thesis that quality assessment or measurement has benefited from the integration of epidemiological principles and methods into theory and practice. Donabedian suggests that epidemiology has contributed to quality assurance in at least four different areas:

1. specifying the standards and criteria of good practice;
2. specifying which characteristics and configuration of providers and settings are associated with good quality;
3. the development of measurement tools; and
4. the design and conduct of monitoring systems.

The first area relates primarily to the field of clinical epidemiology, which is discussed more thoroughly in Chapter 14. Epidemiological studies can inform the clinical decision-making process with regard to choice of diagnostics or therapeutic strategies.

The second area falls into the realm of health services research, inasmuch as the concern is with system design (refer to the discussion of "firms" in Chapter 13, for instance). These investigations determine which attributes or characteristics of individual providers or systems of care are associated with better quality. Epidemiology can certainly make significant contributions to the design and development of new measurement instruments.

Rates and Surveillance

A rate quantifies the number of healthcare events, such as disease or mortality, with reference to a defined population (e.g., 1,000 people) for the purpose of comparison across intervals of time, geographic regions or settings, or different population groups.

The epidemiologist is familiar with rates expressing the mortality or morbidity experience of a population at risk, such as elderly females in the state of Kentucky. For the healthcare organization, the appropriate population at risk would be defined in terms of inpatient episodes (e.g., admissions), units of time (patient days), or enrolled members, in the case of managed care organizations.

Suppose, for example, that a growing managed care organization is interested in comparing preventable hospitalizations over time to determine if a new case manager program is effective. A crude count of these events over time would be misleading because enrollment has been rapidly increasing. The correct measure would be a rate expressing the number of preventable hospital episodes per 1,000 enrolled members. A significant decrease in this rate over time would be a signal that the case manager program has been successful.

Most healthcare organizations have surveillance programs in place that are charged with the responsibility of monitoring key indicators, such as infection rates. The focus should be on targeting infections that are frequent, are preventable, generate high treatment cost, or have serious effects on either morbidity or mortality (Pottinger, Herwaldt, and Peri 1997).

The "building blocks" of surveillance include a systematic collection of relevant data over a specific period; the management, organization, analysis, and interpretation of these data; and the communication of results to decision-makers, at least some of whom will be healthcare managers (Pottinger, Herwaldt, and Peri 1997). Since the purpose of surveillance is to identify problems and intervene if necessary, it becomes the operational vehicle through which the manager delegates at least part of the control function to physicians, nurses, or other members of the epidemiology staff.

The "bread and butter" of surveillance has historically been nosocomial infections, which, by definition, originate from within the hospital setting. The difference between hospital-acquired illness and comorbidities is a difficult but critical distinction. A *comorbidity* is an illness that exists before, or arises after, the hospital stay, and is not related to the stay. *Nosocomial infections*, on the other hand, are hospital-derived, and can become a reasonable measure of quality (if properly adjusted for risk).

The timing of these events is crucial, which is why some have suggested labeling an infection as nosocomial only if it occurs at least two to three days after admission, within ten days after discharge, or with special exceptions for very short (e.g., the gastrointestinal Norwalk virus) or very long (e.g., hepatitis A) incubation periods.

Larson, Oram, and Hedrick (1988) report that approximately one-third of nosocomial infections are preventable and therefore a reflection of quality of care. The remaining two-thirds are "much less amenable to intervention" (678) due to intrinsic patient risk factors, such as age, gender, and chronic comorbidities, as well as differences in the "recognition" of these events.

A strong argument can be made for the surveillance of noninfectious outcomes of care as well, such as high-volume procedures, outcomes that are important to patients, or outcomes that reflect processes of care that are manageable. These could include accidents, or adverse events related to procedures, equipment, or medications.

Fundamentally, surveillance involves collecting data over time to establish thresholds or baseline endemic rates, and determining whether the rates are stable and if they are higher than they should be. A significantly higher rate would trigger investigation, and even a statistically insignificant, but clinically "significant" increase might be worthy of inquiry (Pottinger, Herwaldt, and Peri 1997).

To compare rates over time or to a threshold, they must be intrinsically comparable. Numerators should be based on precise definitions, reflecting the incidence or prevalence of adverse events, such as infection. Denominators should include only the population at risk, or the period during which the population was at risk, which means that these rates should also adjust for both intrinsic and extrinsic patient risk factors. Intrinsic risks

include the presence of comorbidities—immunodeficiency, for instance—
that are patient-specific. Extrinsic risks are related to the hospital environment or exposures to medical interventions such as ventilators.

For instance, duration of time in a hospital is a risk that can be adjusted
by using patient days rather than admissions in the denominator (Pottinger,
Herwaldt, and Peri 1997). The risk of infection associated with surgery or
medical interventions, such as ventilators, can be adjusted by using total surgical procedures, or total patient hours of contact in the operating room (or
with an intervention) in the denominator. For these examples, one is measuring the incidence density rather than the cumulative incidence of these
adverse events over time (Massanari, Wilkerson, and Swartzendruber 1995).

Pottinger, Herwaldt, and Peri (1997) discuss five distinct surveillance methods. *Hospital-wide* or *traditional surveillance* involves a prospective and continuous survey of all medical care areas to identify the total
incidence of nosocomial infections using microbiology reports and medical records as sources of information. *Periodic surveillance* is conducted
routinely, but periodically. For example, the entire hospital may be surveyed one month each quarter, or a different unit may be surveyed each
month. A *prevalence survey*, on the other hand, tabulates the total number of infections that are present and active within a specific period.
Targeted surveillance focuses on specific settings (e.g., critical care units);
services, such as cardiovascular; or groups of high-risk patients. With *outbreak threshold surveillance*, the baseline endemic infection rates are used
as triggers below which no surveillance activity would occur.

Case Study 5.1 illustrates a hospital-wide surveillance program for
MRSA at a 700-bed hospital.

Case Study 5.1. MRSA Surveillance at University Hospital

The increasing rate of methicillin-resistant *Staphylococcus aureus* (MRSA) is
becoming a serious public health threat inasmuch as outbreaks now occur in
both hospital and community settings. Shitrit et al. (2006) describe the results
of an active surveillance program for MRSA in a 700-bed hospital in which they
culture patients who are considered to be at high risk of MRSA (Table 5.1).

QUESTIONS

1. What kinds of patients might be considered "high risk"?
2. By how much did surveillance increase after the intervention?
3. For which kinds of patients did surveillance increase the most?

4. What kinds of precautions or procedures were recommended for patients who tested positive for MRSA?
5. How successful was this intervention strategy?

TABLE 5.1. ACTIVE SURVEILLANCE PROGRAM FOR MRSA

Statistics (per 1,000 admissions)	Before Intervention	After Intervention
MRSA surveillance cultures	51.6	164.0
Patients identified as carriers	31.3	52.2
MRSA surveillance cultures		
Medicine ward	33.5	269.0
Surgical ward	9.1	75.0
ICUs	1,124.0	1,645.0
Geriatric ward	2,573.0	2,882.0
Carriers identified		
Medicine ward	0.9	15.8
Surgical ward	0.16	3.8
ICUs	24.6	55.5
Geriatric	40.5	204.0
Nosocomial MRSA bacteremia	0.74	0.37
Nosocomial MRSA bacteremia (geriatric ward)	8.44	3.16

SOURCE: Data from Shitrit et al. (2006).

ANSWERS

1. Patients were cultured if they (a) transferred from another hospital or another ward in the hospital, (b) transferred from a long-term care facility, (c) were receiving hemodialysis, or (d) were known to be MRSA carriers.
2. Total MRSA cultures more than tripled. Culture rates in the medical and surgical wards increased by a factor of 8. Carrier rates in the ICU and geriatric doubled and quintupled, respectively.
3. Surveillance increased the most in the medical and surgical wards.
4. Patients who tested positive were either placed in isolation in single rooms or double rooms (with a one-bed distance from other patients). Gloves and gowns were required when in contact with these patients. Masks were recommended for contact with ventilated patients. Eradication treatment was prescribed for MRSA carriers who stayed in the hospital.

5. The intervention was successful, because the overall rate of nosocomial MRSA bacteremia was cut in half. Furthermore, in the geriatric ward, in particular, the rate was reduced by nearly two-thirds, despite the fact that the surveillance activity increased by only 12 percent.

Outcomes of Care—Complication Rates

Outcomes of care include terminal outcomes, such as whether the patient died or survived, and intermediate outcomes, such as changes in functional status or the occurrence of complications or adverse events. The process of risk adjusting mortality rates to be used as a measure of quality is discussed in detail in Chapter 6. This section focuses on complications and adverse events as a measure of quality.

The intrinsic and extrinsic risk mentioned earlier suggests that the occurrence of adverse events in healthcare settings is largely driven by factors related to patients, the environment in which they are treated, or the kind of treatment they receive. Fleming (1996) classifies adverse events along three dimensions: (1) whether procedures were good or deficient, (2) whether the disease processes were normal or abnormal, and (3) whether clinician skills were good or deficient. These dimensions represent extrinsic (1, 3) and intrinsic (2) factors that may lead to poor outcomes.

Clearly, an adverse event, like infection, may result from deficient procedure or practice, abnormal disease process (i.e., unexpected disease course or complication), poor clinical skills, or more than one factor. The surveillance system discussed earlier is typically unable to completely disentangle these factors, and it is difficult to make valid judgments about quality of care without knowing the cause of the adverse event.

Nonetheless, there is some evidence from the literature that complication rates may be a useful measure of quality because they are more sensitive and directly related to the process of patient care than other more crude measures of outcome such as mortality rates. DesHarnais and colleagues (1990), for instance, developed risk-adjusted indices of mortality, readmission, and complications based on a sample of 776 short-term hospitals in 1993. The measures were shown to be stable over time and unbiased with respect to hospital size, ownership, and teaching status. The measures accounted for much of the variation across hospitals in the incidence of these adverse events. The complication measure, in particular, was adjusted for the risk associated with age and comorbidities.

More recently, Brailer and colleagues (1996) described a comorbidity-adjusted complication measure that, like DesHarnais, is based on diagnoses reported on hospital claims. The Brailer measure, however, attempts to address at least two problems with some of the earlier measures: (1) the difficulty in distinguishing between a post-admission complication and a comorbidity occurring before or during hospitalization, and (2) the impact of multiple complications. This measure assigns a complication risk to each patient based on the secondary diagnoses recorded on claims data, and the probability that each diagnosis is a complication for a specific admitting diagnosis. For example, if a patient were admitted with simple pneumonia, the probability that congestive heart failure, respiratory failure, and urinary tract infection were complications rather than comorbidities would be 20 percent, 50 percent, and 90 percent, respectively. Brailer and colleagues discuss how this measure is highly correlated with other "gold standards" such as those based on chart review.

Iezzoni and colleagues (1994) identified 27 complications that "raise concern about the quality of care." The list includes such conditions as wound infections and decubitus ulcers. Each complication is assigned to a "risk pool," which represents the patients at risk of those complications. For example, only patients who endure surgery would be at risk for "postoperative complications." Observed-to-expected complication rates were compared across hospitals with the conclusion that larger and major teaching facilities, and those that performed open heart surgery, had higher relative complication rates.

The Iezzoni study is especially relevant in this chapter for at least two reasons. The assignment of each quality indicator, in this case specific complications, to risk pools recognizes the importance of denominators in calculating rates. The incidence of adverse events, such as complications (the numerator), is derived from and must be compared only to the population "at risk" of the event (the denominator).

Table 5.2 lists five complications and their associated risk groups. Notice that some complications, such as aspiration pneumonia, ought to be associated only with a surgical risk group. Others, such as post-operative pneumonia, may arise from a somewhat larger risk group, which also contains patients subject to endoscopy and invasive cardiac procedures. Patients at risk of wound infections, on the other hand, compose the largest group of medical and surgical patients, including those who endure endoscopic or invasive cardiac procedures.

The second reason the Iezzoni study is relevant to the discussions of this chapter is the finding that complications were not significantly related to hospital mortality rates as calculated by the Health Care Financing Administration (now the Centers for Medicare & Medicaid Services). One explanation for this noncorrelation is that the latter measure is either too crude, poorly designed, or not a particularly robust indicator of quality. Critics of this measure are not shy with their disapproval. The larger question is whether mortality even should be correlated with complications, or whether each measure reflects a different dimension of quality of care.

Silber and colleagues (1995) evaluated the complication rate as a measure of quality of care and focused on coronary artery bypass graft

TABLE 5.2
Complications and Associated At–Risk Categories

	Major, Minor, Miscellaneous Surgery	Invasive Cardiac Procedures (e.g., catheterization)	Endoscopy	Medical Patients	Complications Relating to All Patients
Aspiration pneumonia	X				
Postoperative acute myocardial infarction	X		X		
Postoperative pneumonia	X	X	X		
Pulmonary embolism	X	X	X	X	X
Wound infection	X	X	X	X	X

SOURCE: Data from Iezzoni et al. (1994).

surgery (CABG). They compared actual death, complications, and failure to rescue (after complications develop) with expected rates, using variables that had been previously identified as predictive of these outcomes, such as severity of illness. Fifty-seven hospitals were ranked by each of these three measures. The complications that were chosen were those that "increased the risk of dying and those that added complexity to the management of the patient" (Silber et al. 1995, 318). The complication measure correlated poorly with either failure to rescue or mortality, both of which were more often associated with hospital characteristics related to higher quality, such as the presence of a magnetic resonance imaging facility or an approved residency program. The authors suggest that complications may not be a good indicator of quality since they may be measuring something different than either mortality or failure to rescue.

Several of these studies have raised cautionary flags with regard to the utility or validity of complications as a measure of quality, given the poor correlation with other more acceptable measures, such as mortality. What remains unclear is whether complications and these other quality measures should be associated—or should at least move in the same direction—and whether it would even be misleading to applaud organizations with low complication rates and vice versa.

How would an epidemiologic frame of mind enable the health services manager to interpret these puzzling results and glean critical truths to put into the practice of the control function of management? An adverse event, such as a nosocomial infection or complication, is clearly undesirable, because of the cost and suffering involved (Fleming 1996). These events should be monitored over time as rates, with the denominator of each rate representing the patient population at risk of the event (Iezzoni et al. 1994). A more sophisticated surveillance program might include predicted rates, which include patient risk factors, such as age, that are unrelated to quality of care. The lack of association between complications and mortality does not exonerate complications as a cause for concern, but rather suggests that there may be confounding factors that make it difficult to accept complications as an indicator of quality, particularly when comparing across organizations. It may be more useful to compare complication rates among providers or services within an organization, particularly if one can control for patient risk factors.

Case Study 5.2 examines the use of risk-adjusted complication rates in a small rural hospital.

Case Study 5.2. Risk-Adjusted Complication Rates in a Small Rural Hospital

Boondocks Hospital is a small 50-bed hospital located in a little Midwestern town of 10,000 people. Although the hospital has struggled financially over the last ten years or so, it has been able to maintain a 70 percent occupancy. The hospital boasts two operating rooms, an active general surgery service, and an obstetrical service, which has recently partnered with a teaching hospital 25 miles away. The hospital has decided to monitor quality of care with several different measures, including a risk-adjusted measure of complications (Iezzoni et al. 1994). The developers of the measure report observed-to-expected rates of complications for a large sample of hospitals in Table 5.3. Boondocks Hospital calculates an index of 1.2 for minor surgery and 1.1 for medical patients.

QUESTIONS

1. Why might you expect the complications measure to be higher for the large and/or teaching hospital?
2. Describe some plausible explanations for the risk-adjusted complication rates of Boondocks Hospital.
3. What kinds of action should Boondocks take?

TABLE 5.3 RISK-ADJUSTED COMPLICATION RATES FOR BOONDOCKS HOSPITAL

Hospital Type	Major Surgery	Minor Surgery	Medical
Large hospitals	1.15	1.14	1.33
Small hospitals	0.82	0.89	0.94
Teaching hospitals	1.00	1.00	1.10
Nonteaching hospitals	0.89	0.95	0.94

ANSWERS

1. Any risk-adjustment methodology is flawed to the extent that it excludes important risk factors. This measure is based on administrative data and the risk factors that can be derived from such data. Larger hospitals are more likely to handle patients with a higher level of severity or complexity, particularly patients who have been referred from other institutions. These patients may have risk factors that are not easily captured by administrative data but may be present in a review of their medical charts.

2. We must first determine if risk-adjusted rates of 1.2 and 1.1 are statistically significantly different from 1.0. We also need to look at the actual number of complications (numerators) in each of these two measures to see if this might be a "small numbers" problem.

3. If the rates are significantly different than 1.0 and the numerators are stable, but relatively small, Boondocks may want to do a medical audit of the specific patients to determine which processes of care or patient factors may have compromised quality of care.

Managed Care

Managed care organizations (MCOs) require even greater accountability insofar as quality of care is concerned because of the perverse incentives in this form of healthcare delivery. These responsibilities rest heavy on the shoulders of healthcare managers exercising the control function of quality assurance and improvement.

Report cards and physician profiling are becoming commonplace in managed care. A notable example is the Healthcare Effectiveness Data and Information Set (HEDIS) developed by the National Committee for Quality

Assurance (NCQA). The initial version of HEDIS (1.0) was released in 1991, followed by a 2.0 version in October of 1993, and the 3.0 version in early 1997. The most recent version (2007) contains 71 performance measures in eight different areas: effectiveness of care, access/availability of care, satisfaction, health plan stability, use of services, cost of care, informed healthcare choices, and health plan descriptives. Over 90 percent of American health plans voluntarily submitted these data for publication by NCQA. The purpose of HEDIS is to give employers an objective set of performance measures with which to judge the strengths and weaknesses of various managed care organizations.

Physician profiles, on the other hand, are derived from administrative databases and intended to provide feedback to physicians on costs, immunizations, screening, practice patterns, and appropriateness of care (Spoeri and Ullman 1997). Obviously, these profiles are intended to "encourage" physicians to practice medicine within the boundaries and norms established by their colleagues. Managerial control can be exercised directly through financial incentives, or by requiring physicians to justify deviations from these norms. MCOs are particularly interested in specialist referrals and inpatient admissions.

Many hospital episodes may be avoidable, particularly those related to ambulatory care-sensitive conditions (ACSCs), where treatment, monitoring, and follow-up outside the hospital may prevent these episodes from occurring in the first place. Furthermore, one could categorize ACSCs into conditions that are completely preventable (e.g., an immunizable disease such as measles); conditions for which earlier primary care would have prevented hospitalization (e.g., cellulitus); and conditions that require careful monitoring and treatment (e.g., asthma).

All of these conditions are especially relevant under capitation, where the managed care organization bears the financial burden of healthcare services for an enrolled population. With the incentive to underutilize, surveillance of ACSCs would seem particularly appropriate. A reduction in unnecessary hospitalization affects quality, access, and cost. If patients can avoid hospitalization, they evade iatrogenic (Brennan et al. 1991) and other risks associated with care in that environment; in short, quality of care is better if hospitalization can be legitimately avoided. However, this requires that patients have access to ambulatory care services. To the extent that these services prevent, replace, or reduce the duration of a hospital episode, overall costs to the plan would be lower.

A number of studies support these premises. Bigby and associates (1987) report that 9 percent of 686 emergency hospital admissions were potentially preventable, and of these, two-thirds were caused by iatrogenic misadventures. Solberg, Peterson, and Ellis (1990) studied 673 potentially avoidable hospital episodes for patients in 15 clinical conditions and found that hospitalizations could have been avoided at rates ranging from 1 percent of asthma cases to 21 percent for diabetes ketoacidosis cases. Another study compared uninsured to privately insured patients in terms of hospital admission for 1 of 12 potentially avoidable hospital conditions. Uninsured patients were 71 percent more likely to be admitted in Massachusetts and 49 percent more likely to be admitted in Maryland.

Bindman and colleagues (1995) showed that access to care across 250 zip code areas in urban California, as measured by insurance coverage and having a regular source of care, is more strongly related to preventable hospitalization than it is to patient care-seeking behavior or physician practice style. In Maryland, poor children with asthma had 40 percent fewer physician visits, but nearly twice the hospitalization rate and over three times the bed days (Halfon and Newacheck 1993). In another study using Maryland hospital claims data, the hospitalization rate for asthma among black children was nearly three times the rate of white children (Wissow et al. 1988).

Clearly, the size of the preventable hospitalization problem is significant, and the causes are still unclear but coming into focus: they relate to issues of medical competence and accessibility, particularly financial accessibility, and perhaps physical accessibility as well.

The studies mentioned above suggest that quality assurance in a managed care organization should include the surveillance of ambulatory-sensitive conditions as well as preventable hospital episodes that can be traced back to deficient care in the ambulatory setting. Some ambulatory care-sensitive conditions include asthma, cervical cancer, hypertension, perforated/bleeding ulcer, diabetes, and ruptured appendix.

The epidemiological insight in view here is the need to monitor changes in both the at-risk population (those with the ACSC—the denominator) and the adverse outcome (the potentially avoidable hospitalization—the numerator) to calculate cause-specific avoidable hospitalization rates. For example, we need to know the prevalence of enrolled members with diabetes (the at-risk population) as well as the number of avoidable hospital episodes (for coma or ketoacidosis) during that same time. Changes in these cause-specific rates would inform managers about access-of-care barriers for specific clinical conditions. A less useful approach would be to monitor changes in the rate of avoidable hospitalization expressed as the number of these hospital episodes per 1,000 enrolled members. Cause-specific rates would more accurately and specifically measure the ability of an MCO to control diseases that may result in needless hospitalizations.

Quality Indicators

The Agency for Healthcare Research Quality publishes four sets of quality indicators (QIs): Prevention QIs; Inpatient QIs; Patient Safety Indicators; and Pediatric QIs. The purpose of these indicators is to provide quality of care measures that can be derived from readily available claims data. Table 5.4 summarizes the specific indicators in each of these sets.

Each of the 14 prevention QIs measure potentially avoidable hospitalizations for ambulatory care–sensitive conditions. These admission rates have different denominators that are specific to the quality indicator. For example, the diabetes short-term complication rate is expressed as the number of admissions per 100,000 population, whereas the perforated appendix admission rate is calculated as the number of admissions for a perforated appendix per 100 admissions for an appendicitis.

The Inpatient QIs can be categorized into three areas: (1) measures of the volume of inpatient procedures where the link between volume and outcome has been clearly established; (2) measures of in-hospital mortality for common procedures and outcomes; and (3) utilization measures for procedures with questions of overuse, abuse, or underuse. The volume indicators are not rates, but counts of the number of surgical or medical cases, for example, the number of hip replacements or acute stroke cases. Specific benchmarks or thresholds are given for each of these indicators, each based on the link between higher volume and better outcomes. The mortality rates are basically case fatality rates (Chapter 6), where the numerators are the number of deaths and the denominators are the number of discharges for each condition. The utilization measures also have indicator-specific denominators. The cesarean delivery rate is expressed as the number of cesarean deliveries per 100 deliveries, whereas the coronary artery bypass graft surgery is expressed as the number of CABGs per 100,000 population.

TABLE 5.4
Agency for Healthcare Research and Quality (AHRQ) Quality Indicators

Prevention Quality Indictors	Patient Safety Quality Indicators
Diabetes short-term complications admission rate	Complications of anesthesia
Perforated appendix admission rate	Death in low-mortality diagnosis-related groups
Diabetes long-term complications admission rate	Decubitus ulcer
Chronic obstructive pulmonary disease admission rate	Failure to rescue
Hypertension admission rate	Foreign body left during procedure, provider level
Congestive heart failure admission rate	Foreign body left during procedure, area level
Low birthweight rate	Iatrogenic pneumothorax, provider level
Dehydration admission rate	Iatrogenic pneumothorax, area level
Bacterial pneumonia admission rate	Selected infections due to medical care, provider level
Urinary tract infection admission rate	Selected infections due to medical care, area level
Angina without procedure admission rate	Post-operative hip fracture
Uncontrolled diabetes admission rate	Post-operative hemorrhage or hematoma

Prevention Quality Indictors (cont.)

Adult asthma admission rate
Rate of lower-extremity amputation among
    patients with diabetes

Inpatient Quality Indicators

Volume
  Esophageal resection
  Pancreatic resection
  Abdominal aortic aneurysm repair
  Coronary artery bypass graft
  Percutaneous transluminal coronary angioplasty
  (PTCA)
Mortality rate
  PTCA
  Carotid endarterectomy
  CEA mortality rate
  Esophageal resection
  Pancreatic resection
  Abdominal aortic aneurysm repair
  Coronary artery bypass graft
  Craniotomy
  Hip replacement
  Acute myocardial infarction
  Acute myocardial infarction (without transfer cases)
  Congestive heart failure
  Acute stroke
  Gastrointestinal hemorrhage
  Hip fracture
  Pneumonia
Utilization rates
  Cesarean delivery
  Primary cesarean delivery
  Vaginal birth after cesarean (uncomplicated)
  Vaginal birth after cesarean (all)
  Laparoscopic cholescystectomy
  Incidental appendectomy in the elderly
  Bilateral cardiac catheterization
  Coronary artery bypass graft area
  Percutaneous transluminal coronary angioplasty
   area rate
  Hysterectomy
  Laminectomy or spinal fusion

Patient Safety Quality Indicators (cont.)

Post-operative physiologic and metabolic
    derangement
Post-operative respiratory failure
Post-operative pulmonary embolism or deep vein
    thrombosis
Post-operative sepsis
Post-operative wound dehiscence, provider level
Post-operative wound dehiscence, area level
Accidental puncture or laceration, provider level
Accidental puncture or laceration, area level
Transfusion reaction, provider level
Transfusion reaction, area level
Birth trauma—injury to neonate
Obstetric trauma—vaginal delivery with instrument
Obstetric trauma—vaginal delivery without
    instrument
Obstetric trauma—cesarean delivery

Pediatric Quality Indicators

Accidental puncture or laceration
Decubitus ulcer
Foreign body left in during procedure
Iatrogenic pneumothorax (in neonates at risk)
Iatrogentic pneumothorax in non-neonates
Post-operative hemorrhage and hematoma
Post-operative respiratory failure
Post-operative sepsis
Post-operative wound dehiscence
Selected infection due to medical care
Transfusion reaction
Asthma admission rate
Diabetes short-term complications admission
    rate
Gastroenteritis admission rate
Perforated appendix admission rate
Urinary tract infection admission rate
Pediatric heart surgery mortality rate
Pediatric heart surgery volume rate
Postoperative physiologic and metabolic
    derangement
Dehydration admission rate
Bacterial pneumonia admission rate
Craniotomy mortality rate

SOURCES: *Guide to Prevention Quality Indicators: Hospital Admissions for Ambulatory Care Sensitive Conditions.* Department of Health and Human Services, Agency for Healthcare Research and Quality. October 2001, Version 3.1 (March 12, 2007); *Guide to Inpatient Quality Indicators: Quality of Care in Hospitals—Volume, Mortality, and Utilization.* Department of Health and Human Services, Agency for Healthcare Research and Quality, June 2002, Version 3.1 (March 12, 2007); *Measures of Pediatric Health Care Quality Based on Hospital Administrative Data: The Pediatric Quality Indicators.* Department of Health and Human Services, Agency for Healthcare Research and Quality, February 20, 2006; *Guide to Patient Safety Indicators.* Department of Health and Human Services, Agency for Healthcare Research and Quality, March 2003, Version 3.1 (March 12, 2007).

The pediatric healthcare quality indicators include an eclectic mix of patient safety, mortality, and potentially avoidable hospitalization rates. For the patient safety events, these rates are expressed as the number of these potentially preventable events per 1,000 eligible admissions, which in most cases means pediatric admissions less exclusions. For example, the denominator of the decubitus ulcer quality indicator excludes admissions in the denominator for patients with a length of stay less than five days, presumably because these patients were not at risk of this complication. Mortality rates are the typical case fatality rates, expressed as the number of deaths per 100 surgical cases. The potentially avoidable hospitalization rates are expressed as the number of these admissions (e.g., asthma, diabetes with complications, gastroenteritis) per 100,000 population.

The patient safety quality indicators are potentially preventable complications and iatrogenic events that occur in patients treated in the hospital setting. These indicators are rates with specific denominators and exclusions. For example, complications of anesthesia include only surgical patients, whereas decubitus ulcers include all medical and surgical discharges. In some cases, these rates are risk-adjusted by age, sex, diagnosis-related group, and comorbidity categories. Some of these rates are "provider level" indicators, meaning that the denominators refer to the specific hospital in which the patient received care. Other rates are "area level" rates, which capture the risk of these events in a particular geographic area, such as a metropolitan area or county. Case Study 5.3 examines the use of these indicators at Bluegrass Hospital.

Case Study 5.3. Inpatient Quality of Care Indicators for Bluegrass Hospital

Suppose that the Kentucky Hospital Association decided to provide a service to its member hospitals by using the inpatient claims database to calculate inpatient quality of care indicators for each hospital. It provides a report to every hospital comparing each to national norms. Table 5.5 presents some of these indicators for Bluegrass Hospital, a fictional 200-bed hospital located in central Kentucky. Upon receiving this report, Bluegrass Hospital organizes a quality improvement (QI) team to evaluate and develop recommendations.

QUESTIONS

1. From an evaluation of the report card only, Bluegrass Hospital seems to be deficient in which areas?

TABLE 5.5 REPORT CARD FOR BLUEGRASS HOSPITAL COMPARED TO AVERAGE AND STANDARD DEVIATION (SD) OF ALL HOSPITALS

Impatient Quality Indicator	Hospital	Average	Standard Deviation
Volume			
Abdominal aortic aneurysm repair	25	10^a, 32^b	
Coronary artery bypass graft	50	100^c, 200^d	
Percutaneous transluminal			
coronary angioplasty (PTCA)	100	200^e, 400^f	
Mortality rate			
Esophageal resection	25.0	20.2	36.6
Pancreatic resection	16.0	15.4	31.3
Abdominal aortic aneurysm repair	30.4	21.5	26.8
Coronary artery bypass graft	13.3	5.1	6.2
Craniotomy	18.2	16.2	18.5
Hip replacement	1.0	1.2	5.7
Acute myocardial infarction	45.0	24.4	16.1
Congestive heart failure	7.4	7.5	9.5
Acute stroke	21.2	21.3	13.7
Gastrointestinal hemorrhage	4.9	4.6	5.7
Hip fracture	13.9	14.2	16.0
Pneumonia	12.0	13.8	10.2
Utilization rates			
Cesarean delivery	19.0	21.4	8.7
Vaginal birth after cesarean (all)	35.0	33.6	14.8
Larporoscopic cholescystectomy			
(per 100 cholescystectomies)	67.0	66.2	19.2
Incidental appendectomy in the			
elderly	2.8	2.7	3.5
Bilateral cardiac catheterization			
(per 100 cardiac catherizations)	30.0	19.3	20.0
Coronary artery bypass graft area	200.0	180/100,000	571.6/100,000
Percutaneous transluminal	210.0	190.8/100,000	455.6/100,000
coronary angioplasty			
Hysterectomy	440.0	419.4/100,000	323.3/100,000
Laminectomy or spinal fusion	145.2	139.0/100,000	347.5/100,000

a: at this volume, 83.9% of procedures were by high-volume providers; b: at this volume 43.0%, were by high-volume providers; c: at this volume, 98.3% of procedures were by high-volume providers; d: at this volume, 90.7% were by high-volume providers; e: at this volume, 95.7% of procedures were by high-volume providers; f: at this volume, 69% were by high-volume providers

2. Since the report is based on an evaluation of administrative data, what should the first course of action be?
3. After the QI team compares the inpatient quality indicators to an internal chart review, it meets with various clinical departments. What would be the purpose of such meetings?
4. What specific recommendations might the QI team make?

ANSWERS

1. This hospital is a high outlier by at least one standard deviation in coronary artery bypass graft surgery (case fatality rate 13.3% and acute myocardial infarction case fatality rate 45%). It should also be noted that this hospital is below the lowest volume threshold for both coronary artery bypass graft surgery and percutaneous transluminal coronary angioplasty (PCTA). Hannan and colleagues (1994) found that CABG patients were 16% less likely to die (RR = 0.84) in high-volume hospitals (>200 cases per year) compared to low-volume hospitals. The volume of CABG for Bluegrass Hospital was only 50 cases a year. Ritchie and colleagues (1999) found that risk-adjusted hospital mortality and same admission bypass surgery rates were lower in hospitals with a higher volume of cases. Bluegrass Hospital performed only 100 PCTA procedures a year, compared with the lowest threshold of 200.
2. The team compares the data to other "internal" sources of this information. For example, a chart review of a random sample of patients in each condition could determine whether the mortality data were accurate, and whether the death was preventable.
3. The purpose of these meetings would be to discuss the results with each department and determine the extent to which processes of care or patient factors affected outcomes, with a view toward making recommendations for improvement.
4. The team might suggest that the hospital develop risk assessment tools and treatment guidelines for patients at risk of dying, particularly for those who present with symptoms of acute myocardial infarction. The team might suggest that the hospital evaluate referral policies to neighboring institutions that have higher volumes of cardiac operations each year.

Total Quality Management

Many healthcare organizations today have adopted a philosophy of management referred to as total quality management (TQM) or continuous quality improvement. These programs have spread across the medical landscape with a kind of religious zeal, in response to a number of factors, such as the escalation of healthcare costs and the variation in clinical practice (Fleming, Bopp, and Anderson 1993).

A number of key individuals were responsible for transplanting the TQM theories and concepts of earlier visionaries (Juran and Gryna 1988; Berwick, Godfrey, and Roessner 1990) from industrial settings to the healthcare sector. The underlying premise behind these theories is that quality can be improved by eliminating unwanted and nonrandom variation in the processes of healthcare. These techniques of statistical process control from industrial engineering fit nicely with the concepts of epidemiology, as we will see later.

Berwick (1989) discusses the basic principles of total quality management, which include a focus on the processes of healthcare. According to this system, each employee plays the triple role of customer (receiving work from others), processor (adding value), and supplier (giving work to others). The main source of quality problems is with process rather than people, according to TQM theory. To point the finger at a process rather than a "bad apple" (i.e., a hapless and probably innocent employee) was a major development in quality assurance (Berwick 1989). TQM focuses on the most vital healthcare processes, with a scientific and statistical mind-set that encourages total employee involvement. In short, the TQM philosophy fosters employee empowerment with a corporate culture that rewards inquiry.

Organizations that have embraced TQM continuously engage in quality improvement projects through a number of different techniques, such as the Plan, Do, Study, Act cycle. In the Plan phase, the project team diagrams a particular healthcare process with a flow chart, identifies sources of variation, and suggests potential changes. Changes are implemented on a small scale in the Do phase and observed during the Study phase. Final changes are instituted across the organization in the Act phase. A related approach would be to (1) define the process, (2) collect data, (3) redesign the process, (4) implement changes, (5) measure results, and (6) hold the gains. Alternatively, some distinguish between the "diagnostic" and "remedial" journeys involved with quality improvement. TQM projects employing any of these three paradigms can be summarized as "storyboards," which detail the quality improvement process and lessons learned from each experience.

Quality improvement consists of a toolbox of descriptive and analytical techniques heavily grounded in statistics and either directly or indirectly related to epidemiological concepts.

One of the techniques is the *flow chart*, which illustrates each step in a particular healthcare process. It displays the complexities of the process, identifies the decision points, and accentuates the junctures where timing is critical.

Another tool is the cause-effect, or *fishbone*, diagram, which classifies the potential causes of a problem by category, such as the four Ms (method, manpower, material, machinery), the four Ps (policies, procedures, people, plant), or other alternatives (e.g., people, methods, information, materials, or facilities) (Marszalek-Gaucher and Coffey 1993).

FIGURE 5.2
Control Chart
of Catheter–
Associated
Infections

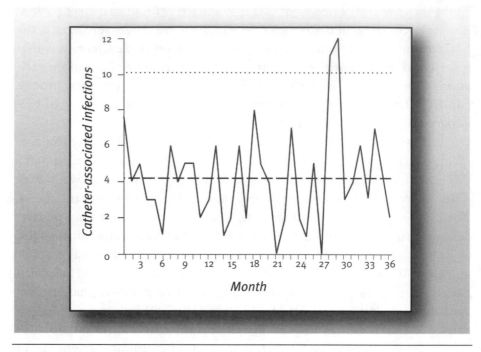

SOURCE: Benneyan (1998). Copyright © 1998, Society of Healthcare Epidemiology of America. Used with permission.

A similar, albeit less fishy, approach, would be to summarize a brainstorming session with an *affinity diagram*, in which potential causes are fit into a classification scheme.

Control charts and *run charts* depict trends over time, with and without confidence intervals, respectively. *Histograms* are simply bar graphs that illustrate frequency by category, and *Pareto charts* are histograms that have been sorted by frequency. *Scatter diagrams* portray the relationship between two variables.

Each of these illustrative tools provides insight into the diagnostic or remedial process of quality improvement, and each has epidemiological relevance.

Figure 5.2 depicts the trend of catheter-associated infections over a three-year period, by month. Notice the mean of 4.22 infections per month and the upper confidence limit (UCL) of three standard deviations from the mean of 10.08. The purpose of TQM is to eliminate nonrandom variation from the process and thereby improve quality. The control chart isolates specific points of nonrandom variation when the trend exceeds the upper (or lower) confidence interval, as is the case during months 28 and 29. Further inquiry into the matter would attempt to identify possible causes and suggest remedial action. The control chart illustrates the essence of what is called *statistical process control* (SPC), and is rich with epidemiological meaning. The purpose of SPC is to monitor a process over time

FIGURE 5.3
Cause–Effect
Diagram for
Falls

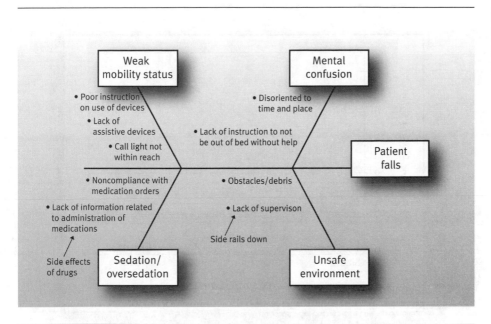

SOURCE: Al-Assaf and Schmele (1993). Used with permission.

(epidemiologists might call this *surveillance*), and distinguish between natural and unnatural variation in that process. With infections, for instance, the interest is in distinquishing between the endemic or underlying rate of disease, and any abnormal (or epidemic) increase in that rate over time, during months 28 and 29, perhaps. The threshold (UCL above) represents an action limit that would trigger further investigation.

One can also use control charts to illustrate non-disease-related trends over time, such as daily emergency room admissions, average waiting time in minutes, or average time until referral in days. In each case, the purpose is to monitor the trend and identify the out-of-control points, which the epidemiologist would call *sentinel events*. The circumstances surrounding these events provide useful insights into potential causes of the problem.

Cause-effect or fishbone diagrams categorize the potential causes of process problems. Figure 5.3, for instance, illustrates a hypothetical cause-effect diagram for patient falls in four categories—weak mobility status, mental confusion, sedation, and environment. Note that the chart does not quantify the degree to which each factor contributes to the breakdown in process but merely illustrates the aggregation of factors into categories and subcategories. Epidemiologists search for the causes of disease, disability, and other human suffering. Although these causes are typically not summarized in a cause-effect diagram, some have elaborate webs of causation for chronic disease. Refer to Timmreck 1998 (pp. 342–344) for webs of causation for coronary heart disease, myocardial infarction, and heart disease. A "web of causation" would advance the cause-effect diagram one step further because it

FIGURE 5.4
Pareto Chart:
Patient Falls

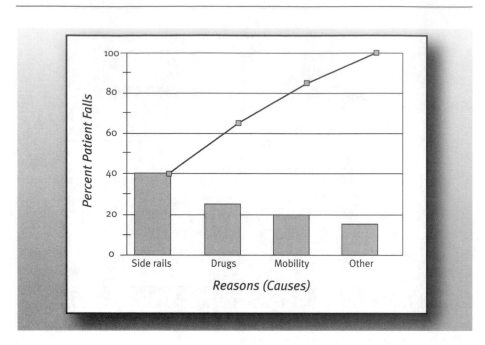

depicts the intricacy of causal relationships among various factors, not simply the categories to which they belong. For example, in Figure 5.3, sedation could also cause mental confusion. Clearly, it would be more efficient to eliminate the root cause rather than the derivative causes of process problems.

A Pareto chart is simply a sorted bar graph that is used to prioritize. Figure 5.4 illustrates a contrived Pareto chart associated with the cause-effect diagram of Figure 5.3. Notice that the top three reasons for falls compose 85 percent of the risk of this process failure. The Pareto chart assumes that each instance of process failure (e.g., patient fall) can be attributed to one distinct cause (e.g., side rails). In fact, these charts are derived by identifying which cause is responsible for each process failure. This is akin to the epidemiologist recognizing one specific agent responsible for disease at a time.

The multi-cause model of chronic disease consists of numerous interrelated risk factors, each of which acts both individually and severally to increase the probability of developing disease. Thus, the attributable fraction (see Chapters 11 and 12) is calculated as a measure of the extent to which a particular risk factor is responsible for disease in the population, given the relative risk and prevalence of the risk factor in the population.

Although this is typically not done, TQM teams could design studies to determine the relative risk (or odds ratio) of each specific cause associated with a process failure. For example, of those patients who are sedated, the study could learn what proportion fall out of the bed. A simple case-control or cohort study would be adequate here.

Ideally the study would control for all proposed causes (i.e., it probably needs to be a multi-variate analysis). Once the relative risk of each specific cause was determined, along with the prevalence of the cause in the population, the attributable fraction of each cause could be calculated. A Pareto chart derived from these results would identify the most important causes of process failure, assuming that each cause does not result in process failure all the time, and that more than one cause may trigger process failure some of the time.

The statistical tools discussed above, and others, are used by TQM teams to determine the cause(s) and remedies for process failures, with an eye toward improving quality. Clearly, epidemiology should play a pivotal role in the design and implementation of these studies. The concepts of causal relationships, risk, rates, and surveillance are fundamental to TQM.

Summary

An epidemiological frame of mind is particularly relevant to the health services manager insofar as the control function is concerned. The focus has been on measuring and managing quality of care using the fundamental principles of epidemiology: (1) the distribution of disease in human populations across time, places, and people; (2) the measurement and study of risk factors that increase the probability of adverse outcomes such as morbidity; and (3) the surveillance, monitoring, and identification of atypical clusters of disease. The concepts of rates and at-risk populations and the definition and measurement of such quality indicators as complications and avoidable hospitalizations have been discussed. Further, we have described how the traditional epidemiological concepts of age adjustment can be extended to include a multi-factorial model of risk adjustment. Finally, the basic principles and tools of quality improvement have been described with an epidemiological interpretation.

Eighty years ago or so, Ernest Amory Codman was engaged in a struggle for recognition and reputation for an idea that brings us back to the future. Codman passionately advocated the idea that physicians be held accountable for the care they provide. The symptoms, main diagnosis, treatment plan, complications, and one-year follow-up for each patient would be summarized on an "end-results card." Codman's passion foresaw what we call "the outcomes movement" and provider report cards. His ideas anticipate clinical quality improvement and clinical practice guidelines, since the end results system would reveal to each doctor (Donabedian 1989, p. 244):

> an undistorted picture of both his successes and failures [from which] he could then learn which cases he could treat better, which cases he should refer to others, and which subjects are deserving of further research...the first inklings of a discovery would appear in the end results attained by individual physicians as they introduced their particular innovations. It

would be the responsibility of the hospital, then, to take note of the events, and to subject those innovations that seemed promising to a more thorough test, always guided by end results. The innovations that survived would be referred to the committee of the college [American College of Surgeons] which, in turn, would select the more worthy ones for further testing at other collaborating hospitals.

Let us remember the foresight of Codman as we close this chapter on the relevance of epidemiology to quality measurement and control. Codman knew that accountability was the key to quality improvement and advancing clinical science, and surveillance of entire patient populations was the essence of innovation.

REFERENCES

Al-Assaf, A. F., and J. A. Schmele. 1993. *The Textbook of Total Quality Management in Healthcare*. Boca Raton, FL: St. Lucie Press.

Benneyan, J. C. 1998. "Statistical Quality Control Methods in Infection Control and Hospital Epidemiology. Part I: Introduction and Basic Theory." *Infection Control and Hospital Epidemiology* 19 (3): 194–214.

Berwick, D. M. 1989. "Continuous Improvement as an Ideal in Health Care." *New England Journal of Medicine* 320 (1): 53–56.

Berwick, D. M., A. B. Godfrey, and J. Roessner. 1990. *Curing Health Care: New Strategies for Quality Improvement*. San Francisco: Jossey-Bass.

Bigby, J., J. Dunn, L. Goldman, J. B. Adams, P. Jen, C. S. Landefeld, and A. L. Komaroff. 1987. "Assessing the Preventability of Emergency Hospital Admissions: A Method for Evaluating the Quality of Medical Care in a Primary Care Facility." *American Journal of Medicine* 83 (6): 1031–36.

Bindman, A. B., K. Grumbach, D. Osmond, M. Komaromy, K. Vranizan, N. Lurie, J. Billings, and A. Stewart. 1995. "Preventable Hospitalization and Access to Care." *Journal of the American Medical Association* 274 (4): 305–11.

Brailer, D. J., E. Kroch, M. V. Pauly, and J. Huang. 1996. "Comorbidity-Adjusted Complication Risk: A New Outcome Quality Measure." *Medical Care* 34 (5): 490–505.

Brennan, T. A., L. L. Leape, N. M. Laird, L. Hebert, A. R. Localio, A. G. Lawthers, J. P. Newhouse, P. C. Weiler, and H. H. Hiatt. 1991. "Incidence of Adverse Events and Negligence in Hospitalized Patients: Results of the Harvard Medical Practice Study." *New England Journal of Medicine* 324 (6): 370–76.

DesHarnais, S. I., L. F. J. McMahon, Jr., R. T. Wroblewski, and A. J. Hogan. 1990. "Measuring Hospital Performance: The Development and

Validation of Risk-Adjusted Indices of Mortality, Readmission, and Complications." *Medical Care* 28 (12): 1127–41.

Donabedian, A. 1980. *The Definition of Quality and Approaches to Its Assessment.* Chicago: Health Administration Press.

———. 1985. "The Epidemiology of Quality." *Inquiry* 22 (Fall): 282–92.

———. 1989. "The End Results of Health Care: Ernest Codman's Contribution to Quality Assessment and Beyond." *Milbank Quarterly* 67 (2): 233–67.

Drucker, P. F. 1986. "If Earnings Aren't the Dial to Read." *Wall Street Journal,* October 30, 32.

Fleming, S. T. 1996. "Complications, Adverse Events, and Iatrogenesis: Classifications and Quality of Care Measurement Issues." *Clinical Performance and Quality Health Care* 4 (3): 137–47.

Fleming, S. T., K. D. Bopp, and K. G. Anderson. 1993. "Spreading the 'Good News' of Total Quality Management: Faith, Conversion, and Commitment." *Health Care Management Review* 18 (4): 29–33.

Ginter, P. M., L. E. Swayne, and W. J. Duncan. 1998. *Strategic Management of Health Care Organizations.* Malden, MA: Blackwell.

Halfon, N., and P. W. Newacheck. 1993. "Childhood Asthma and Poverty: Differential Impacts and Utilization of Health Care Services." *Pediatrics* 91 (1): 56–61.

Hannan, E. L., D. Kumar, M. Racz, A. L. Siu, and M. R. Chassin. 1994. "New York State's Cardiac Surgery Reporting System: Four Years Later." *Annals of Thoracic Surgery* 58 (6): 1852–57.

Iezzoni, L. I., J. Daley, T. Heeren, S. M. Foley, J. S. Hughes, E. S. Fisher, C. C. Duncan, and G. A. Coffman. 1994. "Using Administrative Data to Screen Hospitals for High Complication Rates." *Inquiry* 31 (1): 40–55.

Juran, J. M., and F. M. J. Gryna, eds. 1988. *Juran's Quality Control Handbook,* 4th ed. New York: McGraw-Hill.

Larson, E., L. F. Oram, and E. Hedrick. 1988. "Nosocomial Infection Rates as an Indicator of Quality." *Medical Care* 26 (7): 676–84.

Marszalek-Gaucher, E. J., and R. J. Coffey. 1993. *Total Quality in Healthcare: From Theory to Practice.* San Francisco: Jossey-Bass.

Massanari, R. M., K. Wilkerson, and S. Swartzendruber. 1995. "Designing Surveillance for Noninfectious Outcomes of Medical Care." *Infection Control and Hospital Epidemiology* 16 (7): 419–26.

Pottinger, J. M., L. A. Herwaldt, and T. M. Peri. 1997. "Basics of Surveillance: An Overview." *Infection Control and Hospital Epidemiology* 18 (7): 513–27.

Rakich, J. S., B. B. Longest, and K. Darr. 1992. *Managing Health Services Organizations.* Baltimore, MD: Health Professions Press.

Ritchie, J. L., C. Maynard, M. K. Chapko, N. R. Every, and D. C. Martin. 1999. "Association Between Percutaneous Transluminal Coronary

Angioplasty Volumes and Outcomes in the Healthcare Cost and Utilization Project, 1993–1994." *American Journal of Cardiology* 83 (4): 493–97.

Shitrit, P., B. S. Gottesman, M. Katzir, A. Kilman, Y. Ben-Nissan, and M. Chowers. 2006. "Active Surveillance for Methicillin-Resistant Staphylococcus Aureus (MRSA) Decreases Incidence of MRSA Bacteremia." *Infection Control and Hospital Epidemiology* 27 (10): 1004–8.

Silber, J. H., P. R. Rosenbaum, J. S. Schwartz, R. N. Ross, and S. V. Williams. 1995. "Evaluation of the Complication Rate as a Measure of Quality of Care in Coronary Artery Bypass Graft Surgery." *Journal of the American Medical Association* 274 (4): 317–23.

Solberg, L. I., K. E. Peterson, and R. W. Ellis. 1990. "The Minnesota Project: A Focused Approach to Ambulatory Quality Assessment." *Inquiry* 27 (4): 359–67.

Spoeri, R. K., and R. Ullman. 1997. "Measuring and Reporting Managed Care Performance: Lessons Learned and New Initiatives." *Annals of Internal Medicine* 127 (8): 726–32.

Timmreck, T. C. 1998. *An Introduction to Epidemiology.* Boston: Jones and Bartlett.

Wissow, L. S., A. M. Gittelsohn, M. Szklo, B. Starfield, and M. Mussman. 1988. "Poverty, Race, and Hospitalization for Childhood Asthma." *American Journal of Public Health* 78 (7): 777–82.

MORTALITY AND RISK ADJUSTMENT

Steven T. Fleming and F. Douglas Scutchfield

"It is appointed unto men once to die, but after this the judgment." Hebrews 9:26 Authorized (King James) Version

Mortality has a sobering theological meaning and context, as evidenced by this quotation. However, the mortality experience is "judged" in a number of other settings as well. In the acute care setting, physicians routinely assemble for "mortality and morbidity" presentations, which are part educational, and part remedial. Mortality data are routinely collected by most developed countries. Comparisons and judgments can be made across countries with these critical vital statistics, with regard to the burden of disease and the availability of and access to healthcare resources. Mortality rates, if properly standardized, also are a useful measure of quality of care with which hospitals, nursing homes, and individual physicians and surgeons can be graded on performance.

Mortality statistics are particularly useful for epidemiologic surveillance or research, because these data are widely available as part of the vital records of most developed countries. In the United States, these data are typically collected by state health departments and derived from death certificates (Figure 6.1). Such documents include personal identifiers, demographic information such as age and race, and cause(s) of death. The certificate identifies the immediate cause of death, several underlying causes of death, and other significant conditions. For example, the immediate cause of death may be a ruptured myocardium due to two underlying conditions (acute myocardial infarction and ischemic heart disease), with influenza and pneumococcal pneumonia listed as other conditions.

The validity of data derived from death certificates may not be entirely accurate, depending on who identifies cause of death (usually a physician, resident, pathologist, or sometimes coroner), the degree to which the true underlying cause of death can be discerned, and other nonmedical factors. For example, AIDS was underreported as the cause of death for a number of years, perhaps due to the social stigma associated with the disease. Stroke was an overreported cause of death, a reflection of the difficulty in making accurate judgments as to the true sequence of events that leads to death.

Epidemiologists and historians are interested in changes in the leading causes of death over the years. This information reflects the burden of

FIGURE 6.1
Standard
Certificate
of Death

NAME OF DECEDENT
For use by physician or institution

U.S. STANDARD CERTIFICATE OF DEATH

LOCAL FILE NO.   STATE FILE NO.

To Be Completed/Verified By: FUNERAL DIRECTOR

1. DECEDENT'S LEGAL NAME (Include AKA's if any) (First, Middle, Last)   2. SEX   3. SOCIAL SECURITY NUMBER

4a. AGE-Last Birthday (Years) | 4b. UNDER 1 YEAR [Months | Days] | 4c. UNDER 1 DAY [Hours | Minutes] | 5. DATE OF BIRTH (Mo/Day/Yr) | 6. BIRTHPLACE (City and State or Foreign Country)

7a. RESIDENCE-STATE   7b. COUNTY   7c. CITY OR TOWN

7d. STREET AND NUMBER   7e. APT. NO.   7f. ZIP CODE   7g. INSIDE CITY LIMITS? □ Yes   □ No

8. EVER IN US ARMED FORCES? □ Yes □ No   9. MARITAL STATUS AT TIME OF DEATH □ Married □ Married, but separated □ Widowed □ Divorced □ Never Married □ Unknown   10. SURVIVING SPOUSE'S NAME (If wife, give name prior to first marriage)

11. FATHER'S NAME (First, Middle, Last)   12. MOTHER'S NAME PRIOR TO FIRST MARRIAGE (First, Middle, Last)

13a. INFORMANT'S NAME   13b. RELATIONSHIP TO DECEDENT   13c. MAILING ADDRESS (Street and Number, City, State, Zip Code)

14. PLACE OF DEATH (Check only one: see instructions)
IF DEATH OCCURRED IN A HOSPITAL: □ Inpatient □ Emergency Room/Outpatient □ Dead on Arrival   IF DEATH OCCURRED SOMEWHERE OTHER THAN A HOSPITAL: □ Hospice facility □ Nursing home/Long term care facility □ Decedent's home □ Other (Specify):

15. FACILITY NAME (If not institution, give street & number)   16. CITY OR TOWN, STATE, AND ZIP CODE   17. COUNTY OF DEATH

18. METHOD OF DISPOSITION: □ Burial □ Cremation □ Donation □ Entombment □ Removal from State □ Other (Specify):   19. PLACE OF DISPOSITION (Name of cemetery, crematory, other place)

20. LOCATION-CITY, TOWN, AND STATE   21. NAME AND COMPLETE ADDRESS OF FUNERAL FACILITY

22. SIGNATURE OF FUNERAL SERVICE LICENSEE OR OTHER AGENT   23. LICENSE NUMBER (Of Licensee)

To Be Completed By: MEDICAL CERTIFIER

ITEMS 24-28 MUST BE COMPLETED BY PERSON WHO PRONOUNCES OR CERTIFIES DEATH   24. DATE PRONOUNCED DEAD (Mo/Day/Yr)   25. TIME PRONOUNCED DEAD

26. SIGNATURE OF PERSON PRONOUNCING DEATH (Only when applicable)   27. LICENSE NUMBER   28. DATE SIGNED (Mo/Day/Yr)

29. ACTUAL OR PRESUMED DATE OF DEATH (Mo/Day/Yr) (Spell Month)   30. ACTUAL OR PRESUMED TIME OF DEATH   31. WAS MEDICAL EXAMINER OR CORONER CONTACTED? □ Yes □ No

CAUSE OF DEATH (See instructions and examples)

32. PART I. Enter the chain of events--diseases, injuries, or complications--that directly caused the death. DO NOT enter terminal events such as cardiac arrest, respiratory arrest, or ventricular fibrillation without showing the etiology. DO NOT ABBREVIATE. Enter only one cause on a line. Add additional lines if necessary.

Approximate interval: Onset to death

IMMEDIATE CAUSE (Final disease or condition resulting in death) → a. ____ Due to (or as a consequence of):

Sequentially list conditions, if any, leading to the cause listed on line a. Enter the UNDERLYING CAUSE (disease or injury that initiated the events resulting in death) LAST
b. ____ Due to (or as a consequence of):
c. ____ Due to (or as a consequence of):
d. ____

PART II. Enter other significant conditions contributing to death but not resulting in the underlying cause given in PART I.   33. WAS AN AUTOPSY PERFORMED? □ Yes □ No

34. WERE AUTOPSY FINDINGS AVAILABLE TO COMPLETE THE CAUSE OF DEATH? □ Yes □ No

35. DID TOBACCO USE CONTRIBUTE TO DEATH? □ Yes □ Probably □ No □ Unknown

36. IF FEMALE: □ Not pregnant within past year □ Pregnant at time of death □ Not pregnant, but pregnant within 42 days of death □ Not pregnant, but pregnant 43 days to 1 year before death □ Unknown if pregnant within the past year

37. MANNER OF DEATH □ Natural □ Homicide □ Accident □ Pending Investigation □ Suicide □ Could not be determined

38. DATE OF INJURY (Mo/Day/Yr) (Spell Month)   39. TIME OF INJURY   40. PLACE OF INJURY (e.g., Decedent's home; construction site; restaurant; wooded area)   41. INJURY AT WORK? □ Yes □ No

42. LOCATION OF INJURY: State: City or Town:
Street & Number: Apartment No.:   Zip Code:

43. DESCRIBE HOW INJURY OCCURRED: 44. IF TRANSPORTATION INJURY, SPECIFY: □ Driver/Operator □ Passenger □ Pedestrian □ Other (Specify)

45. CERTIFIER (Check only one):
□ Certifying physician-To the best of my knowledge, death occurred due to the cause(s) and manner stated.
□ Pronouncing & Certifying physician-To the best of my knowledge, death occurred at the time, date, and place, and due to the cause(s) and manner stated.
□ Medical Examiner/Coroner-On the basis of examination, and/or investigation, in my opinion, death occurred at the time, date, and place, and due to the cause(s) and manner stated.
Signature of certifier:

46. NAME, ADDRESS, AND ZIP CODE OF PERSON COMPLETING CAUSE OF DEATH (Item 32)

47. TITLE OF CERTIFIER   48. LICENSE NUMBER   49. DATE CERTIFIED (Mo/Day/Yr)   50. FOR REGISTRAR ONLY- DATE FILED (Mo/Day/Yr)

To Be Completed By: FUNERAL DIRECTOR

51. DECEDENT'S EDUCATION-Check the box that best describes the highest degree or level of school completed at the time of death.
□ 8th grade or less
□ 9th - 12th grade; no diploma
□ High school graduate or GED completed
□ Some college credit, but no degree
□ Associate degree (e.g., AA, AS)
□ Bachelor's degree (e.g., BA, AB, BS)
□ Master's degree (e.g., MA, MS, MEng, MEd, MSW, MBA)
□ Doctorate (e.g., PhD, EdD) or Professional degree (e.g., MD, DDS, DVM, LLB, JD)

52. DECEDENT OF HISPANIC ORIGIN? Check the box that best describes whether the decedent is Spanish/Hispanic/Latino. Check the "No" box if decedent is not Spanish/Hispanic/Latino.
□ No, not Spanish/Hispanic/Latino
□ Yes, Mexican, Mexican American, Chicano
□ Yes, Puerto Rican
□ Yes, Cuban
□ Yes, other Spanish/Hispanic/Latino (Specify) ____

53. DECEDENT'S RACE (Check one or more races to indicate what the decedent considered himself or herself to be)
□ White
□ Black or African American
□ American Indian or Alaska Native (Name of the enrolled or principal tribe) ____
□ Asian Indian
□ Chinese
□ Filipino
□ Japanese
□ Korean
□ Vietnamese
□ Other Asian (Specify) ____
□ Native Hawaiian
□ Guamanian or Chamorro
□ Samoan
□ Other Pacific Islander (Specify) ____
□ Other (Specify) ____

54. DECEDENT'S USUAL OCCUPATION (Indicate type of work done during most of working life. DO NOT USE RETIRED).

55. KIND OF BUSINESS/INDUSTRY

U.S. (2004)	World (2003)	U.S. (1900)
Diseases of the heart	Ischemic heart disease	Pneumonia and influenza
Malignant neoplasms	Cerebrovascular disease	Tuberculosis
Cerebrovascular disease	Lower respiratory	Gastritis, enteritis, colitis
Chronic lower respiratory disease	HIV/AIDS	Heart diseases
Accidents (unintentional injuries)	Chronic obstructive pulmonary disease	Senility, ill-defined conditions
Diabetes mellitus	Diarrheal disease	Vascular lesions affecting central nervous system
Alzheimer's disease	Tuberculosis	Chronic nephritis and renal sclerosis
Influenza and pneumonia	Malaria	Unintentional injuries
Nephritis, nephrotic syndrome, and nephrosis	Cancer of trachea/bronchus/lung	Malignant neoplasms
Septicemia	Road traffic accidents	Diphtheria

TABLE 6.1
Leading Causes of Death U.S., World, and 1900.

SOURCE: Deaths: Preliminary Data for 2004; The World Health Report, 2003, The World Health Organization (WHO); U.S. Bureau of Census.

various diseases in that time period, and the ability of the public health and medical care systems to recognize and cope with those diseases.

Table 6.1 presents the ten leading causes of death across the world in 2003 and in the United States in 1900 and 2004. Whereas heart disease, cancer, and stroke were the leading causes of death in the United States in 2004, such was not the case at the turn of the twentieth century, when pneumonia, influenza, tuberculosis, and gastrointestinal disorders were the leading causes of mortality. It is interesting to note the differences between United States and worldwide mortality, where the burden of cancer is replaced by respiratory diseases and AIDS.

Measuring Mortality with Rates

Mortality is usually measured by a rate. A rate must contain three parts: a numerator (the number of deaths), a denominator (the population in which people are at risk of dying), and a multiplier (usually some power of 10). Mortality rates are usually expressed within a certain time frame, a given locality, and for certain kinds of people, as in the 2007 mortality rate for 65- to 74-year-olds in the state of Kentucky.

The mortality rate is an expression of probability, as both affected and unaffected individuals are in the denominator. It expresses the risk that someone in a population will die. The purpose of a multiplier is to convert an unwieldy fraction into a whole number for comparison purposes. It is important to ensure that the numerator and denominator refer to a similar population; for example, if the numerator is white males only, then the denominator should also be white males only (the population at risk). It is important also to recognize that the population may be something other than a geographic population.

To illustrate the concept of rate, consider the various kinds of mortality rates that can be calculated for a reference population (Table 6.2). In this case the event is death. For the most part, there are three kinds of rates: (1) crude rates, (2) specific rates, and (3) adjusted rates.

The annual death rate, which is an example of a *crude rate*, is simply the number of deaths that occurred during a period, such as a year, divided by the population at risk of death (e.g., U.S. or state population) times the multiplier, in this case usually 100,000.

With *specific death rates*, the number of deaths is within certain age groups or disease categories, as in elderly mortality rates (for those ≥ 65), or rates for certain kinds of diseases (e.g., cardiovascular disease). For example, case fatality rates refer to the number of deaths from a specific disease divided by those diagnosed with the disease.

Notice that the at-risk population (the denominator) varies with the situation. In the annual death rate, the population is all the people in a population at risk of death; in the case of age-specific death rates, the at-risk population is a particular age group. In case fatality rates, the at-risk population includes only those diagnosed with a particular disease.

The infant mortality rate is, in one sense, a specific death rate, because it applies to infants only, and is calculated as the number of deaths that occur in infants less than a year old divided by the number of live births, with a multiplier of 1,000. In 1990, for example, African Americans had more than double the infant mortality rate of whites: 18.0/1,000 compared with 7.9/1,000. (In Figure 6.2, the two different perinatal mortality rates depend on whether the perinatal period [intrauterine] is defined as 20 or 28 weeks gestation with a corresponding extrauterine period of 7 days and 28 days, respectively.)

Another kind of mortality rate is one that has been adjusted for differences in certain characteristics of the population, such as age, gender, or a patient characteristic, such as severity of illness or the presence of certain types of comorbidities.

TABLE 6.2
Common
Rates Used by
Epidemiologists

Crude mortality rate	Deaths among residents during a calendar year/midyear population × 100,000
Cause-specific mortality rate	Deaths due to a specific cause (e.g., heart disease) in a given year/midyear population × 100,000
Age-specific mortality rate	Deaths in persons in a certain age range/midyear population in that same age range × 100,000
Proportionate mortality rate	Proportion of deaths attributed to a specific cause such as cardiovascular disease
Case fatality rate	Number of deaths assigned to a cause/total number of cases occurring × 100
Infant mortality rate	Number of deaths of those less than one year of age/number of live births × 1,000
Perinatal mortality rate	Number of deaths less than 30 days old/number of live births × 1,000
Post-neonatal mortality rate	Number of deaths age 30 days to one year of age/number of live births × 1,000
Maternal mortality rate	Number of deaths assigned to puerperal causes/live births × 1,000
Perinatal mortality rate	(Fetal deaths + postnatal deaths)/(fetal deaths + live births) × 1,000

Comparing Mortality Across Time, Place, and Person

Mortality rates can be compared across time, place, or population groups, which are the three dimensions from which epidemiologists describe important patterns and make inferences regarding risk factors, disease, and longevity (see Chapter 7 for more detail). Mortality rates can be tracked across time, both in the short and long term. Figures 6.3 and 6.4 represent changes in cancer mortality over a 72-year period for various

FIGURE 6.2
Mortality
Rates
Among the
Very Young

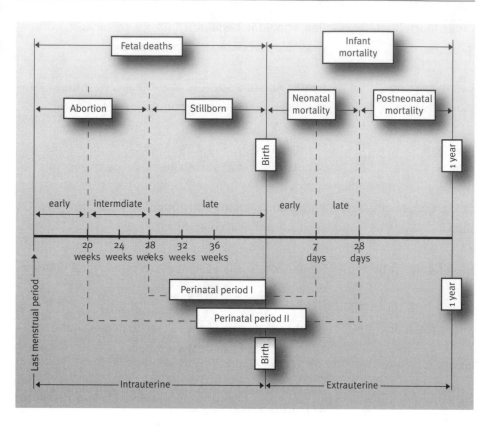

SOURCE: Timmreck, *An Introduction to Epidemiology*, 3rd Ed., (2002). Jones and Bartlett Publishers, Sudbury, MA.www.jbpub.com. Reprinted with permission.

sites of cancer, and for men and women, respectively. For men, we notice constant and large increases in lung cancer mortality rates, peaking around 1990 and then declining. For women, the rise in lung cancer mortality occurs about 25 years later. We see decreases in cancers of the stomach and uterus for women over the years, and a steady increase, leveling off, and then decrease in prostate cancer among men. Because these graphs are age-adjusted, we must look to something other than aging population to explain these trends, such as rates of cigarette smoking over the years, changes in dietary habits, food preservation, or successful medical treatments for cancer.

Secular trends in mortality are those that occur over a relatively long period, such as the cancer mortality statistics reported earlier. We must exercise some caution while interpreting these statistics, and discern between real and artifactual differences in mortality (Lilienfeld and Stolley 1994, 78). Real differences include changes in the age distribution of the population for each year that is being reported, changes in survival—due perhaps

FIGURE 6.3
Age-
Adjusted
Cancer
Death Rates,
Males

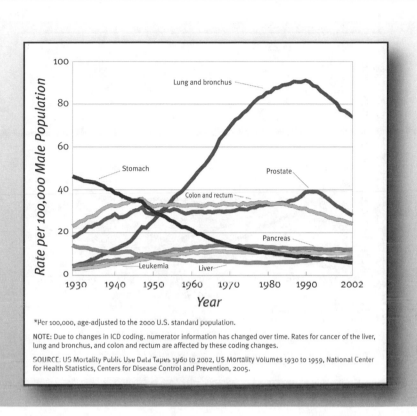

*Per 100,000, age-adjusted to the 2000 U.S. standard population.

NOTE: Due to changes in ICD coding. numerator information has changed over time. Rates for cancer of the liver, lung and bronchus, and colon and rectum are affected by these coding changes.

SOURCE. US Mortality Public Use Data Tapes 1960 to 2002, US Mortality Volumes 1930 to 1959, National Center for Health Statistics, Centers for Disease Control and Prevention, 2005.

to clinical or technical innovation in treatment—and changes in the incidence of disease as a result of environmental or genetic factors, such as a change in living habits or environmental conditions (e.g., global warming). Artifactual differences may be due to changes in how the disease is recognized—improved imaging, for example—changes in cause of death classification, or changes in the accuracy of determining age at time of death.

Figure 6.5 illustrates the importance of correcting for "real" differences in mortality rates. Notice that the crude mortality rates in the United States over the 44-year period declined only about 10 percent. When these rates are adjusted for the real differences in the age distribution of the population over the 44-year period, the rates declined by about 40 percent. The small decline in crude rates is deceiving; the real change in age distribution presents a more accurate view.

Mortality rates can also be compared across geographic regions or "places," such as countries, states, or counties. The purpose of such comparisons is to detect important patterns that can be useful for understanding factors that are likely to influence mortality, such as environmental hazards, behaviors or attitudes specific to certain geographic regions, or medical care resources.

FIGURE 6.4
Age–
Adjusted
Cancer
Death Rates,
Females

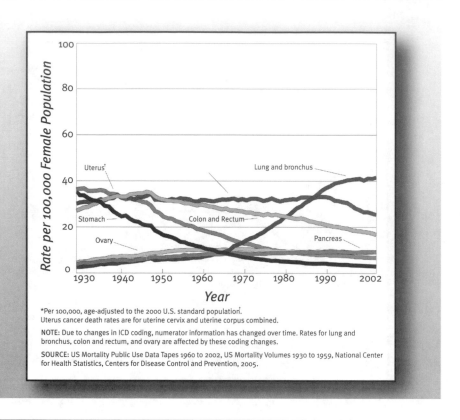

*Per 100,000, age-adjusted to the 2000 U.S. standard population.
Uterus cancer death rates are for uterine cervix and uterine corpus combined.

NOTE: Due to changes in ICD coding, numerator information has changed over time. Rates for lung and bronchus, colon and rectum, and ovary are affected by these coding changes.

SOURCE: US Mortality Public Use Data Tapes 1960 to 2002, US Mortality Volumes 1930 to 1959, National Center for Health Statistics, Centers for Disease Control and Prevention, 2005.

FIGURE 6.5
Crude and
Age–
Adjusted
Death Rates:
United
States,
1960–2004

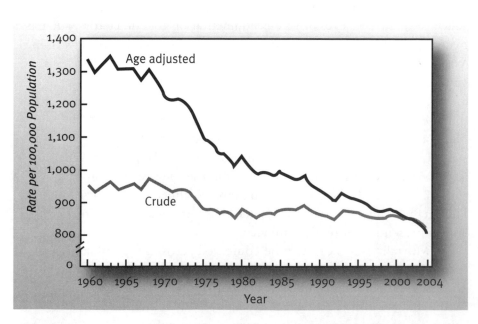

SOURCE: CDC/NCHS, National Vital Statistics System, Mortality.

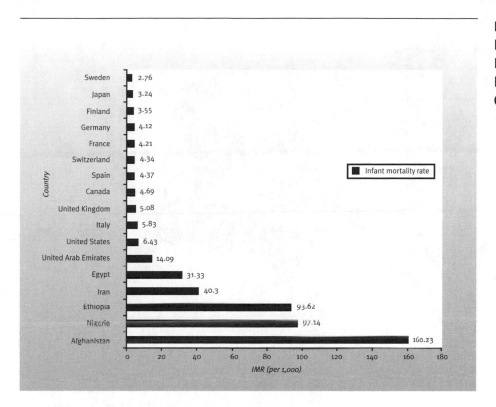

FIGURE 6.6
Infant
Mortality
Rates, 17
Countries

SOURCE: Central Intelligence Agency, *World Factbook* (2006).

Figure 6.6 compares infant mortality rates across 17 countries. There are huge disparities, with the infant mortality rate in Afghanistan over 50 times the rate in Sweden. Even the United States has over twice the rate of Sweden. While the ravages of war may play a large role in the very high Afghanistan rate, and socialized medicine may be a reason why the United States falls behind some of the Scandinavian and European countries, there are certain to be other environmental and cultural factors behind these differences.

Figure 6.7 shows heart disease death rates in the late 1990s for those 35 and older, by county in the United States, with the highest rates in the southeastern United States, including most of Louisiana and Mississippi, eastern Arkansas, southeastern Missouri, and western Tennessee. Rates are also high in West Virginia and Oklahoma. Causes for these high rates could be either environmental, for example hardness of the water, or cultural. Figure 6.8 shows a similar map for stroke mortality rates. The high-risk areas are somewhat similar, although they also include the southeastern coastal states.

Mortality rates can also be compared across population groups to see if there are specific differences in these rates that might be explained by genetic, environmental, or behavioral factors specific to each of these groups.

FIGURE 6.7
Heart
Disease
Death Rates,
1996–2000,
Adults Age
35 Years
and Older,
by County

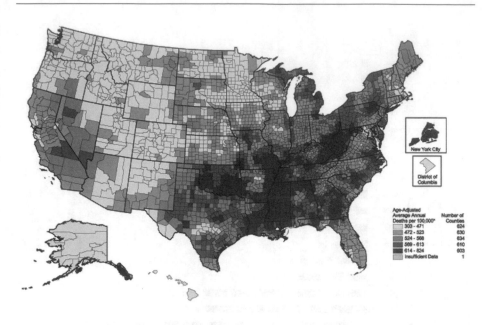

SOURCE: U.S. Census Bureau; National Vital Statistics System.

For example, low socioeconomic status is related to higher mortality rates (Bassuk, Berkman, and Amick 2002). Lilienfeld and Stolley (1994) describe how three dimensions of socioeconomic status ultimately affect health outcomes: (1) Wealth affects access to healthcare and dietary choices, which have an impact on detection and treatment of disease, and the risk of obesity, high blood pressure, and high cholesterol levels; (2) Education affects knowledge, attitudes, and behavior about diet, smoking, alcohol, exercise, sex, and drug abuse. Such knowledge and attitudes have an impact on risk factors for heart disease, lung cancer, AIDS, and high-risk pregnancies; (3) Occupational choices affect exposure to hazards, psychological stress, and physical activity, all of which influence rates of cancer, heart disease, accidents, miscarriages, and birth defects.

Migration studies are a useful approach to understanding differences between environmental and behavioral causes of disease. The ultimate question is whether migrating population groups acquire the incidence of disease (and risk of mortality from that disease) from the areas to which they migrate. If they maintain the same incidence of disease as the population from which they migrate, one could argue that the etiology is mostly genetic. If, on the other hand, they assume a risk of disease similar to the population to which they migrate, one could make the argument for an environmental etiology.

The study of mortality rates among immigrants adds another dimension of complexity. The mortality rate can be used instead of the incidence

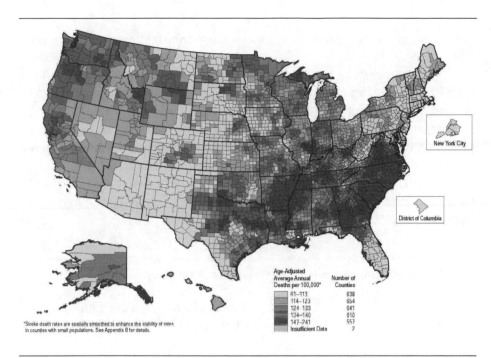

FIGURE 6.8
Stroke Death Rates, 1991–1998, Adults Age 35 Years and Older, by County

SOURCE: Casper et al. (2003).

rate, where the latter may be unavailable or difficult to obtain, though this works best for diseases with a high case fatality rate.

If the mortality rate is used in migration studies, one must also recognize the impact of differences in the public health and medical care systems across countries, and the degree to which these differences influence mortality rates. Case Study 6.1 examines breast cancer mortality rates of immigrants to either Australia or Canada.

Case Study 6.1. Breast Cancer Mortality Rates and Migration

Kliewer and Smith (1995) published an article entitled "Breast Cancer Mortality Among Immigrants to Australia and Canada," the purpose of which was to compare mortality rates among people who moved from 30 other countries to either Australia or Canada. The question was the extent to which "native" breast cancer mortality rates shift to the rates of either Australia or Canada.

The underlying issue was the degree to which breast cancer mortality (or by implication, incidence) was caused by environmental or genetic factors. If immigrants maintain the rates of their native countries, the cancer is more likely to be genetically related. If they assume the risk of the country to which they immigrate, then the cancer is more likely to have an environmental etiology. The degree of shift is therefore a measure of relative contribution of environmental factors.

The authors calculated direct age-standardized mortality rates for each of the 30 native countries and rates for each of the immigrant groups in both Australia and Canada. Table 6.3 below is adapted from this work, and presents the native country breast cancer mortality rates as well as the rates of 5 of the 30 countries from which residents immigrated to either Australia or Canada. Table 6.4 shows two age-standardized rate ratios calculated as (1) the ratio of the native country rate to native-born rates of either Australia or Canada and (2) the ratio of the immigrants rate to native born rates of either Australia or Canada.

TABLE 6.3. AGE-STANDARDIZED MORTALITY RATES (PER 100,000)

Country	Native	Australian Immigrants	Canadian Immigrants
Australia	48.0	—	58.7
Canada	55.9	55.0	—
United States	53.1	79.1	64.1
Sweden	41.7	92.2	46.5
Romania	32.0	84.7	59.8
France	44.9	49.5	36.0
UK/Ireland	67.3	56.7	60.7

SOURCE: Kliewer and Smith (1995). By permission of Oxford University Press.

QUESTIONS

1. Table 6.3 provides age-standardized breast cancer mortality rates for native Canadians, Australians, and natives from five other countries, as well as these rates for immigrants who migrated to either Australia or Canada. Calculate age-standardized rate ratios (ASRRs) using native or immigrant rates in the numerator and either Australian or Canadian native rates in the denominator.

2. What is the interpretation for an ASRR greater than 1.0?
3. If the etiology of breast cancer were entirely environmental, what would you expect to happen to these rates?

ANSWERS

1. Table 6.4 presents ASRRs for immigrants to either Australia or Canada.
2. For the first ASRR measure (columns A1 and C1), a ratio greater than 1.0 implies that the breast cancer mortality rate in the native country is greater than the breast cancer mortality rate in either Australia or Canada. For the second ASRR measure (columns A2 and C2), a ratio greater than 1.0 implies that the breast cancer mortality rate of immigrants is greater than native-born Australians or Canadians.
3. We would expect the rates of the second measure, columns A2 and C2, to converge to 1.0 for each country, which would indicate that immigrants to Australia develop cancer at the same rate as natives, meaning environment is the key factor. For example, the ASRR for Romanian immigrants to Australia was 1.07. In their homeland, the Romanian residents' ASRR was only 0.57, so there was significant movement toward the native Australian breast cancer mortality rate. In fact, the extent of convergence overall (as reported by the authors) was 50 percent in Australia and 38 percent in Canada, indicating that environmental and lifestyle factors associated with a new place of residence do influence breast cancer mortality rates of immigrants.

TABLE 6.4. AGE-STANDARDIZED RATE RATIOS FOR IMMIGRANTS TO AUSTRALIA AND CANADA

Country	ASRR Native/Australia (A1)	ASRR Immigrants/ Australia (A2)	ASRR Native/Canada (C1)	ASRR Immigrants/Canada (C2)
Australia	1.0	—	0.86	1.05
Canada	1.16	1.15	1.0	—
United States	1.11	1.65	0.95	1.15
Sweden	0.87	1.92	0.75	0.83
Romania	0.67	1.76	0.57	1.07
France	0.94	1.03	0.80	0.64
UK/Ireland	1.40	1.18	1.20	1.09

SOURCE: Kliewer and Smith (1995). By permission of Oxford University Press.

Standardization of Mortality Rates

Rates can occasionally appear confusing. For example, if the crude death rate for Miami, Florida, is 990 per 100,000 and that for Lexington, Kentucky, is 975 per 100,000, one might conclude that Miami is inherently less healthy than Lexington. However, an easy alternative explanation is that the people in Miami, on average, are older because many people retire to Florida. The mechanism for allowing comparisons among divergent groups is called *standardization*. The most common example is standardization for age, but other attributes, such as sex or race, may be the source of standardization, thus allowing for better comparisons of rate. Rates also may be adjusted for the risk of death associated with diagnosis, comorbidities, and other clinical factors.

Remember that the main purpose of standardization is to enable us to compare two or more population groups that differ on the basis of age, sex, race, or other factors that influence mortality. In short, standardization "levels the playing field" in the interest of making valid comparisons. Two principle standardization methods are used to adjust mortality rates on the basis of age: direct and indirect standardization.

With the *direct method of standardization*, age-specific death rates from the two population groups to be compared are each applied to a third reference group, or standard population. This can be any population; however, for this example, we use the entire U.S. population for 2005. We calculate the expected number of deaths in the standard population using rates from each of the two comparison groups.

For example, suppose we are comparing the mortality experience between Florida and Alaska. We want to take into consideration that Florida has more elderly citizens who are at an increased risk of dying. We take age-specific rates for both Florida and Alaska and apply these rates to a third reference population, say, the U.S. population. The number of expected deaths in the U.S. population is calculated for both Florida and Alaska. In other words, we calculate the number of the people in the United States who would be expected to die if the entire population of the country were dying at the rate of Florida and of Alaska, respectively. The expected deaths can be calculated this way: (rate × population)/100,000. Table 6.5 illustrates this concept and shows that Alaska has a somewhat lower age-adjusted mortality rate than Florida.

Through use of the *indirect method of standardization*, on the other hand, age-specific mortality rates from a standard population (e.g., the entire United States) are applied to the specific age groupings of the two comparison groups (e.g., Florida and Alaska). The numbers of expected deaths in each of the two comparison populations are calculated using the rates of the standard population. For example, here we estimate the number of people who would be expected to die in both Florida and Alaska as if they were dying at the same rate as people across the entire country. A

Age	Age-Specific Mortality Rate (Florida) per 100,000	Age-Specific Mortality Rate (Alaska) per 100,000	Reference Population (U.S. 2005)	Expected Deaths (Florida)	Expected Deaths (Alaska)
0–44	150	130	186,500,000	279,750	242,450
45–64+	760	550	72,800,000	553,280	400,400
65+	4,400	4,200	36,700,000	1,614,800	1,541,400
Total			296,000,000	2,447,830	2,184,250

TABLE 6.5
Direct Method of Standardization Comparing Florida and Alaska

Age-adjusted death rate (Florida)
2,447,830/296,000,000 (pop. U.S.) × 100,000 = 827/100,000.
Age-adjusted death rate (Alaska)
2,184,250/296,000,000 (pop. U.S.) × 100,000 = 738/100,000.

Age	U.S. Mortality Rates	Population Florida (2005)	Population Alaska (2005)	Expected Deaths (Florida)	Expected Deaths (Alaska)
0–44	110	10,000,000	446,000	11,000	491
45–64+	650	4,500,000	170,000	29,250	1,105
65+	5,030	3,000,000	44,000	150,900	2,213
Total		17,500,000	660,000	191,150	3,809

TABLE 6.6
Indirect Method of Standardization Comparing Florida and Alaska

Actual deaths (Florida) 185,000.
Actual deaths (Alaska) 3,600
SMR (Florida)= 185,000/191,150 × 100 = 97
SMR (Florida)= 3,600/3,809 × 100 = 95

standardized mortality ratio (SMR) is then calculated as the ratio of actual to expected deaths in the two comparison populations times 100. If the ratio is more than 100, it means that actual deaths exceeded expected deaths, or that the comparison population was dying at rates in excess of the standard population. A ratio less than 100 implies that the comparison group had fewer deaths than expected, or that the rate was less than that of the standard population group. The SMRs for the two groups (Florida and Alaska) are directly comparable: the lower the SMR, the lower the mortality rate, taking age mix into consideration.

Table 6.6 illustrates the indirect method of standardization. Alaska has a somewhat lower SMR than Florida, although both states have lower mortality rates than the nation as a whole, as evidenced by SMRs less than 100.

If the total actual deaths are given to be 185,000 for Florida and 3,600 for Alaska, then the SMR is calculated as (actual deaths/expected deaths × 100) or 97 for Florida and 95 for Alaska. Case Study 6.2 uses direct standardization with both age and gender to compare the cardiovascular mortality of two managed care organizations.

Case Study 6.2. Age and Gender Adjustment in Two Managed Care Organizations

The purpose of standardization is to make two or more populations "similar" along dimensions in which they differ. Earlier, we demonstrated two methods of age adjustment. For example, we know that Florida has proportionately more older folks, and older folks die at higher rates than younger folks. To compare the mortality rate of Florida to Alaska, we needed to control for this disparity by adjusting for differences in the age mix of the two states.

Conceptually, we can adjust for more than one dimension. For example, we can adjust for age and gender, if we know that the age and gender mix will be different in those populations, and also know that some disease-specific mortality rates depend on both age and gender.

Such is the case with cardiovascular disease in two large managed care organizations (MCOs), Bluegrass East (BGE) and Bluegrass West (BGW), the former with 100,000 members, and the latter with 120,000 members. Suppose that BGE has a higher proportion of older folks and a higher proportion of women than BGW. Assume that the crude disease-specific mortality rate for cardiovascular disease is 300 (per 100,000) in BGE and 150 (per 100,000) in BGW.

QUESTIONS

1. From these statistics alone, which MCO has the higher cardiovascular mortality rate?
2. The member mix in BGE and BGW is quite different. In BGW, 90 percent of the population is less than 55 years old, compared to 77 percent in BGE. Refer to Table 6.7 to guide the calculation of age-adjusted cardiovascular mortality rates using the direct age-adjustment technique and the U.S. population as the standard. With age-adjusted rates, which MCO has the higher mortality rate?
3. Now assume that 53 percent of the members in BGW are men compared to 47 percent in BGE. Men have higher cardiovascular mortality rates than women. Refer to Table 6.8 to calculate age- and gender-adjusted cardiovascular mortality rates. With age- and gender-adjusted rates, which MCO has the higher cardiovascular mortality rate?

ANSWERS

1. BGE has twice the mortality rate as BGW, so it would seem like people have twice the risk of dying from cardiovascular disease in BGE as they do in BGW.

2. Table 6.7 summarizes the age-adjusted rate calculations. We can now calculate the age-adjusted rates for BGW and BGE: (968,800/280,000,000) × 100,000 = 346 per 100,000 for BGW, and (956,200/280,000,000) × 100,000 = 341.5 per 100,000 for BGE. Thus, after adjusting for differences in the age mix for BGW and BGE, it would appear that BGW has a higher cardiovascular mortality rate than BGE.

TABLE 6.7. DIRECT AGE ADJUSTMENT OF CARDIOVASCULAR MORTALITY FOR BLUEGRASS EAST (BGE) AND BLUEGRASS WEST (BGW) MANAGED CARE ORGANIZATIONS

Age	Age-Specific Mortality Rate BGW	BGE	U.S. Mix (2000)	BGW Expected	BGE Expected
1–54	23	22	210,000,000	48,300	46,200
55+	1,315	1,300	70,000,000	920,500	910,000
Total			280,000,000	968,800	956,200

TABLE 6.8. DIRECT AGE AND GENDER-ADJUSTED CARDIOVASCULAR MORTALITY FOR BLUEGRASS EAST (BGE) AND BLUEGRASS WEST (BGW) MANAGED CARE ORGANIZATIONS

Age	Age-and-Gender-Specific Mortality Rate BGW	BGE	U.S.	BGW Expected	BGE Expected
Males					
1–54	33	33	105,000,000	34,650	34,650
55+	1,450	1,400	35,000,000	507,500	490,000
Females					
1–54	11	13	100,000,000	11,000	13,000
55+	1,165	1,200	40,000,000	466,000	480,000
Total			280,000,000	1,019,150	1,017,650

3. Table 6.8 summarizes the age- and gender-adjusted rate calculations. We can now calculate the age- and gender-adjusted cardiovascular rates for BGW and BGE as follows: (1,019,150/280,000,000) × 100,000 = 364 per 100,000 for BGW,

and (1,017,650/280,000,000) × 100,000 = 363 per 100,000 for BGE. Thus, after adjusting for differences in the age and gender mix for BGW and BGE, it would appear that BGW has a slightly higher rate of mortality than BGE.

Risk-Adjusted Mortality Rates

Epidemiologists have long been interested in the study of mortality rates inasmuch as death is usually an easily defined event that is well-documented across cultures, and its incidence is routinely collected as part of the vital statistics collected by health departments. The cause of death can be studied with insurance claims data or with death certificates. Epidemiologists typically adjust mortality rates either directly or indirectly by age to compare trends across time, settings, or people (see Chapter 7). The concept of "risk adjustment" adds multiple dimensions to this process by recognizing that many factors, in addition to age, affect the likelihood of mortality.

Epidemiologists have long been interested in the study of mortality rates inasmuch as death is usually an easily defined event that is well-documented across cultures, and its incidence is routinely collected as part of the vital statistics collected by health departments. The cause of death can be studied with insurance claims data or with death certificates. Epidemiologists typically adjust mortality rates either directly or indirectly by age to compare trends across time, settings, or people (see Chapter 7). The concept of "risk adjustment" adds multiple dimensions to this process by recognizing that many factors, in addition to age, affect the likelihood of mortality.

The theory and methods of risk adjustment have been elaborated by Iezzoni (1997a, 1997b) and others. Conceptually, risk adjustment is an extension of age-adjustment techniques that have graced epidemiologic tradition for years, in the sense that they are trying to "level the playing field" for the purposes of comparison. The process of adjusting for age, either directly or indirectly, facilitates a comparison of mortality rates across time, settings, or people by accounting for differences in age mix that would otherwise confound the comparisons.

Adjusting for risk extends this theory to include multiple risk factors, each of which potentially affects mortality rates. According to Iezzoni, risk adjustment can be used to "calculate the so-called algebra of effectiveness" (Figure 6.9), in the sense that patient outcomes, such as mortality, are a function of clinical attributes (i.e., risk factors), random factors, quality, and effectiveness. The epidemiologist compares age-adjusted rates across time to detect any significant temporal differences unrelated to age. Clinicians and health services researchers use risk-adjusted rates to detect any significant differences across providers, settings, or patient groups that are unrelated to patient risk factors (i.e., presumably they are related to healthcare quality or effectiveness).

Iezzoni (1997a, 1997b) documents and explains the important risk factors that affect patient outcomes as follows. Age affects mortality rates to the extent that older people have lower "physiological reserve" and may be treated less aggressively. Gender affects mortality in that life expectancy and response to treatment may vary with anatomic, physiological, and hormonal differences. Moreover, some suggest a "gender bias" that affects the kinds of treatments made available to one or the other

FIGURE 6.9
The
Algebra of
Effectiveness

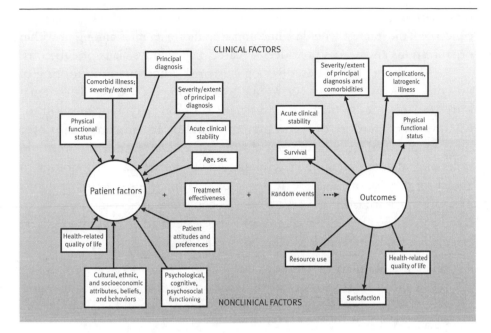

SOURCE: Iezzoni (1997a).

gender. Clinical attributes include acute clinical stability, principal diagnosis, disease-specific severity, comorbidities, and functional status. Acute clinical stability refers to physiological functioning, as indicated by vital signs and serum electrolytes, for instance. Principal diagnosis represents a hypothesis of illness, a focal point of treatment, and the cause for making contact with the healthcare system, and as such it relates to the probability of survival. Disease-specific severity is a risk factor for mortality because it represents the intensity or seriousness of illness within a distinct category of disease. Comorbidities increase the risk of mortality in that they represent an additional disease burden that may complicate treatment, recovery, or prognosis. A permanent or temporary limitation in the ability to function—measured by functional status—influences mortality to the extent that everyday behavior affects one's sense of well-being and quality of life. Cultural, racial, ethnic, and socioeconomic factors may influence mortality through barriers to access (e.g., lack of insurance coverage), care-seeking behaviors, diet, and compliance, among others.

Mortality is probably affected by other risk factors that are as difficult to measure as those just described, for instance, psychological, cognitive, and psychosocial functioning; health status; quality of life; and patient attitudes and preferences.

Iezzoni (1997a) describes the "ideal" risk-adjustment process that would probably include most of the factors likely to affect mortality. Remember that the purpose of all of this is to gain the ability to compare outcomes across time, settings, and people. So far as the control function of the manager is concerned, the interest would be in comparing mortality rates among or within organizations and across providers of care, such as physicians or surgeons.

Blumberg (1986) describes a generic risk adjustment monitoring of outcome (RAMO) system where one would compare expected-to-actual outcomes of care by hospital, physician, surgeon, payment method, or whatever. The purpose of such a system would be to measure trends over time or to investigate unexpected clusters of adverse events: the nuts and bolts of epidemiologic inquiry. This system would need a methodology to adjust for the risk of death, such as one of the numerous severity-of-illness measures that are on the market today. These measures could be categorized into those based on claims and those derived from clinical data. According to Blumberg, RAMO steps would include:

1. select the population to study;
2. select the clinical subjects within that population to study, for example, Medicare patients who undergo coronary arterial bypass graft surgery (CABG);
3. choose the outcome measure, for example, mortality;
4. list patient attributes that may be risk factors for adverse outcomes;
5. review data sources to see which attribute measures are available;
6. select cases to serve as the standard population, for example state of New York CABG patients;
7. select estimation model, for example contingency table or multivariate method;
8. estimate probability of adverse outcome in each case;
9. see if the model predicts outcomes (predictive validity); and
10. see if the model is biased.

Because the competing methods of risk-adjusted outcomes are not well correlated when they are used to rank hospitals on the basis of risk-adjusted mortality, each risk-adjustment method, it is suggested, may lead to a different judgment about a hospital's overall performance (Iezzoni 1997a, 1997b).

The former Health Care Financing Administration, now the Centers for Medicare & Medicaid Services, published annual risk-adjusted mortality statistics by hospital from 1986 until 1993, when the practice was discontinued. The statistics were the subject of intense criticism and controversy over the years, and the focus of contention was the Achilles' heel of most risk-adjusted measures: severity of illness. The measure had evolved considerably over the years; the final version was an elegant hazard function based on both short- and long-term risk, and patients were classified into 23 analytical categories (Fleming, Hicks, and Bailey 1995). It was argued, nonetheless, that this measure, which was based entirely on claims data, did not adequately adjust for severity of illness. Clearly, one cannot refute the limitations of claims-based data that are designed primarily for insurance purposes and not clinical decisions. However, there is some evidence that the measure could have been a useful screening tool to flag potential problem areas and prompt further investigation (Fleming, Hicks, and Bailey 1995).

More recently, both New York and Pennsylvania have published "report cards" for cardiovascular surgery. Since 1992, the Pennsylvania Health Care Cost Containment Council has published risk-adjusted in-hospital mortality rates for CABG. The rates compare in-hospital mortality to a range of expected rates by individual surgeon and hospital. The risk-adjustment methodology includes both severity of illness and comorbidities. The state of New York has also published risk-adjusted mortality rates for CABG since 1990, with a methodology that includes clinical risk factors, such as body mass index and ejection fraction, as well as comorbid illness.

Both programs are intended to improve quality of care, in light of the choices that consumers and physicians can make regarding treatment or referrals based on these outcome scores. These programs have generated a fair amount of controversy. In fact, the New York State Department of Health was forced to release surgeon-specific risk-adjusted mortality rates through litigation, despite physician protests and the well-worn argument that the measures do not adequately adjust for severity of illness. The concern is not whether physicians like these measures—or even should like them, for that matter—but whether they find them credible and useful tools in decision making. A related issue is the extent to which managers would consider these measures informative and empowering in dealing with the medical staff. Finally, to what extent should consumers be involved in choosing a surgeon on the basis of a report card score, the methods of which neither the patient nor the surgeon probably understands?

In terms of clinical utility, Schneider and Epstein (1996) surveyed a 50 percent randomized sample of Pennsylvania cardiologists and cardiac surgeons to assess the clinical impact of the Pennsylvania program. Only 10 percent of the sample said the mortality rates were "very important" in assessing surgical skills, and 87 percent reported that the "guide" had little or minimal influence on referral decisions. The majority of respondents questioned the inadequate risk adjustment, the absence of other quality indicators, and the lack of data reliability.

A compelling side-effect of the report card was that 63 percent of the cardiac surgeons agreed that—because of the report cards—they would be less willing to operate on severely ill patients. In fact, 59 percent of the cardiologists reported an increased difficulty in finding surgeons willing to perform CABG on severely ill patients.

The reluctance of surgeons to treat high-risk patients is a concern of the New York program as well (Green and Wintfeld 1995). The issue is whether report cards such as these can adversely affect access to care for the severely ill. This effect on access should occur only if cardiac surgeons are not convinced that the measures accurately reflect the risk of surgery for these patients. Remember that the calculus of report cards depends on both actual and expected deaths. These scores can be improved in two ways: positive changes in quality (i.e., fewer actual deaths) or higher expected deaths (i.e., a sicker case mix). If surgeons believe the measures do not accurately take into account the risk of treating severely ill patients, they may be tempted to improve their score by eschewing these patients. On the other hand, a more extensive coding of severity-related conditions would improve report card scores by increasing the expected number of deaths from the more severely ill patients. If this occurs, we should see an increase in prevalence over time of conditions associated with higher severity of illness, for example, unstable angina. Anecdotal evidence would suggest that this has occurred (Green and Wintfeld 1995).

It appears that the New York program had a clinical impact in terms of mortality rates, as reported by Hannan and associates (1995). Cardiovascular surgeons were categorized into high, middle, and low groups based on mortality ranking. Over a four-year period, each group showed improvement in risk-adjustment mortality, with the largest improvement being attributed to the group with the poorest outcome scores. The authors are willing to acknowledge a nationwide reduction in CABG mortality as partial explanation, but a more encouraging argument is that hospitals used the information to make strategic changes in process and personnel that reduced preventable deaths (Chassin, Hannan, and DeBuono 1996).

In another study, Hannan and colleagues (1995) describe shifts in surgical utilization among New York cardiovascular surgeons. These include a decrease in low-volume cardiac surgeons and in the percentage of operations performed by low-volume cardiac surgeons, and increases in both high-volume cardiac surgeons and the operations they performed. This apparent shift from low- to high-volume surgeons is applauded, given the lower risk-adjusted mortality rates among high-volume surgeons.

Other report cards are sure to appear in different settings, and for physicians other than cardiac surgeons. Clearly, the impact of these programs, in terms of "real" changes in quality, depends on the credibility of the risk-adjustment methodology, the ability of providers to "game" the system, and the willingness of managers and clinicians to implement the hard choices regarding the practice of medicine. Case studies 6.3 and 6.4 demonstrate risk-adjusted mortality using contingency table and multivariate approaches.

Case Study 6.3. Risk Adjustment with Contingency Tables—State of Pennsylvania

Pennsylvania adopted the contingency method of risk adjustment to report mortality statistics for 16 different conditions:

1. chronic obstructive pulmonary disease;
2. congestive heart failure;
3. heart attack—medical management;
4. pneumonia;
5. septicemia;
6. stroke—hemorrhagic;
7. stroke—nonhemorrhagic;
8. abdominal aortic aneurysm repair;
9. gallbladder removal—laparoscopic;
10. gallbladder removal—open;
11. colorectal procedures;
12. heart attack—angioplasty/stent;
13. hysterectomy—abdominal;
14. hysterectomy—vaginal;
15. prostatectomy—radical; and
16. prostatectomy—transurethral.

The contingency table was based on three dimensions: (1) admission severity score, (2) cancer status, and (3) age category. This method is similar to the indirect method of risk adjustment discussed earlier, except instead of using just standard age-specific mortality rates, the rates are specific to the three dimensions mentioned above.

Table 6.9 represents the contingency table for congestive heart failure for a specific hospital. There would be contingency tables for each of the other 16 different conditions, and in each case for every hospital or physician to which this methodology applies.

QUESTIONS

1. How do the statewide mortality rates compare along each of the three dimensions?
2. Table 6.9 reports 13 expected deaths for patients 80 and above with no cancer, and admission severity level 3. What does this number 13 mean?
3. What is the expected mortality rate for congestive heart failure for hospital A?
4. What additional information is necessary to calculate an SMR?
5. Are there other ways of comparing observed-to-actual mortality statistics?

TABLE 6.9. CONTINGENCY TABLE FOR CONGESTIVE HEART FAILURE, PENNSYLVANIA, 2001

Admission Severity Group	Cancer Status	Age Category	Number of Patients Treated at Hospital (a)	Statewide Mortality Rate (b)	Expected Number of Deaths for Hospital A a × b
0	No cancer	Under age 65	2	0.019608	0.0392
1	No cancer	Under age 65	10	0.004388	0.0439
		Age 65–79	5	0.004261	0.0213
		Age 80 and over	1	0.017094	0.0171
2	No cancer	Under age 65	20	0.009498	0.1900
		Age 65–79	80	0.013526	1.0821
		Age 80 and over	70	0.020612	1.4429
	Malignant neoplasm or cancer in situ	Under age 65	1	0.055901	0.0559
		Age 65–79	5	0.039179	0.1959
		Age 80 and over	3	0.030471	0.0914
	History of cancer	Age 80 and over	5	0.009050	0.0452
3	No cancer	Under age 65	10	0.069703	0.6970
		Age 65–79	50	0.075641	3.7821
		Age 80 and over	150	0.086699	13.0049
	Malignant neoplasm or cancer in situ	Under age 65	1	0.135135	0.1351
		Age 65–79	7	0.110887	0.7762
		Age 80 and over	12	0.090056	1.0807
	History of cancer	Under age 65	2	0.000000	0.0000
		Age 65–79	4	0.032338	0.1294
		Age 80 and over	6	0.064350	0.3861
4	No cancer	Under age 65	2	0.266667	0.5333
		Age 65–79	5	0.343096	1.7155
		Age 80 and over	7	0.406471	2.8449
	History of cancer	All age categories combined	5	0.250000	1.2500
Total			463		29.5601

SOURCE: The Pennsylvania Health Care Cost Containment Council. A Hospital Performance Report: Common Medical Procedures and Treatments. Technical Notes for Western Pennsylvania, Central and Northeastern Pennsylvania, and Southeastern Pennsylvania. Calendar Year 2001. December 2002. http://www.phc4.org/reports/hpr/01/docs/hpr2001technotes.pdf

ANSWERS

1. Notice that the statewide mortality rates increase, as expected, as age increases, severity increases, and cancer status changes. For example, for patients with the highest level of admission severity and no cancer, the statewide mortality rate is 27 percent for those under 65 years of age but 41 percent for those 80 and above. For those 65–79 years of age at severity level

3, the statewide mortality rates for those with and without cancer are 7.6 percent and 11.1 percent, respectively.

2. This represents the number of patients in this hospital with these characteristics who we would expect to die if mortality in this hospital were similar to mortality across the state.

3. The expected mortality rate is calculated as $29.56/463 \times 100 = 6.38$ percent.

4. We would need to know the actual number of deaths for congestive heart failure patients in this hospital. On that basis we could sum the actual and expected deaths for all 16 conditions and calculate an SMR.

5. Pennsylvania used a binomial test to determine if the difference between observed and expected mortality is too large to be due to chance alone.

Source: State of Pennsylvania. http://www.phc4.org/reports/hpr/01

Case Study 6.4. Risk Adjustment with Multivariate Techniques—State of New York

The state of New York has reported risk-adjusted mortality statistics for coronary artery bypass graft surgery for a number of years, as discussed earlier in the text. New York uses the second major approach to risk adjustment, a multivariate model. Such models control for different kinds of patient characteristics that are likely to influence mortality. Table 6.10 reports the multivariate model used to calculate this risk-adjusted measure.

QUESTIONS

1. Which factors are supposedly related to CABG mortality?
2. Which factors are most strongly related to CABG mortality?
3. How could one derive an expected mortality rate from the multivariate model?

ANSWERS

1. Presumably, demographic factors, such as age and gender, hemodynamic state, comorbidities, severity of atherosclerotic process, ventricular function, and previous open heart operations are related to the risk of CABG mortality.

2. The odds ratio (discussed in more detail in Chapter 11) is a measure of the relative risk of mortality for patients with and without the characteristic. Patients with hepatic failure have about 21 times the odds of mortality compared to those without this comorbidity. Notice the dose-response relationship between ventricular function and mortality—the risk of dying increases as ejection fraction decreases.

3. Once we agree on the statistically significant covariates, as reported in Table

6.10, we can use the model coefficients to calculate a "predicted value" for each patient, which can be transformed to a "probability of death." If we sum the probabilities of death across each hospital or surgeon's case load, we derive the total expected deaths for each hospital or surgeon. Dividing the expected deaths by the number of patients and multiplying by 100 would give an expected mortality rate (per 100).

TABLE 6.10. MULTIVARIATE APPROACH TO RISK ADJUSTMENT, NEW YORK, 1998

Patient Risk Factor	Prevelance (%)	Logistic Regression		
		Coefficient	P-Value	Odds Ratio
Demographic				
Age	—	0.0671	< 0.0001	1.069
Female Gender	28.92	0.5105	< 0.0001	1.666
Hemodynamic state				
Unstable	1.32	1.0423	< 0.0001	2.836
Shock	.045	1.8458	< 0.0001	6.333
Comorbidities				
Diabetes	30.91	0.3607	< 0.0010	1.434
Malignant ventricular arrhythmia	2.28	0.9759	< 0.0001	2.654
COPD	15.97	0.5012	< 0.0001	1.651
Renal failure (dialysis), creatinine > 2.5	1.89	0.9213	< 0.0001	2.513
Renal failure requiring dialysis	1.27	1.7384	< 0.0001	5.688
Hepatic failure	0.10	3.0535	< 0.0001	21.190
Severity of atherosclerotic process				
Aortoiliac disease	5.42	0.5481	0.0006	1.730
Stroke	7.01	0.4775	0.0016	1.612
Ventricular function				
Ejection fraction < 20	1.77	1.4235	< 0.0001	4.151
Ejection fraction 20–29	7.40	0.8183	< 0.0001	2.267
Ejection fraction 30–39	14.49	0.6186	< 0.0001	1.856
Previous open heart operations	5.98	0.6800	< 0.0001	1.974

Intercept = −9.4988
C Statistic = 0.793

SOURCE: New York State Department of Health. *Coronary Artery Bypass Surgery in New York State 1996-1998.* January 2001.

Summary

The focus of this chapter has been on how mortality measures can be developed and used to describe and compare the burden of death across periods, population groups, or geographic areas and settings of care. We discussed the standardization of mortality rates by age, and the rationale for using such an approach to compare these rates across geographic regions that may have very different age mixes. We then moved to the next level and demonstrated how mortality rates can be standardized along more than one dimension, for example, age and gender. Finally, we introduced the concept of risk-adjusted mortality, as the final extension to this approach, where the idea is to standardize mortality rates along numerous patient-related dimensions so that providers with different patient mixes can be compared.

The purpose of any of these measures is to make judgments regarding whether the "burden" of mortality is excessive. That is, why do some countries have higher mortality rates than others, or why do some hospitals or surgeons have higher risk-adjusted mortality rates than others? Such judgments involve an evaluation of the relative success of one "region," or provider, versus another. With the former, we might be interested in understanding higher rates of mortality in terms of risk factors in the population or inadequacies of public health or medical care systems. With the latter, these are judgments of relative quality or effectiveness of one provider versus another.

References

Bassuk, S. S., L. F. Berkman, and B. C. Amick III. 2002. "Socioeconomic Status and Mortality Among the Elderly: Findings from Four U.S. Communities." *American Journal of Epidemiology* 155: 520–33.

Blumberg, M. S. 1986. "Risk-Adjusting Health Care Outcomes: A Methodological Review." *Medical Care Review* 43:351–93.

Casper, M. L., E. Barnett, G. I. Williams Jr., J. A. Halverson, V. E. Braham, and K. I. Greenlund. 2003. *Atlas of Stroke Mortality: Racial, Ethnic, and Geographic Disparities in the United States.* Atlanta, GA: U.S. Department of Health and Human Services, Centers for Disease Control and Prevention.

Chassin, M. R., E. L. Hannan, and B. A. DeBuono. 1996. "Benefits and Hazards of Reporting Medical Outcomes Publicly." *New England Journal of Medicine* 334 (6): 394–98.

Donabedian, A. 1989. "The End Results of Health Care: Ernest Codman's Contribution to Quality Assessment and Beyond." *Milbank Quarterly* 67 (2): 233–67.

Fleming, S. T., L. L. Hicks, and R. C. Bailey. 1995. "Interpreting the Health Care Financing Administration's Mortality Statistics." *Medical Care* 33 (2): 186–201.

Green, J., and N. Wintfeld. 1995. "Report Cards on Cardiac Surgeons: Assessing New York State's Approach." *New England Journal of Medicine* 332 (18): 1229–32.

Hannan, E. L., D. Kumar, M. Racz, A. L. Siu, and M. R. Chassin. 1994. "New York State's Cardiac Surgery Reporting System: Four Years Later." *Annals of Thoracic Surgery* 58 (6): 1852–57.

Hannan, E. L., A. L. Siu, D. Kumar, H. Kilburn, Jr., and M. R. Chassin. 1995. "The Decline in Coronary Artery Bypass Graft Surgery Mortality in New York State: The Role of Surgeon Volume." *Journal of the American Medical Association* 273 (3): 209–13.

Iezzoni, L. I. 1997a. *Risk Adjustment for Measuring Healthcare Outcomes.* Chicago: Health Adminstration Press.

———. 1997b. "The Risks of Risk Adjustment." *Journal of the American Medical Association* 278 (19): 1600–07.

Kliewer, E. V., and K. R. Smith. 1995. "Breast Cancer Mortality Among Immigrants in Australia and Canada." *Journal of the National Cancer Institute* 87 (15): 1154–61.

Lilienfeld, D. E., and P. D. Stolley. 1994. *Foundations of Epidemiology,* 3rd ed. New York: Oxford University Press.

Schneider, E. C., and A. M. Epstein. 1996. "Influence of Cardiac Surgery Performance Reports on Referral Practices and Access to Care." *New England Journal of Medicine* 335 (4): 251–56.

Timmreck, T. C. 2002. *An Introduction to Epidemiology,* 3rd ed. Boston: Jones and Bartlett.

DESCRIPTIVE EPIDEMIOLOGY: TIME, PLACE, PERSON

Steven T. Fleming and Jeffery Jones

"Whoever wishes to investigate medicine properly, should proceed thus: in the first place to consider the seasons of the year, and what effects each of them produces for they are not at all alike, but differ much from themselves in regard to their changes." Hippocrates, On Air, Waters, and Places 400 B.C. *(Translated by Francis Adams)*

Many years ago, Hippocrates understood the importance of people and places in describing and treating disease. He recognized that there were certain "diseases peculiar to the place" and that the inhabitants of various areas have distinct physical characteristics, behaviors, and predisposing diseases. Modern-day epidemiologists also recognize the importance of understanding disease patterns over time, across various geographic places, and among various population groups. Koepsell and Weiss (2003) argue that disease is not random, and because of this, differences across these three dimensions are inevitable. Such descriptive epidemiology may ultimately lead to a better understanding of disease etiology, and better methods of prevention and control. It has been said that clinicians are concerned with what disease a person has (because this dictates treatment), whereas epidemiologists are concerned with what person a disease has (because this suggests risk factors and etiology).

Descriptive Epidemiology: The Person

Each person has characteristics and behaviors that make him or her more or less likely to develop disease. These factors can be broadly categorized into those that are modifiable, such as behaviors and habits and socioeconomic status, and those that are relatively stable. Smoking and overeating are examples of the former, while gender and race are examples of the latter. Age is unmodifiable, but progressive.

Age is clearly related to the risk of disease and mortality, as evidenced by differences in age-specific morbidity and mortality rates. Koepsell and Weiss (2003) discuss various attributes or diseases associated with age, such as immunological status, human development, slow progressive diseases, and variations in lifestyle.

For example, newborns are blessed with maternal immunity for weeks or months after birth; they are susceptible to disease once it wanes. At the other end of the spectrum are the elderly who may have a lowered immunological status due to drugs or treatment.

Human development, or what Dever (2006) calls "life-stage," is another explanation behind the relationship between age and disease patterns. As we age, we progress through various stages, some of which make us particularly susceptible to certain kinds of diseases. Unintentional injuries are the leading cause of death in the 1–34 age group. Suicides are the second leading cause of death in the 15–24 age group. Cancer, heart disease, and stroke are heavy burdens on the elderly. The morbidity and death associated with pregnancy are obviously linked to the childbearing phase of a woman's life. The slow progressive diseases, such as heart disease or cancer, may take decades to develop to the point where they are measured and classified as a morbidity, thus older age is associated with a steep rise in the prevalence of these diseases. Finally, there are variations in lifestyle risk that are associated with age, such as the risk of sexually transmitted diseases and the risk of motorcycle collisions.

Gender is another personal characteristic with which we can observe differences in morbidity and mortality rates. For example, women have markedly lower cancer incidence and mortality rates than men. Koepsell and Weiss (2003) differentiate between biological and nonbiological factors behind these disparities. Women have a different balance of hormones than men, which explains why they are 100 times more likely than men to get breast cancer, a disease for which estrogen is a clear risk factor. There are anatomical differences between men and women beyond the obvious sexual ones. For example, women have smaller coronary arteries that men, a characteristic that affects case fatality rates for coronary artery bypass graft surgery. Women are blessed with childbearing, but some must bear the burden of certain related morbidities, such as pregnancy-induced hypertension (pre-eclampsia) and gestational diabetes. The non-biological factors include those that relate to gender-specific roles, including differences in employment opportunities and the level of stress associated with such activities. For example, the dramatic rise in female employment over the last half century has put more women at risk of stress-related morbidity.

Race is another stable characteristic that has been associated with different patterns of disease and mortality. There may be some biological (or genetic) factors behind such disparities. For example, African Americans have much lower rates of melanoma (skin cancer) than whites, with skin pigmentation being the key factor there. On the other hand, African Americans have much higher rates of sickle-cell anemia as a result of a genetic defect. Non-biological factors would include behaviors, habits, or attitudes that are associated with culture, and the society in which we live. For example, according to the Youth Risk Behavior Surveillance System (Centers for Disease Control and Prevention 2004), white female high school students smoke at two and one-half times the rate of African American female high school students.

African Americans, however, have much higher rates of diabetes and hypertension, conditions that are associated with obesity and diet, and have consistently experienced nearly double the infant mortality rate of whites.

Table 7.1 illustrates the extent to which cancer mortality rates differ among African Americans and whites. African American men have a 40 percent higher

TABLE 7.1
Cancer Sites in Which African American Death Rates Exceed White Death Rates,* U.S., 1997–2001

Site	African American	White	Ratio of African American/ White
Men			
All sites	347.3	245.5	1.4
Prostate	70.4	28.8	2.4
Larynx	5.4	2.3	2.3
Stomach	13.3	5.8	2.3
Myeloma	9.0	4.4	2.0
Oral cavity and pharynx	7.5	3.9	1.9
Esophagus	11.7	7.4	1.6
Liver/Intrahepatic bile duct	9.3	6.1	1.5
Small intestine	0.7	0.5	1.4
Colon and rectum	34.3	24.8	1.4
Lung and bronchus	104.1	76.6	1.4
Pancreas	16.0	12.0	1.3
Women			
All sites	196.5	165.5	1.2
Myeloma	6.6	2.9	2.3
Stomach	6.3	2.8	2.3
Uterine cervix	5.6	2.6	2.2
Esophagus	3.2	1.7	1.9
Larynx	0.9	0.5	1.8
Uterine corpus	6.9	3.9	1.8
Pancreas	12.8	8.9	1.4
Colon and rectum	24.5	17.1	1.4
Liver/intrahepatic bile duct	3.8	2.7	1.4
Breast	35.4	26.4	1.3
Urinary bladder	2.9	2.3	1.3
Oral cavity and pharynx	2.0	1.6	1.3

*Per 100,000, age-adjusted to the 2000 U.S. standard population.

SOURCE: National Cancer Institute (2004).

mortality rate for all cancer sites compared with white men. For African American women the rate is 1.2 times higher. African American men have 2.4 times the mortality rate from prostate cancer, compared with white men, and African American women (compared with white women) have over twice the mortality rate from either myeloma, stomach cancer, or cervical cancer.

In some cases, there may be multiple factors behind racial disparities. For example, African American women have 1.3 times the mortality rate from breast cancer compared to white women, with 75 percent five-year survival, compared to 89 percent five-year survival for white women. The incidence of breast cancer, however, has been higher for whites for the last 30 or more years. Thus, it may be that proportionately more African American women are diagnosed at an advanced stage of cancer, perhaps because of lack of mammography screening or problems with accessing the medical care system.

Socioeconomic status (SES) is another factor associated with morbidity and mortality, and one could argue SES is modifiable. Although one will rarely find variables that directly measure this characteristic, it is typically associated with such factors as income (or wealth), education, and employment. Each of these factors is associated with attitudes, preferences, and behaviors that affect the risk of disease. For example, an adequate daily intake of fruits and vegetables may be affordable only to those of a certain income level, preferences for cancer screening may be partly driven by education, and exposure to hazardous chemicals is a risk of certain employment settings.

The evidence is clear that those of a higher SES enjoy higher levels of health, and consider themselves healthier than those of a lower SES. For example, Dever (2006) reports age-adjusted death rates for both men and women in the 25–64 age group based on data from the National Center for Health Statistics. Men with less than 12 years of education have nearly triple the death rate of men with 13 or more years of education, and women in the first category have over twice the rate. Moreover, Dever (2006) also summarizes a 1999 Australian study that reports disparities in cause-specific mortality rates across SES levels. Compared with "professionals," "unskilled" laborers have six times the age-adjusted standardized mortality ratio (SMR) from diabetes, nearly three times the SMR from lung cancer, nearly seven times the SMR from bronchitis, and a 30 percent higher SMR from coronary heart disease.

Marital status is another modifiable factor associated with differences in morbidity and mortality rates. In general, single people tend to have higher mortality rates, which may be related to poorer health, risky behavior, or differences in lifestyle (Dever 2006).

Most "modifiable risk factors" to which a person is exposed are the behaviors and habits that have been linked with disease. Smoking is an obvious and well-documented risk factor that has been linked with lung cancer, pancreatic cancer, heart disease, bronchitis, and a number of other morbidities. Certain dietary habits also play a role. Saturated fat intake and the consumption of fruits and vegetables are associated with an increased and decreased risk of disease, respectively. Clearly, sexual behavior can affect the risk of sexually transmitted diseases.

The risk factors for breast cancer are illustrative of some characteristics that are modifiable, and some that are not (McPherson, Steel, and Dixon 2000). Age and gender are unmodifiable risk factors—older women have higher rates of breast cancer than younger women, and women have much higher rates than men. Age at menses and menopause are unmodifiable risk factors, with a younger age at menses, and an older age at menopause, being associated with a higher risk. The number and timing of pregnancies are somewhat modifiable, with more and earlier pregnancies being associated with a lower risk of breast cancer. Diet may be a modifiable factor in the risk of breast cancer, and induced abortion may be associated with a slight increase in the risk of the disease. Case Study 7.1 illustrates racial disparities in infant mortality rates.

Case Study 7.1. Infant Mortality Disparities by Race

Infant mortality rates have been decreasing over the last several decades for both African Americans and whites, although the disparity between African American and white infant mortality rates has persisted despite the widespread growth of neonatal intensive care units in many hospitals. Figure 7.1 illustrates the trend in African American and white infant mortality rates from 1980 through 2000. Such an observation in descriptive epidemiology can be used to more fully understand risk factors and suggest possible prevention and control programs. A *National Vital Statistics Report* is summarized in Table 7.2.

FIGURE 7.1. AFRICAN AMERICAN AND WHITE INFANT MORTALITY RATES, 1980–2000

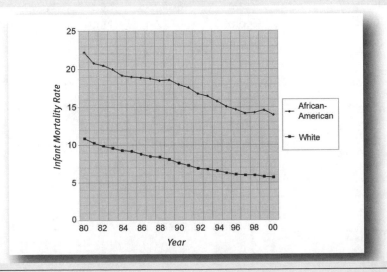

SOURCE: "Mortality and Morbidity Weekly Report (MMWR)." *Infant Mortality and Low Birth Weight Among Black and White Infants—United Sates, 1980-2000.* 51(27): 589–592. July 12, 2002.

TABLE 7.2 INFANT MORTALITY RATES (PER 1,000 LIVE BIRTHS) AND LIVE BIRTHS BY RISK FACTORS, 2000

Risk Factor	African American Infant Mortality Rate	Live Births	White Infant Mortality Rate	Live Births
Total	13.5	622,621	5.7	3,194,049
Birth weight				
<1,500 grams (very low)	266.9	19,369	232.7	36,828
1,500–2,499 grams (low)	15.8	61,747	16.0	172,649
>2,500 grams	3.9	541,244	2.2	2,982,366
Age of mother				
<20 years	13.8	122,763	8.5	337,462
20–24 years	13.1	202,598	6.2	772,818
25–29 years	13.1	141,974	5.1	874,190
30–34 years	13.8	94,815	4.7	764,721
35–39 years	14.5	49,299	5.4	368,714
40–54 years	15.1	11,172	7.0	76,144
Marital status[a]				
Married	11.5	195,962	4.9	2,327,678
Unmarried	14.4	426,659	7.8	866,371
Prenatal care[a]				
First trimester	12.2	444,515	5.1	2,649,248
No prenatal care	50.0	14,545	25.7	28,068
Maternal smoking during pregnancy[a]				
Smoker	19.8	52,852	10.7	360,981
Nonsmoker	12.7	529,582	6.5	2,372,979

NOTE: a = Totals in these categories will not add up to 100 percent of live births because of omitted items in each category.

SOURCE: Centers for Disease Control and Prevention (2002).

QUESTIONS

1. Is there a relationship between newborn birth weight and infant mortality?
2. Is the prevalence of low infant birth weight higher among African Americans?
3. Is there a relationship between teenaged motherhood and infant mortality?

4. Are proportionately more African American mothers teenagers?

5 Is there a relationship between unmarried motherhood and infant mortality?

6. Are proportionately more African American mothers unmarried?

7. Is there a relationship between prenatal care and infant mortality?

8. What is the prevalence of prenatal care (in the first trimester) among African American mothers compared to white mothers?

9. Is there a relationship between maternal smoking during pregnancy and infant mortality?

10. Is the prevalence of maternal smoking during pregnancy higher among African Americans?

11. What intervention(s) might you suggest to reduce the infant mortality rate among African Americans?

ANSWERS

1. Consider the following three categories of birth weight: (1) normal, ≥2,500 grams (5.5 lbs); (2) low, 1,500–2,499 grams (3.3 lbs–5.5 lbs); and (3) very low, <1,500 grams (3.3 lbs). For whites, the birth weight–specific mortality rates (per 1,000 live births) in 1999 in these three categories was 2.2, 16.0, and 232.7, respectively. For African Americans, the rates were 3.9, 15.8, and 266.9, respectively (Iyasu and Tamashek 2002).

2. In 2000, African Americans had nearly twice the rate of low birth weight infants compared to whites (9.9 percent of live births versus 5.4 percent of live births), and over two and one-half times the rate of very low birth weight infants (3.1 percent of live births versus 1.15 percent of live births).

3. For whites in 2000, infant mortality rates (per 1,000 live births) for mothers under 20 years, 20–24 years, 25–29 years, and 30–34 years were 8.5, 6.2, 5.1, and 4.7, respectively. For African Americans, the rates were 13.8, 13.1, 13.1, and 13.8, respectively. We could test for statistically significant differences in these rates, but it would appear that age of the mother is related to infant mortality in white, but not African American, infants.

4. In 2000, 19.7 percent of all live births among African Americans were to those under 20 years old. Among whites, the proportion was 10.6 percent. Infant mortality among African Americans is higher than in whites, for all ages of the mothers.

5. Unmarried mothers have higher infant mortality rates (per 1,000 live births) than married mothers: 7.8 versus 4.9 (for whites) and 14.4 versus 11.5 (for African Americans).

6. In 2000, 68.5 percent of all live births among African American women were to those who were unmarried. Among whites, the percentage was 27.1 percent.

7. In 2000, the infant mortality rates (per 1,000 live births) for women with no prenatal care were 25.7 and 50.0 for whites and African Americans, respectively. This compares with rates of 5.1 and 12.2 for whites and African Americans who obtained prenatal care in the first trimester of pregnancy.

8. In 2000, 82.9 percent of live births were among white women who obtained prenatal care in the first trimester. Among African American women, the rate was 71.4 percent.

9. In 2000, maternal smokers had higher infant mortality rates (per 1,000 newborns) than nonsmokers: 19.8 versus 12.7 (for African Americans) and 10.7 versus 6.5 (for whites).

10. In 2000, 8.5 percent of all live births were to African American women who smoked compared to 11.3 percent of all live births to white women smokers.

11. Reducing the proportion of low and very low birth weight among African American newborns should be a focus. Reducing the rate of teenaged pregnancies may be a more critical factor for whites than African Americans because the difference in mortality rate between teenaged and older mothers is higher for whites. Smoking cessation programs should probably be focused on both races, although proportionately more white women smoke during pregnancy. Clearly, programs to promote prenatal care would be important, given the much higher rates among those who do not obtain prenatal care.

Descriptive Epidemiology: Time

Epidemiologists are also interested in how the incidence and prevalence of disease vary across the dimension of time, both in the short and long term. Chapter 2 discussed how an "epidemic curve" illustrates the incidence of disease for a specific disease outbreak by showing how the incidence of disease (on the y-axis) varies over time, either hours or days, on the x-axis. Such a curve can be useful in characterizing an epidemic, in terms of the magnitude of the outbreak (height of the curve) and the duration of the outbreak (breadth of the curve). It can also provide insight into the identity of the causative agent, by showing the "incubation period" once time of exposure is known.

Short-term and long-term trends may provide an understanding of both the risk factors and etiology of disease, and the means or methods of transmission. For example, some diseases are characterized by cyclical or seasonal trends. Figure 7.2 illustrates the seasonal cycle for Lyme disease. If we did not understand how this disease was transmitted, such a graph would suggest some kind of vector to which subjects are exposed during leisure activities outside.

Long-term or secular trends illustrate how the incidence or prevalence of disease varies across a longer period, years or decades. For example, figures 6.3 and 6.4 from the last chapter show how cancer mortality has changed for men and women in the United States from 1930 to 2002. Such trends may also provide helpful clues into the etiology of disease. Figure 7.3 illustrates secular trends for both lung cancer mortality and cigarette consumption. One might infer a link between the exposure (cigarettes) and the outcome (lung cancer) by observing the relationship between the two trends.

FIGURE 7.2
Season Cycle for Lyme Disease

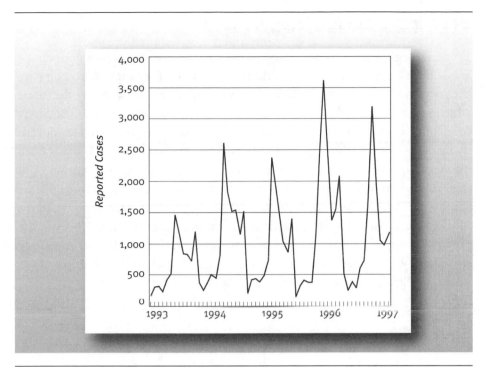

SOURCE: *Morbidity and Mortality Weekly Reports*: 42 (53): 10/21/94; 43 (53): 10/6/95; 44 (53): 10/25/96; 45 (53): 10/31/87; 46 (54): 11/20/98.

FIGURE 7.3
Lung Cancer Mortality and Cigarette Consumption

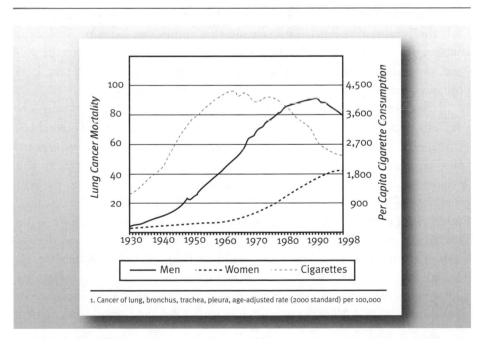

1. Cancer of lung, bronchus, trachea, pleura, age-adjusted rate (2000 standard) per 100,000

SOURCES: (1) Wingo et al. (2003). "Long-Term Trends in Cancer Mortality in the United States, 1930–1998." *Cancer* 97 (12, Suppl.): 3133–275. (2) Reducing the Health Consequences of Smoking: 25 Years of Progress. A report of the Surgeon General 1989. (3) Tobacco Outlook/TBS-262/April 24, 2007, Economic Research Service, USDA. (4) Tobacco Situation and Outlook/TBS-244/September 1999. Economic Research Service, USDA.

Descriptive Epidemiology: Place

Epidemiologists are also interested in the disease patterns across geographic areas, both large and small. It would be interesting, for example, to compare the incidence of HIV/AIDS across the various countries in the world to see which regions of the world have the highest burden of this disease. Case Study 6.1 from the previous chapter examined differences in breast cancer mortality rates for women who migrated into, and out of, Australia and Canada from numerous other countries. The conclusion was that breast cancer risk has both genetic and environmental components, since immigrants do not entirely assume the risk of the country to which they migrate. Intra-country patterns of disease are also interesting, such as shown in figures 6.7 and 6.8 from the previous chapter. Differences in mortality rates from cardiovascular disease or stroke may be attributed to environmental causes, such as the hardness of the water, or differences in other behaviors, such as dietary choices.

Spot Maps

Spot maps illustrate the cases of disease within a specific geographic area, such as a city. The purpose of such maps is to identify clusters of cases in space, which may help determine disease etiology.

Figure 7.4 illustrates the results of John Snow's outstanding work with cholera in the mid-1800s. In this case, the spots are stackable bars with the height of the bar representing the number of cases of cholera at that particular location. Note that spot maps report the incidence of disease, not the incidence rate of disease, since there is no way to take into consideration population at risk with these kinds of maps.

Spot maps can also be used to identify the location of cases within a smaller geographic area, such as a hotel or hospital. Panackal and colleagues (2006) report on an outbreak of fungal infections (*Aspergillus ustus*) among transplant patients in a large tertiary care hospital. Figure 7.5 represents the spot map showing the locations of six patients who were infected on the seventh and eighth floors during 2001 (left panel) and 2003 (right panel). Patient 3 is not reported because she (he) was in the outpatient clinic at the time of diagnosis. Patients 5 and 6 stayed in the same rooms at different times. Patients 2, 4, and 5 moved around to a number of different rooms. The authors conclude that "a common source for the *A. ustus* infections appears possible, since the case-patients clustered in space and time" (406).

Clusters

Another useful epidemiologic technique is to evaluate time-place clusters. Epidemiologists use this approach regularly to study epidemics. By definition,

FIGURE 7.4
Spot Map
Around the
Broad Street
Pump,
London,
1839, John
Snow

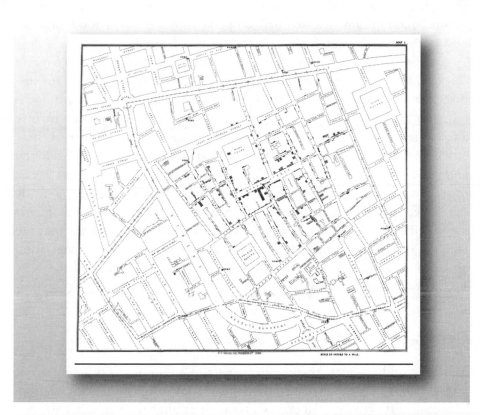

SOURCE: John Snow website, UCLA, School of Public Health, http://www.ph.ucla.edu/EPI/snow.html

FIGURE 7.5
Spot Map of
Transplant
Patients
with
*Aspergillus
ustus*
Infections

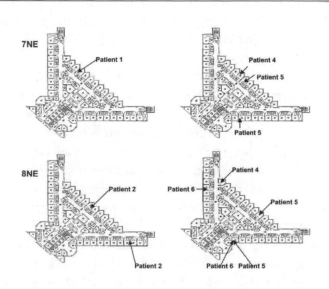

SOURCE: Panackal et al. (2006).

an epidemic is an unusually high occurrence of disease, at a particular point in time, and typically in a well-defined geographic area. The foodborne illness outbreak at a church picnic is the classic example.

Time-place clusters may also be useful as a surveillance tool for rare diseases, such as some cancers. Such analyses identify risk factors for diseases that may be associated with a particular region, such as environmental pollutants. The challenge with these analyses, since they often involve a few cases of a very rare disease, is to determine if the incidence of these rare events exceeds that which might ordinarily occur by chance. Kulldorff and colleagues (1997), for example, examine mortality rates from breast cancer in counties in the northeastern United States. They use a newly developed spatial scan statistic that tests whether the mortality rate in any identified cluster is higher than would be expected, and conclude that the elevated breast cancer mortality that has been reported in the Long Island area is part of a much larger cluster that includes large parts of the New York City–Philadelphia metropolitan area.

Geographic Information Systems

Managers and researchers can look at data in a number of different ways: a spreadsheet, a graph, a textual description, or via statistical manipulation. Mapping and other spatial analysis tools offer another way of transforming data to see patterns and meaning. A geographic information system (GIS) provides a sophisticated tool for such spatial analysis.

GIS systems can map a single data variable, or perform more complex analytical functions by overlaying different variables or computing new variables. While ESRI's ArcView is the most widely used GIS software, there are a number of other GIS software packages, including MapInfo and the U.S. Centers for Disease Control and Prevention's (CDC) Epi Map software. Newer online applications such as Google Earth and Google Earth Plus also provide some of the GIS layering and mapping capabilities.

Commercial GIS systems such as ArcView can cost hundreds of dollars and require training to operate. Hardware investments in scanners or other equipment to digitize new base maps for use on a computer can run into the thousands. Fortunately, ESRI and other software makers provide short classes and accessible manuals for using their software's more basic mapping capabilities. Thousands of existing base maps are also available free via the Internet for international, state, county, and other boundaries. Furthermore, a user can download for free the CDC's Epi Map software. A user can also produce quick and free basic maps via Google Earth or buy the extended Google Earth Plus software for functionality such as *geocoding* (where the software can map street addresses in a spreadsheet provided by a user to the software's preloaded street and road coordinates).

If training and cost considerations deter individuals or agencies from using GIS, another possible way to access mapping and other spatial analyses is by seeking local GIS referrals. Many larger urban and regional planning agencies have GIS systems and workers trained in their use. Likewise, universities and colleges teaching GIS skills in geography, public health, mining, and other disciplines usually require students to complete GIS projects. A number of such academic instructors team up with local agencies to map their data needs while giving students opportunities to use real-world data in a GIS application. Thus, for managers or agencies with limited spatial analysis needs, outsourcing data to trained, local GIS users may be an economical and time-saving practice.

Some people have the perception that a computer-generated map constitutes GIS. While many people use GIS to produce maps, GIS software can also provide more sophisticated analysis functions such as layering various spatial variables and querying for defined parameters. Thus, rather than only producing static maps, GIS can provide interactivity. For example, if the user has previously compiled a GIS library of various data layers, a user can query the system to find any combination of data from various layers. A user could then, for example, use a GIS system to look for the largest concentration of Hispanic seniors living in a particular city, or compute areas where there are housing units reporting repeated cases of children exposed to lead. GIS systems can also measure not only the direct distance between a neighborhood and its nearest hospital, but also the actual driving distance via an existing road network. GIS thus offers two important tools beyond its capabilities to make quality maps: (1) GIS can provide fast, interactive querying of data and (2) GIS can compute new data from existing variables. As such, GIS provides a flexibility to adapt data to new questions as a community's planning needs and analytical questions change.

GIS also provides the foundation for a host of related technologies. For instance, the emergency 911 locator and dispatch system utilizes a GIS framework. Cell phone networks, online interactive maps, and wrist-worn locator services worn by some Alzheimer patients also are built from a GIS spatial system linking location and data. As such, the impact of GIS in the public health and healthcare arena extends beyond the immediate software application, and into a broad range of technologies linking people and places.

As with any powerful tool, GIS raises issues of ethical use. Many researchers utilize GIS in public health planning. From studying the distribution of dentists in Ohio to analyzing seniors' pharmaceutical usage in Canada, such studies often look for access barriers defined by distance and travel times to care facilities. In these cases, GIS is used as a top-down planning tool. While most studies aim to improve the quality of life of patients, the controlled access and use of spatial information by policymakers can also carry tones of authoritarianism and control. In *Ground Truth,* John

Pickles (1995) probes questions around the ethics of GIS. For example, what are the ethical issues of a large transnational corporation using satellite images and GIS to define areas of potential mineral deposits in a developing country? Is it fair to offer information about these locations to a poor developing country's government only if the transnational corporation has exclusive access to mine the deposits? Sarah Elwood's (2002) work on community empowerment expands on this theme and the ways in which GIS can consolidate existing power groups and disenfranchise others. These authors warn that, as with any tool, GIS can be used to the benefit or disadvantage of individuals and groups.

More recently, geographers have begun to write about using GIS to empower individuals and communities by providing access to information. In her study, Elwood (2002) first summarizes the various ways empowerment has been conceptualized:

- *Distributive*: Individuals or communities empower themselves by gaining greater access to goods, information, and services.
- *Procedural*: Empowerment comes from greater involvement in decision making, from the planning process through implementation.
- *Capacity building*: Empowerment comes from individuals and communities having greater abilities to advocate for and make decisions for themselves.

Elwood documents the experiences of a Minneapolis neighborhood association and its efforts to utilize GIS in its planning process. In this example, community members gave input into what data were collected and what questions were asked. A small group of GIS-trained residents produced the data products, and they were widely distributed to community members. Thus, the neighborhood residents were empowered via greater access to data products (distributive), input into data collection and analysis (procedural), and a greater awareness of the availability and uses of spatial analysis (capacity building). For public health and healthcare practitioners seeking to define how to empower communities and use GIS as an empowerment tool, Elwood's work provides a framework for goal-setting and implementation.

How can GIS be used in the health sector? The following examples offer some uses of basic mapping to visualize data and present it more effectively:

1. *Linking patient and provider*: The map in Figure 7.6 shows the county of residence of adult survivors of childhood cancers who are seeking follow-up care appointments with regional cancer hospitals. The North Carolina Children's Hospital's market area for such patients covers a broader area than similar clinics in Ohio, Illinois, and New Jersey. Such maps can be useful in a number of ways, such as determining a location for a satellite clinic or planning an advertising campaign.

   In an interesting case study in Laura Lang's (2000) *GIS for Health Organizations,* Jewish Hospital HealthCare Services (JHHS) uses ArcView to link patients to closer clinics. JHHS's goals in this analysis are to link more patients to a neighborhood clinic and better define a patient base for each clinic's ideal service area. Operating nine clinics in the greater Louisville, Kentucky area, JHHS corporate planning gathered several pieces of information from patient records:

a. Patient's residence
b. Patient's worksite
c. Clinic generally used by the patient
d. If the patient is using any specialty care offered only at a particular clinic

These variables produced interesting maps that helped JHHS better understand their clients' distribution. More importantly for JHHS, these variables and mapped layers were then used to find patients who were not using the clinic closest to their home. In some cases, a patient was utilizing a clinic closer to his/her worksite or using specialty services offered at a particular clinic. Individuals meeting these criteria were filtered out. The remaining patients consisted of individuals who were going to more distant clinics when a closer one could meet their needs. JHHS then reassigned these patients to clinics closest to their homes.

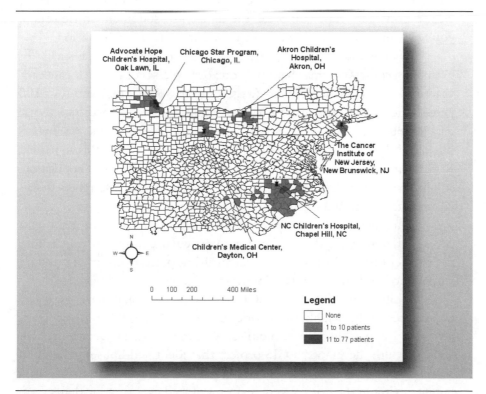

FIGURE 7.6
County of Residence for Adult Survivors of Childhood Cancers Who Are Seeking Follow-up Care

SOURCE: Jeff Jones, PhD, University of Kentucky College of Public Health, 2007.

2. *Epidemiology:* From the time of Dr. Snow's spatial analysis of cholera incidents in London, epidemiologists have utilized maps to study the origin, diffusion, and incidence of disease. The map in Figure 7.7 shows the age-adjusted annual death rate from lung cancer for the years 2000 to 2004. The map clearly illustrates clusters of higher lung cancer mortality rates in impoverished southeastern Kentucky.

In this map, the cartographer divided the rates for Kentucky's 120 counties into three categories (plus a fourth for a county with insufficient cases to establish a stable mortality rate). Counties with lung cancer death rates at or below the state median rate of 79.95 make up the lightest shaded category. The medium shaded category represents counties whose death rates range from the median to 20 points higher. The darkest shaded category shows counties whose rates are from 100 to 138.1 (the state's highest mortality rate, which is found in Lee County).

This breaking of data is critical in determining the type of pattern produced. The same mortality rates broken into five, six, or more categories would show a more highly resolved pattern. Likewise, breaking the data by standard deviations, equal intervals, or other categorization criteria would produce a different map and pattern. As with any representation of data, a presenter can manipulate data to convey different impressions. Care must be taken to represent data in an accurate and fair manner. In such cases, fair representation often involves having a clear rationale for how you break the data and a statement to viewers of your rationale and possible bias in your particular representation.

In some cases where the incidence of a particular disease is small (for example, a county that may have only one or two cases of Lyme disease each year) and thus prone to variability (a rise from one to two cases creates a 100 percent increase in Lyme disease for that county), it may be necessary to use data for multiple years, as in Figure 7.7. In this particular example, researchers calculated these rates for data from 2000 to 2004. Even with this approach, Robertson County, a northeastern Kentucky county with a small population, still had too few incidences of lung cancer deaths for the researchers to calculate a stable rate and to ensure confidentiality of the existing cases.

Another means of addressing such limitations is smoothing, a process that averages data values for a particular county with the values for each county adjacent to it. The resulting pattern smooths outlying values and tends to produce more recognizable regional patterns.

While planners often use GIS to analyze regional patterns, it can also be used at the neighborhood or even household level. Neal Rosenblatt, a GIS project manager/epidemiologist with the Kentucky Department for Public Health, developed a GIS project that identified houses generating repeated reports of high levels of lead exposure in children. In many cases, families living in the homes were unaware of lead exposure incidents from years before. This program helped the Louisville Metro Health Department focus on particular repeat offender residences for lead abatement.

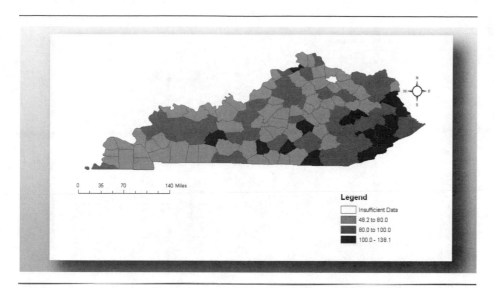

FIGURE 7.7
Lung Cancer Mortality Rates in Kentucky— 2000–2004

Legend
☐ Insufficient Data
▨ 48.2 to 80.0
▨ 80.0 to 100.0
■ 100.0 - 138.1

SOURCE: Jeff Jones, PhD, University of Kentucky College of Public Health, 2007.

3. *Emergency planning*: The ability of GIS to quickly take large amounts of spatially defined data and graphically present individual or combined variables makes GIS extremely valuable in emergency planning and response efforts. Greene's *Confronting Catastrophe: A GIS Handbook* (2002) examines how planners are using GIS to identify, mitigate, respond to, and recover from natural and manmade disasters. Whether identifying low-lying areas around Houston Bay most susceptible to hurricane storm surges or using thermal mapping data to identify smoldering fires in the World Trade Center debris after 9/11, a well-managed GIS library can quickly call up a variety of prepared maps or map layers displaying utility lines, fire hydrants, nearby hospitals, typical wind flows, administrative boundaries, and a host of other information.

4. *Managed care and compliance*: While the actual types of tests performed have been fictionalized in the map shown in Figure 7.8 for privacy issues, this map shows how GIS can be used to track and compare different data streams. In this case, one data stream—invoices to the state Medicaid office for tests performed—is considerably higher in number than the stream showing test results reported to the Kentucky Department for Public Health.

   This map helped illustrate three clusters of counties where testing results reports were far below Medicaid payments for such tests, which indicated that labs were billing Medicaid for tests but not properly reporting the test results to the state. Once these clusters were identified as corresponding primarily to three large health districts, the state was able to work with the labs doing the local testing to improve reporting and compliance. In turn, the state agency in charge of working with families testing positive on these tests hoped to be able to reach more

FIGURE 7.8
Medicaid
Test Claims
Not Linked to
Database—
Kentucky,
2005

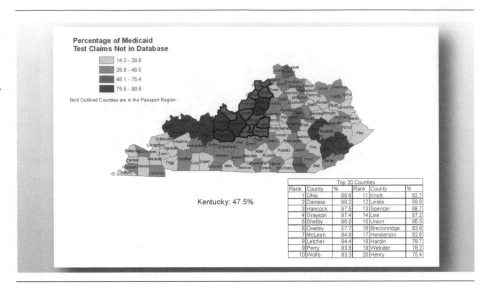

Percentage of Medicaid
Test Claims Not in Database

	14.3 - 28.8
	28.9 - 46.0
	46.1 - 75.4
	75.5 - 99.6

Bold Outlined Counties are in the Passport Region

Kentucky: 47.5%

Top 20 Counties					
Rank	County	%	Rank	County	%
1	Ohio	99.6	11	Knott	92.7
2	Daviess	99.2	12	Leslie	89.9
3	Hancock	97.5	13	Spencer	88.7
4	Grayson	97.4	14	Lee	87.2
5	Shelby	96.0	15	Union	86.3
6	Owsley	57.7	16	Breckinridge	83.9
7	McLean	94.6	17	Henderson	82.6
8	Letcher	94.4	18	Hardin	78.7
9	Perry	93.8	19	Webster	78.2
10	Wolfe	93.3	20	Henry	75.4

SOURCE: Hypothetical data and map created by Kate Jones.

such families with free state services. Before being able to gather and compare these two different data sets from two different agencies, the health agency felt it was not getting results from all the tests in the state, but could not easily identify how many or where they should be coming from. GIS was able to answer this question.

Earlier we mentioned that GIS has layering capabilities that facilitate interactivity. Case Study 7.2 illustrates the use of multiple layers to determine the location of an HIV clinic in the state of Kentucky.

Case Study 7.2. HIV Clinics in Kentucky

Imagine you work for the Kentucky Department of Public Health and are assigned the responsibility of finding a location for a new HIV clinic. Although currently (2007), there are only four clinics in the state, a number of northern Kentuckians also utilize a fifth clinic located across the Ohio River in Cincinnati. You decide to use GIS to help you find the best location for the new clinic.

Figure 7.9 shows four maps with increasing layers of variables. The first map (panel A) shows Kentuckians living with AIDS as of 2007, according to the Kentucky Department for Public Health's HIV/AIDS Branch. It does not include Kentuckians living with HIV who have not been diagnosed with AIDS. HIV-only data are currently not available for Kentucky. Notice the clusters of clients in some of the larger metropolitan areas. The second map (panel B) adds a layer revealing the locations of existing HIV clinics as well as medical colleges that could provide residents with specialty care. The third map (panel C) illustrates major roads linking clients to potential and existing clinic sites. Finally, the

FIGURE 7.9. DECIDING WHERE TO LOCATE AN HIV CLINIC IN KENTUCKY, USING GIS

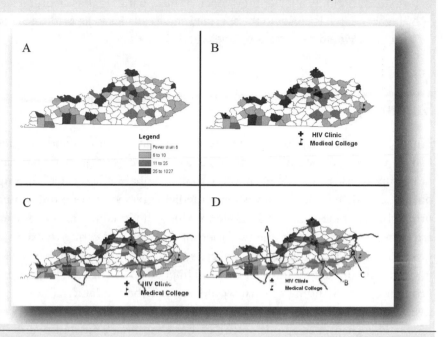

fourth (panel D) map shows three potential clinic sites based on clients' residences, existing clinics, and transportation networks.

QUESTIONS

1. What criteria should be used to locate a new clinic?
2. Are there other criteria and data not presented in the example that would help locate a new clinic?
3. Write a rationale for the site (A, B, or C) that would be best for locating the new clinic.

ANSWERS

1. The location of a new clinic should depend on the prevalence of AIDS in the population. You would like to locate a clinic in an area where there is a relatively high prevalence of people living with AIDS. You also want to choose an area that does not currently have a clinic that serves this population, and an area that is relatively close to specialized hospital services.
2. Since people who are HIV-positive are at risk of developing AIDS, the prevalence of HIV-positive residents in each of the counties would be helpful.
3. Site A (Bowling Green) has a high prevalence of AIDS patients, has good access by highways, and is a couple of hours away from the closest existing clinic and the nearest medical college. Site B (Somerset) has a high prevalence of AIDS patients, has good access by highways, and is a couple of hours

away from the closest existing clinic and the nearest medical college. Site C (Prestonsburg) has a lower prevalence of AIDS patients, has poorer access by highways, but is closer to the specialty services of Pikeville Medical School. The choice would be a "toss up" between sites A and B.

Summary

Hippocrates knew 2,400 years ago that variation in seasons and geography had an impact on the "diseases peculiar to the place or the particular nature of common diseases." He even knew that personal behavior had an impact on disease, for he said "to investigate medicine properly" one must, among other things, understand "the mode in which the inhabitants live, and what are their pursuits, whether they are fond of drinking and eating to excess, and given to indolence, or are fond of exercise and labor, and not given to excess in eating and drinking." In other words, Hippocrates seemed to have an almost prophetic understanding of what would become the fundamentals of descriptive epidemiology: variation in disease patterns across time, place, and person.

This chapter has built on the earlier chapters of morbidity and mortality with the purpose of seeing the ways in which disease patterns can vary by characteristics of the host—such as age and race—across short and long intervals of time, and across small and large geographic regions. Geographic information systems are an excellent tool to facilitate the recognition and discernment of geographic patterns of disease. Remember that the purpose of descriptive epidemiology is not just to characterize disease patterns, but also to recognize risk factor/disease associations that could ultimately lead to disease prevention and control.

References

Centers for Disease Control and Prevention. 2002. *National Vital Statistics Report* 50 (12), August 28.

———. 2004. "Youth Risk Behavior Surveillance System, 2003." Chronic Disease Prevention and Health Promotion. Atlanta, GA: Centers for Disease Control and Prevention.

Dever, G. E. Alan. 2006. *Managerial Epidemiology: Practice, Methods, and Concepts.* Boston: Jones and Bartlett.

Elwood, S. A. 2002. "GIS Use in Community Planning: A Multidimensional Analysis of Empowerment." *Environment and Planning A* 34: 905–22.

Greene, R. W. 2002. *Confronting Catastrophe: A GIS Handbook.* Redlands, CA: ESRI Press.

Iyasu, S., and K. Tamashek. 2002. "Infant Mortality and Low Birth Weight

Among Black and White Infants—United States, 1980–2000." *Morbidity and Mortality Weekly Report* 51 (27): 589–92.

Koepsell, T. D., and N. S. Weiss. 2003. *Epidemiologic Methods: Studying the Occurrence of Illness.* New York: Oxford University Press.

Kulldorff, M., E. J. Feuer, B. A. Miller, and L. S. Freedman. 1997. "Breast Cancer Clusters in the Northeast United States: A Geographic Analysis." *American Journal of Epidemiology* 146 (2): 161–70.

Lang, L. 2000. *GIS for Health Organizations.* Redlands, CA: ESRI Press.

McPherson, K., C. M. Steel, and J. M. Dixon. 2000. "ABC of Breast Diseases. Breast Cancer—Epidemiology, Risk Factors, and Genetics." *British Medical Journal* 32 (7261): 624–28.

National Cancer Institute. 2004. "Surveillance, Epidemiology, and End Results Program, 1975–2001." Bethesda, MD: Division of Cancer Control and Population Sciences, National Cancer Institute.

Panackal, A. A., A. Imhof, E. W. Hanley, and K. A. Marr. 2006. "Asperigillus Ustus Infections Among Transplant Recipients." *Emerging Infectious Diseases* 12 (3): 403–7.

Pickles, J. 1995. "Representations in an Electronic Age: Geography, GIS, and Democracy." In *Ground Truth: The Social Implications of Geographic Information Systems,* edited by J. Pickles, 1–30. New York: Guilford.

EPIDEMIOLOGY AND FINANCE

The two chapters of this section focus on the application of epidemiologic principles to financial management. Chapter eight deals specifically with financial management. The chapter has a heavy emphasis on managed care and capitation, because managed care has brought attention to populations, or more specifically the "health maintenance" of a defined population. This paradigm shift in the way health insurers view risk has made an understanding of epidemiology principles critically important to the healthcare manager. Chapter nine summarizes cost-effectiveness analysis (CEA), a decision-making technique for evaluating the relative effectiveness of alternative programmatic choices in an era of constrained resources. The process of CEA includes both economic and financial principles; this chapter demonstrates clearly in both text and case studies how epidemiologic principles should be woven into such analyses.

8

EPIDEMIOLOGY AND FINANCIAL MANAGEMENT

Keith E. Boles and Steven T. Fleming

> *"I had no ill-luck myself, but none of my cousins escaped. There were eight of them, and at one time and another they broke four-teen arms among them. But it cost next to nothing, for the doctor worked by the year—$25 for the whole family." Mark Twain, My Autobiography*

The healthcare landscape is ever changing, making it necessary to view the finance function through a wide-angle lens. Managed care, specifically, has broadened the horizon of financial managers, and the landscape is not without faults and crevices. New risks need to be considered for managed care to succeed and for the health of the population to improve.

The new healthcare landscape has several features that stand out. The first is risk: most of this chapter will discuss the implications of the changing risk "topography" for the financial manager. The second feature is the need for information. The identification, measurement, and management of risk require a great deal of information. More information supplied on a timely basis can lead to a greater reduction in risk—or a greater degree of planning activity. We will not discuss the validity of information per se; for our purposes we will assume that information is accurate and timely. The science of decision making has always been based on the premise that more information is better than less and that decisions are better made when the information is more accurate and timely. This premise is becoming ever more critical in the health industry.

Healthcare Delivery: Reactive or Proactive?

Healthcare costs are driven by the healthcare needs of the population. Historically, these needs have been determined by the occurrence of disease. This disease-based approach to medical care has been the cornerstone philosophy of medical schools, in which physicians are trained to diagnose and treat disease. Thus, the primary focus of educating health providers, regardless of type, is "reactive." The healthcare provider reacts to the healthcare needs presented in the office—when the patient has specific signs and symptoms, what is the disease?

Within the historical context of the health system, the individual man, woman, or child has been referred to as a patient. This has seemed appropriate, since an individual entered the health system only when the need for health services arose, that is; when specific signs and symptoms signaled that the individual should take action. After the disease was successfully treated, the patient left the healthcare system until another event occurred. These behaviors, on the part of both the healthcare provider and the individual consumer of health services, determined the growth and development of the healthcare field through most of the twentieth century. These behaviors have changed with the advent of managed care.

The primary objective of the illness or sickness system, misnamed the healthcare system, is to heal the sick and injured. This system is meant to be reactive in form and is designed with that objective in mind. This objective is taught in the medical schools, and most systems have been constructed to engage in a battle with disease after it develops. But the primary objective of a health system should be to emphasize individual health and, in so doing, to maximize the health of the population. This statement recognizes the interaction and interdependencies among people. The health status of one individual may have an impact on the health status of others.

Costs in the health system are driven by a variety of factors. The most obvious are those associated with the direct delivery of health services. These costs usually derive from a physical structure, with state-of-the-art equipment and supplies, and with plenty of labor to provide the services. The factors include: drugs, primary care physicians, specialty physicians, nurses, therapists, pharmacists, dentists, behavioral health specialists, magnetic resonance imagers, lithotripters, and so on.

Under managed care, the primary emphasis has shifted from battling disease to maximizing the health of a population. This redirected emphasis changes the focus of the system described earlier, and it requires a different way of looking at the world—through that wider-angle lens. This new approach is "proactive," one where all parties (consumers and providers) are involved in maintaining health. This means the individual previously described as a patient is now a client or a consumer of health, and must become a coproducer in the health production function. Maximizing the health of individuals is probably not entirely congruent with maximizing the health of a population, which implies that reactive and proactive approaches to health may be different production functions.

This approach also requires a much broader view of what is inclusive and exclusive to the health system. Earlier we described costs as being driven by physical structures and medical practices designed to react to sick individuals accessing the healthcare system. With managed care and the focus on the health status of a population, the view of the world has changed. This new vista includes a variety of other risks, and these risks play a much greater role in the determination of health system costs than the physical equipment and personnel factors previously addressed.

Healthcare Risks

Cost drivers and associated risks can be separated into four categories: (1) genetic risks, (2) biological risks, (3) behavioral risks, and (4) environmental risks (Figure 8.1). This paradigm, suggested by the National Cancer Institute (2008), is particularly relevant for chronic diseases such as cancer. One can define *exposure* as anything that increases or decreases the probability of disease or injury. All of these risk categories are types of exposure. Furthermore, the four risk categories straddle the agent, host, and environment triad. Genetic, biological, and behavioral risks are associated with the host, whereas environmental risks are clearly associated with the environment.

Genetic risks are congenital and often are passed down from generation to generation. The Human Genome Project is engaged in research to identify the extent to which genes play a role in the human body: physical shape, metabolism, susceptibility to disease, and immunological defensive posture. Genetic risks are genetic predispositions to certain acute or chronic diseases. It is known that diabetes, asthma, hypertension, cardiovascular disease, some forms of cancer, and Alzheimer's tend to be familial.

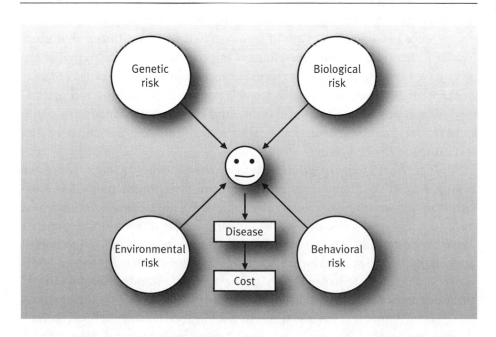

FIGURE 8.1
Healthcare Risks

This form of risk is believed to account for approximately 20 percent of total health system costs. All percentages associated with risk forms must be taken skeptically, since none of these risks are independent of the others. That is, the extent to which genetic risks become actualized is determined by behavioral risks, biological risks, and environmental risks.

Biological risks are physical characteristics that make us more or less likely to develop disease, such as gender, age, race, skin complexion, height, and weight. For example, males are more likely to develop cardiovascular disease than females, whereas women have a higher risk of breast cancer than men. African Americans are more likely to suffer from diabetes, and the men are at increased risk of prostate cancer. A light skin complexion puts one at increased risk of skin cancer. Short men have an increased risk of heart disease, while tall women are at increased risk of breast cancer. Finally, obesity is a significant risk factor for coronary heart disease.

Behavioral risks are believed to account for 50 percent of total health system costs and are assumed to be under the control of the individual. We will sidestep the debate surrounding the extent to which genes are responsible for certain behaviors. Some individuals engage in behaviors known to be risky because they have been linked to disease, such as smoking, eating and drinking to excess, engaging in unprotected and prolific sexual activities, using illicit drugs, and leading a sedentary lifestyle. Some behaviors are known to exacerbate conditions linked to genetic risk, such as eating a high-fat diet if one has a gene for hypercholesterolemia. Some behaviors delay or eliminate the onset of disease—for example, exercise reduces heart disease. Other behavioral risks include those that may result in trauma should an accident occur, such as skydiving, flying an airplane, scuba diving, hang gliding, driving fast, drinking to excess, and so on.

Since behavioral risks are often associated with conditions that must be dealt with by the health system, it is important to recognize that these risks have both internal and external components. The internal components are those that have an effect on physiological functions and pathology—blood pressure, cholesterol levels, and other bodily functions—while the external components are more likely to result in external causes of distress, such as broken bones.

The fourth form of risk is called *environmental risk*, and it originates from a number of different sources. One form of environmental risk is associated with the commonly recognized forms of pollution: air, water, and even sound. These risks, derived from living in our modern industrialized world, include radiation (both solar and otherwise), smog, ozone depletion, global warming, and any other form of pollution that is relatively universal and difficult to avoid. Many of these risks fall under the purview of the Environmental Protection Agency.

Environmental risks also arise from a number of other venues, including the workplace, the home, the roads, and wherever recreation activity occurs. The workplace introduces risk through stress, poor ventilation, exposure to noxious or poisonous fumes, and unsafe work conditions. Many of these risks are regulated through the Occupational Safety and Health Administration.

Risks occurring in the home are not regulated to any great extent, except in cases where children or others are at risk of disease or injury. These risks include many of those associated with the workplace, in addition to others, such as physical and/or mental abuse.

Although many of these environmental risks are often regulated to some extent, they still result in healthcare costs. These risks can be categorized as those primarily having internal implications (i.e., pathogenesis) and those more likely to result in bodily distress from the outside (e.g., injury or trauma).

Environmental risk is also introduced by external factors, such as roads, railways, and other routes for transportation. Road design is responsible for some accidents, while lack of railway infrastructure creates risks of eroding rail beds and of poorly maintained bridges and other structures. Increasing airline travel that outpaces the capacity of the infrastructure may result in increased congestion, stress, and potential for incidents.

It appears that few aspects of life exist that do not have an impact on health risks and costs, at least to some extent. The dilemma concerns the degree to which we formally acknowledge and assimilate these risks into healthcare financing activity, and how we do it. This is where the role of epidemiology comes into play. Accurate and convincing data regarding these risks permit us to correlate these risks with health status and health system costs. This information provides the basis for negotiations, management controls, cost estimation, and most important, the development of proactive health management strategies to address as many of these forms of risk as possible.

The Role of Epidemiology in Finance

What is the role of epidemiology in this discussion? It should be obvious that the use of epidemiologic data and information can help the financial manager forecast the costs associated with taking care of a defined population. More important, these data are capable of providing information that redirects the focus to activities of health promotion to areas that may have the greatest potential for health improvement and cost reduction.

The financial manager should use this information judiciously to evaluate areas with the greatest cost implications. It is important, at this juncture, to put on the wide-angle lenses discussed earlier and recognize the expanded role of the healthcare system. This expanded role means that, without exception, all aspects of life that have an impact on health must be considered in the health services equation. These include genes, individual behaviors, the physical and social environment, highways, intersections, roads without sidewalks, dangerous curves, speeding vehicles, and so on. The modern financial manager, who sees a much wider landscape of risk than his or her predecessors, must be able to forecast the costs associated with maximizing the health of a defined population and devise a reasonable pricing mechanism and structure to use in contract negotiations. This is no simple task.

It is extremely important for the financial manager and all key decision makers in the organization to have a clear objective in mind when negotiating contracts. If that objective is to maximize the health of the population, two premises must be acknowledged. First, all components of the health system are coproducers in the production of health. The payers, the providers, and the clients all play integral roles in the production function. They are a team, and must act as a team, in the production of health. Second, all parties to the transaction react to the incentives with which they are faced. This is rational, economic behavior. Therefore, it is important to ensure that any pricing and regulatory mechanism is evaluated with regard to appropriate incentives, so that incentives do not stand in the way of achieving the desired result.

Managed care has developed a long list of tools. This list includes utilization review, protocols and guidelines, preadmission certification, discharge planning, case management, capitation, and numerous other mechanisms. These mechanisms might appropriately be categorized as regulatory, legalistic, or financial. They create conditions wherein different parties to the interaction have incentives to act in specific ways. Most of them are designed to influence the behavior of the providers (guidelines, protocols, case management, formularies, capitation, fee schedules, and so on). Some are designed to influence the behavior of the client (copayments, use of gatekeepers, emergency room use restrictions) or the behaviors of the health plan or third-party payers.

One of the tools of managed care is capitation. This is the payment of a fixed amount on a per-member-per-month (PMPM) basis. Unfortunately, this tool has been used inappropriately to provide incentives that are sometimes at odds with the objectives of managed care. Capitation is designed to shift at least a portion of the financial risk associated with the health needs of a client onto the provider of health services. Capitation can be paid to a primary care physician or a specialist for a defined set of services, to a hospital, to a behavioral health organization, to a dentist, or to one or more of these in combination. When the capitation is paid separately to the different providers, incentives are created that may be at odds with the team requirements of managed care.

The future of capitation, at this point (2008), is unclear. Some would argue that it is on its deathbed, gasping for air, hoping to survive in some managed care markets. Others would argue that capitation needs a transplant, or intensive care, or something to rejuvenate the enthusiasm that characterized the 1990s. Still others would suggest that capitation simply needs a facelift, or augmentation, to make it more attractive to consumers of healthcare. The uncertainty of capitation notwithstanding, it is an approach to healthcare finance worthy of considerable study, particularly with regard to how epidemiology should be embraced. In short, we still need to "follow the risk," and capitation is an excellent case study, regardless of whether the exercise is historical, contemporary, or prophetic.

Capitation: An Introduction

Clearly, the move to capitation has sent ripples through the healthcare delivery system, not only in terms of financing, but also in patterns of delivery, access to care, and quality of outcomes. These effects are driven by provider incentives to perform healthcare services within a fixed PMPM budget constraint. The incentives encourage providers to use fewer resources (physician visits, diagnostic testing, hospital days) than are paid for by PMPM revenues. This can be accomplished in a number of ways, including process-of-care efficiencies and selection of risks. Newhouse (1998) argues that price competition in managed care should be based more on the former—efficient delivery of services—than on the latter—choosing less risky patients or procedures.

The process of enrolling in a capitated healthcare plan involves two kinds of choices: (1) choice of one plan from among a limited menu of plans by the consumer and (2) selection of members by capitated plans. Both kinds of choices can lead to selection bias, to the extent that patients with more or less risk of incurring healthcare costs either choose, or are chosen by, a capitated healthcare plan. Newhouse and colleagues (1989) distinguish between active and passive selection by the capitated plan. *Active selection* occurs as the plan proactively chooses lower-risk patients through the process of "cream skimming" or selective disenrollment strategies. *Passive selection* occurs if the plan is organized or marketed in such a way as either to attract lower-risk patients or repel higher-risk patients. This process of actively or passively segmenting risks (Giacomini, Luft, and Robinson 1995) implies conscious effort and activity to "choose" more profitable (or less costly) patients.

Giacomini, Luft, and Robinson (1995) suggest that plans can be made attractive to lower-risk patients by locating facilities in healthier areas and by featuring lower premiums (made possible by higher copays, less comprehensive services, exclusions for preexisting conditions, and restricted networks rather than free choice of providers). To the extent that this occurs, there can be favorable risk selection.

Adverse selection, on the other hand, occurs if capitated plans attract higher-than-average-risk patients because of the types of services offered, the cost-sharing arrangements, and the delivery network, in terms of choice and location of physicians and facilities.

Adverse selection is fueled by two concepts: moral hazard and information asymmetry. *Moral hazard* refers to the relationship between insurance and utilization. It poses a hazard to the insurance companies inasmuch as patients use more services if they have insurance. Whether this is amoral or immoral will be left up to the reader. Thus, the principle of moral hazard dictates that patients often choose insurance plans on the basis of expected use (Luft 1995). A high-risk patient will probably choose a capitated plan with comprehensive benefits and low cost-sharing based on the anticipation of using services in the future.

Adverse selection is also fueled by *information asymmetry*, in that not all parties to the relationship or interaction have access to the same kind and quality of information. To the extent that the patient and the capitated plan have access to a different level and quality of information regarding past and present health status, adverse selection may occur. Patients may withhold information regarding preexisting conditions, for instance, to secure enrollment in a healthcare plan at a premium that probably does not reflect their risk of using services.

The literature is unclear about whether capitation plans, such as health maintenance organizations (HMOs), experience adverse or favorable selection. Certainly, healthier patients are less likely to have forged strong ties with their providers and are more likely to switch to an HMO plan with which their physician may not be affiliated (Lubitz 1987). But the comprehensive nature and low cost-sharing of many HMO benefit packages are definitely attractive to the higher-risk patients.

A literature review by Hellinger (1987) concludes that HMOs do not experience favorable selection. Furthermore, measurement issues may cloud the results. The better health status of individuals enrolled in HMOs vis-à-vis fee-for-service plans means either favorable selection or successful health improvement activities directed to current members (Lubitz 1987).

The fear of adverse selection may also result in perverse effects on healthcare delivery. The chronically ill would benefit greatly from the coordinated care of many capitated plans. Unfortunately, these patients are viewed as high-risk patients whom the plan would prefer to avoid. Moreover, the temptation to compete on the basis of what Donabedian would refer to as "structure" quality (e.g., the new heart unit) is dampened by the harsh reality that patients may self-select into the plan with a view toward using these expensive services (Lubitz 1987).

The historical underpinnings of these selection issues are embodied in the "community rating" versus "experience rating" literature.

Community rating was the basis on which the original Blue Cross plans were founded. Under this approach, a single premium is based on the experience of all policyholders within a group, and they are all provided the same benefit package. The idea here is that low-risk groups or individuals subsidize high-risk groups. The result is not only a sharing of risks across individuals, but a transfer of income from the low-risk groups to the high-risk groups.

Community rating may be undesirable to low-risk individuals because the premium "price" to low-risk individuals is likely greater than the marginal costs of services consumed. The smart and healthy consumer will avoid this type of insurance—he or she may find a better value elsewhere. Community rating may be equitable if income redistribution is a policy objective and if one assumes that the high-risk groups tend to be poorer than the low-risk groups—although this is not always the case (Cave, Schweitzer, and Lachenbruch 1989).

Experience rating, on the other hand, purports to adjust premiums based on expected use, with the high-risk groups being charged higher rates than the low-risk groups. However, even if all relevant risk factors are identified and incorporated into premium differentials, random variation still occurs. After all, that is what insurance is all about.

The debate with experience rating is one of "actuarial fairness," that is, whether premiums should reflect expected use (Luft 1995). Actuarial fairness may come into conflict with our notions of equity, with what is fair and just and the right thing to do. Is it right for healthy people to pay less for their insurance than sickly people, or should all people pay the same price in order to support those members of society who need insurance the most? Adding to the debate is the notion that individuals are personally responsible for some risks—tobacco use or frequency of exercise, for example—but not for others—genetics, for example.

So how do these discussions of selection and risk segmentation affect the financial manager, who is responsible for negotiating capitated risk contracts? And how can an epidemiologic perspective be part of the solution?

If actuarial fairness is the operating assumption, then experience rating is the prescription. Premiums should be adjusted on the basis of expected use. This can be done three ways: retrospectively, using historical patterns of utilization; concurrently, based on morbidity profiles of the enrolled population; or prospectively, using risk factors for disease, such as high blood pressure, inactivity, lipids, and cholesterol. These will be discussed further in this chapter under the topic of risk adjustment.

On the other hand, equity may be an important policy objective of the organization. This would mean the organization desires to subsidize those with a heavy burden of illness by reducing their healthcare premiums below the actuarially fair level. If this were to occur only within and not across healthcare plans, this community rating solution would place some healthcare plans (i.e., those that attract high-risk patients) at a serious disadvantage. Their rates would likely be unattractive to healthier patients. On the other hand, if the burden were shared across healthcare plans, the risks could be spread around. Extra money could somehow be captured from the higher-risk populations and distributed to the plans according to their share of high-risk patients. In this case, a much larger group would bear the burden of serious illness and the community-rated premiums would be more tolerable to the healthy. Under this approach it would be necessary for the healthcare plan to apply the tools of epidemiology to assess the morbidity and risk factors of its enrolled population, with a view to identifying the high-risk pool and capturing extra money from it.

A number of policy or management tools might be useful in limiting the extent to which risk selection occurs across healthcare plans (Kronick, Zhou, and Dreyfus 1995). A third-party agency may be necessary to manage enrollment while enforcing guaranteed issue and renewability provisions. This would provide the checks and balances among plans regarding enrollment and reenrollment applications. The same agency could monitor disenrollment to prevent plans from dumping their sickest members. A standardized benefit package would prevent plans from designing benefits specifically to attract the healthier risks or to discourage high risks. Community rating of some sort would ensure that plans do not avoid the higher-risk population by charging exorbitant premiums. Oversight of marketing strategies would ensure that plans are not intentionally catering to the better risks while discouraging the sickest. Finally, the publication of consumer satisfaction and quality information would promote accountability.

Community and experience rating may involve social policy questions, which will not be discussed further. However, the adjustment of capitation rates to reflect different population risk characteristics is pertinent. The following sections will discuss capitation and methods of risk adjustment.

Capitation Basics

The revenues generated by a capitated healthcare plan are derived from fixed monthly premiums (PMPM) collected from enrollees or their employers. Financial solvency, therefore, depends on keeping per capita costs at or below these levels. Per capita costs are driven by at least three factors: population risk, efficiency, and quality of services (Giacomini, Luft, and Robinson 1995). Thus, costs can be lowered by enrolling a healthier population (lower population risk), increasing efficiency, or modifying quality.

Selective enrollment was discussed earlier—strong financial incentives exist to enroll the healthier patients. The value of information about the client cannot be overstated in this instance. The more information about enrollees the organization has, the better it can forecast health status, establish mechanisms for providing for health, and plan for the associated costs.

Efficiencies may involve providing more cost-effective services or eliminating marginally less-effective services. It may also involve substituting less costly but equally effective resources—nurse practitioners for physicians, for instance.

Striving for efficiency is hazardous when the necessary and marginally effective services are eliminated, either intentionally or in ignorance. Therein lies the well-known dilemma: how to distinguish between essential and superfluous services.

This issue also encompasses prevention activities. In the past, the refrain was always, "No one pays for prevention." In a capitated environment, however, preventive programs such as smoking cessation and weight loss are profitable if these programs result in lower costs to the managed care organization in the long run. A related, yet important, issue is the question of how much long-term benefit an HMO can capture from preventive activities, given the proclivity of employers to switch insurers over time. If half of a plan's smokers switch insurers every five years, will the HMO find it financially worthwhile to offer free smoking cessation courses to members?

Per capita costs are also related to quality, although the relationship is far from simple (Fleming 1991; Fleming and Boles 1994). Improvements in quality may be costly, particularly if they involve substituting new technologies.

In addition, in this chapter we have been stressing the additional risks to be dealt with on a proactive basis: genetic risks, biological risks, behavioral risks, and environmental risks. These risks pose the danger of additional costs, together with opportunities for cost reduction.

Because the focus of this chapter is on the use of epidemiology in healthcare finance, we will not describe in detail the concepts of efficiency, quality, and cost, although the excellent work of Donabedian, Wheeler, and Wyszewianski (1982) would be the place to start.

Population risk, however, should be explored in more detail, for it is a major purpose of epidemiology. Manton, Tolley, and Vertrees (1989) discuss financial risk within the context of health maintenance organizations, making the distinction between random and systemic variation. *Random variation* represents the totally unexplainable and unpredictable acts of God, for which the concept of insurance was originally designed. One cannot control or adjust for random variation, only expect and prepare for it. Stop-loss, risk-pooling, and reinsurance mechanisms are three ways in which the industry copes with this kind of uncertainty.

Systemic variation, on the other hand, refers to the potentially explainable uncertainty that relates to beneficiary characteristics (e.g., age, sex, and comorbidities), as well as to differences in treatment strategies, provider costs, and treatment location (Manton, Tolley, and Vertrees 1989). Differences in treatment strategies have been well-studied by Wennberg

(Wennberg and Gittelsohn 1973) and others, resulting in specific methodologies for small area variation studies. Provider costs depend on the cost of resource inputs and on the efficiencies with which they are combined; for instance, location determines local wage level, among other things.

Our concern, from an epidemiologic point of view, is with beneficiary characteristics and the extent to which these characteristics can predict resource use. A critical question is the proportion of total financial risk (and associated costs) that is predictable. Newhouse and colleagues have estimated that we can expect to explain only 20 percent (Newhouse 1982) or 14.5 percent (Newhouse et al. 1989) of healthcare expenditures unless they are outpatient expenditures, in which case the proportion is higher, up to 50 percent (Newhouse et al. 1989). We believe that a greater percentage can be predicted when we approach the management of the different risk forms proactively. At the present time, however, this is only a hypothesis to be tested. In the meantime, we present a capitation calculation model that can be used to determine this risk adjustment. The following section discusses the use of risk information to adjust capitation rates.

Risk Adjustment: The Basics

Giacomini, Luft, and Robinson (1995) describe *risk* as a population's innate need for, and propensity to use, healthcare services, whereas Hornbrook and Goodman (1991) describe risk in a more traditional economic sense as the "expected value of the distribution of per capita costs of efficiently produced preventive, diagnostic, and therapeutic healthcare services delivered to a defined group of enrollees for a specific future period." Earlier we described four kinds of risk: genetic, biological, behavioral, and environmental.

In any case, risk represents "burden" to the capitated system in terms of future expenditures. The question here is whether, and how, one can use population-based and epidemiologically derived risk factors to "adjust" capitation payments to reflect the burden of present and future illness. The purpose of risk-adjusting capitation payments would be to "level the playing field" with regard to patients and force capitated plans to concentrate on efficiencies and quality of care rather than on the selection of healthier patients.

A population can be broken down into four basic groups (Robinson 1993), each with different epidemiologic features: (1) healthy people using few if any medical services, (2) relatively healthy people who are not hospitalized, but use some ambulatory services, (3) people who are hospitalized for routine or nonrecurrent admissions, and (4) high-cost users of inpatient and outpatient services.

Although each of these groups consists of a heterogeneous mix of clinical conditions, a similar epidemiology may exist within groups, and different ways of capturing the burden of illness may occur across groups.

Group 4, for instance, is likely to be composed of many people with chronic illness, for whom inpatient diagnoses may be important predictors of future expenditures. It is important, however, to attempt to identify the most likely future candidates for group 4 in order to take actions to delay or eliminate their entry into group 4. These diagnoses may be less important in predicting group 3 expenses, given the nonrecurrent or "acute" nature of the hospital episode. It may be very difficult to predict the expenses for group 1, whose illnesses would fall within the category of random rather than systemic variation, as discussed earlier.

Clinical conditions within these four groups are categorized as preventable and nonpreventable. Preventable exposures, such as those associated with food and waterborne illness and communicable diseases, can all be managed to some extent. Trauma cases might be reduced through a variety of actions, discussed previously.

It is also important to recognize that the population of each of the four categories is not stable—that is, over time, individuals move from one category to the next. The lowest-cost category is the first, the highest the last. It could very well be, however, that increased expenditures on individuals in the first category may slow their progression into the higher-cost categories.

Manton, Tolley, and Vertrees (1989) describe a number of distinct beneficiary characteristics that are probably related to utilization of services and that potentially could be used to risk-adjust capitation payments. These include health-related characteristics, demographic and social characteristics, prior use of health services, and mortality (as an index of severity).

Health-related characteristics are those that pertain to the mix of diseases and disorders of an enrolled population—call them disease pro files. The case-mix measure used by the Medicare prospective payment system provides one example, where a resource-related weight is assigned to each hospitalized patient on the basis of diagnosis-related group (DRG), and the case-mix index is simply the average of all of these weights.

Conceivably, one could develop case-mix weights for a capitated population on the basis of the "burden of illness" as it relates to expected resource use. Ideally, this measure should go beyond the presence or absence of a set of diagnoses to include such things as severity of illness and response to treatment (Manton, Tolley, and Vertrees 1989). An elderly patient may have a physiological response to illness that is different from that of a younger patient—the former reflected in higher resource use. Demographic characteristics could include such classic epidemiologic variables as age and sex, which are consistently predictive of both resource use and patterns of illness. Socioeconomic status is a rich variable that reflects a complex set of environmental risks and behavioral risks, such as neighborhood environment, housing, and preferences for and access to healthcare. Prior use of healthcare is related to its future use as a proxy for chronicity of illness. The employment of prior use as an adjuster to capitated rates, however, is not without its critics. Past inefficient patterns of healthcare delivery may be perpetuated if capitated plans are rewarded for such behaviors, i.e., if overuse of physician services, such as follow-up visits, represents inefficiency in the delivery of care and not burden of illness. Mortality can be used to adjust capitation rates as an index of illness severity and to recognize the high cost of end-of-life care.

Other beneficiary characteristics of interest should include health status factors, obtained perhaps through health status surveys, and clinical risk factors, such as smoking and genetic screenings, that are precursors to illness (Giacomini, Luft, and Robinson 1995).

Health status surveys are useful for to obtaining information from the patient. Hornbrook (1999) discusses surveys, but cautions that they may be subject to misrepresentation or gaming. Clearly, patients have an incentive to overestimate their health status if they are facing the burden of a higher premium. Patients have been misrepresenting preexisting conditions for years to avoid higher premiums. Alternatively, Hornbrook asserts, patients may be coached by providers to deflate health status scores if that results in a larger third-party payment to the provider (e.g., from Medicare). Thus, any attempt to incorporate self-reported health status scores may result in a kind of "health status creep," similar in concept to the "DRG creep" that occurred during the 1980s, where the "case mix" among some hospitals crept into DRGs for which reimbursement was higher.

Clinical risk factors may also be used to adjust capitated payments. However, only some of these may be available on existing databases or patient records. From an epidemiologic standpoint, risk factors represent an "upstream" rather than a "midstream" kind of adjustment. According to Figure 8.2, risk factors lead to the onset of disease in a certain proportion of cases. This is captured by the epidemiologist's notion of relative risk—how many times more likely you are to have cardiovascular problems if you are a smoker, for example. Cardiovascular disease as a morbidity in prevalence data is then associated with the risk of future inpatient and ambulatory care services. Presumably then, capitated payments can be adjusted upward to reflect both increased risk factor burden and increased disease burden.

Schauffler, Howland, and Cobb (1992) suggest that chronic disease risk factors, such as cigarette smoking (behavioral risk), systolic blood pressure (genetic risk, environmental risk), cholesterol level (genetic risk, behavioral risk), and blood glucose level (genetic risk, behavioral risk) may be used to adjust Medicare capitation. Using Framingham data on 1,162 persons, these authors explained 5 to 6.5 percent of the variance in Medicare Parts A and B payments with chronic risk factors alone. They suggest that these measures are strongly associated with chronic disease and are predictive of future expenses. They can be objectively measured and verified, although there may be a perverse incentive for managed care organizations to reduce health promotion and prevention in the elderly if capitation is somehow tied to the prevalence of these chronic risk factors. The challenge is to develop a way to risk-adjust capitation by taking into consideration chronic risk factors (that should be predictive of future expense) while, at the same time, rewarding those providers whose programs decrease the prevalence of these risk factors among enrollees.

Figure 8.2 also suggests that morbidity is a beneficiary characteristic that is related to future costs and can be used to risk-adjust capitated payments. Morbidity is an epidemiologic concept, and prevalence is the direct measure of disease burden. One would expect chronic illness to be a better predictor of future expense than acute illness, unless, of course, the acute illness has been found to result in long-term complications or future morbidity (for example, strep throat and rheumatic fever). One can measure morbidity by inpatient and ambulatory diagnoses that are recorded on insurance claims. These data are a rich source of morbidity information that are routinely collected by third-party payers such as Medicare. Since the data are a secondary source of information collected by others, primarily for the purpose of documenting financial information, they are subject to a number of biases related to the methods by which they are collected and to underlying incentives. In short, claims data are not without problems and limitations (Fleming and Kohrs 1998).

In a literature review of risk factors, Giacomini, Luft, and Robinson (1995) reported that 1 to 4 percent of the variances in healthcare expenditures were explained by age and gender; 3 to 6 percent by self-reported health status; 5 to 11 percent by physiologic measures; and 4 to 21 percent by prior use, which included inpatient diagnoses. Using up to three years of hospital diagnoses would improve predictability even more, according to a study of the Netherlands Sickness Fund by Lamers (1999).

Hornbrook (1999) suggested that ambulatory diagnoses should be even more predictive of expenses than hospital diagnoses, for several reasons.

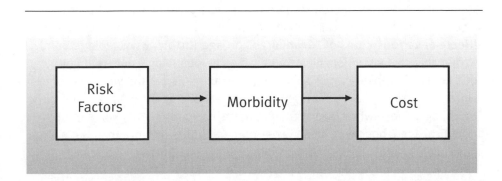

FIGURE 8.2
Risk Factors, Morbidity, and Cost

First, the diagnoses represent a burden of disease that may be missed by inpatient claims only. Second, there is probably less variation in ambulatory expenses vis-à-vis inpatient expenses because ambulatory care is more frequent and typically less expensive. And, finally, many chronic diseases involve continuing care patterns, a large part of which occur in an ambulatory setting.

Newhouse (1998) describes a number of reasons why risk adjustment is difficult to accomplish. First, insurers are reluctant to charge higher premiums to high-risk members. Although this is the crux of experience rating, our charitable nature goes against forcing those with chronic disease or preexisting conditions to pay exorbitant premiums. Second, if we want the bad risks and good risks to pay the same premium, then some fourth party is needed to redistribute money from healthcare plans with proportionately fewer bad risks to those with proportionately more of them. Furthermore, it may be costly to get reliable data that predict spending, and, even if these adjusters can be obtained, they may distort provider behavior. For example, inpatient diagnoses may be more reliable than ambulatory ones, but we would not want to create incentives to hospitalize patients for the purpose of boosting capitation. Also, to the extent that risk adjusters are derived from fee-for-service (FFS) claims databases, they may not reflect optimal patterns of care in non-FFS settings. Moreover, if physicians or healthcare plans have just slightly more information on enrollee health status than the risk-adjustment formula has, there remains considerable incentive to profit through cream skimming or dumping patients. Finally, with regard to geographic variation in treatment costs, it may be difficult to disentangle true health status differences in the population from differences in practice patterns. Case Study 8.1 examines various kinds of risk factors that might be included in capitation rates.

Case Study 8.1. Incorporating Health Risks into Capitation Rates

Apparently it is possible to estimate the effects of malicious and protective exposures on survival by calculating a "real age," which takes into account the effects of various kinds of "exposures" on age (http://www.realage.com). Presumably, these relationships are based on epidemiologic data that link various kinds of exposures with survival. For example, a person who sleeps, on average, 6.5 to 7.5 hours per night can subtract one year from his or her biological age. Those who sleep 7.5 to 8.5 hours can subtract 0.5 years from the biological age. Those who sleep fewer than 6.5 hours or more than 8.5 hours must add 0.5 and 1.5 years to the biological age, respectively (Roizen 2000).

Because many of these exposures are related to increased morbidity as well, managed care organizations may want to consider the extent to which capitation should be adjusted for members with some of these exposures. Suppose the chief financial officer of a managed care organization plans to incorporate health risks into its capitation rates.

QUESTIONS

1. Categorize some of the exposures in the box below as genetic, biological, behavioral, and environmental risk factors (find at least one in each category).
2. Which of these exposures are linked to both morbidity and mortality?

Exposures that affect real-age calculation

General health/demographics
self-reported health
   status
educational level
employment status
income
amount sleep
height
weight

Nutrition
breakfasts per week
breads, rice, pasta
fiber
fruits
vegetables
dairy products
red meats
tomato-based foods
fish
nuts
soy products
vitamins

Stress and social support
caregiver or give med-
   ical advice
marital status
pets
no. close friends
no. in household
no. children in household
satisfied with sex life
attend church
stressful events
unemployed, etc.
group membership
parents divorced,
   separated?

Medications
aspirin daily
no. prescriptions daily
no. over-the-counter
   drugs daily

Physical activities
aerobics, etc.
strength training
flexibility training
other strenuous
   training
sore joints

Medical history
parents age when died
heart rate
blood pressure
cholesterol
HDL cholesterol
weight fluctuations
ever have or treated
   for clogged arteries
asthma
heart attack
stroke
cirrhosis
diabetes
kidney disease
periodontal disease
list of other medical
   conditions
lifestyle and safety

SOURCE: http://www.realage.com.

3. For which of these exposures can the member be held liable in terms of increased premiums?
4. How can the managed care organization guarantee the accuracy of the reporting of these exposures?
5. How can the managed care organization know if a member has changed an exposure level in some area?

ANSWERS

1. Genetic risk factors include age when parents died. Biological risk factors include such exposures as height and weight. Behavioral risk factors include activities such as attending church, aerobics, nutrition, wearing seat belts, driving a motorcycle, and smoking. Environmental risk factors include secondhand smoke. Some of these exposures could be classified in more than one category, such as cholesterol level, which is influenced by both genetic and behavioral factors.
2. Many of these exposures are linked to either morbidity or mortality in the literature. Some links are obvious, such as the relationship between cholesterol and heart disease, or smoking and lung cancer. Others are associated with the risk of injury (and mortality), such as the use of seat belts, air bags, or motorcycles. Fruits, vegetables, fiber, and fish have been associated with a lower risk of some diseases, while dairy products and meats have been associated with an increased risk of disease. Social variables, such as education level, employment status, and marital status have also been studied with regard to the risk of disease.
3. The debate over which risk factors could be included in premium structures is based in part on whether you believe that healthcare is a right or privilege, and in part on whether you think that consumers should be penalized for both unhealthy behaviors and unhealthy conditions, such as either biological or genetic risk factors. Most would probably agree that consumers ought not to be penalized for conditions over which they have no control, such as a faulty gene associated with cancer. Some would argue that consumers ought to be penalized for behaviors over which they have some control, such as smoking. The gray area of dispute is on health conditions with both genetic and behavioral components, such as obesity and high cholesterol.
4. These data would probably be difficult and expensive to obtain. A periodic survey instrument is one possibility. It would be extremely challenging, however, for the organization to guarantee the accuracy of these data. There would be a motive to game the system by underreporting unhealthy behaviors and other factors when it becomes clear that these exposures affect premiums.
5. It would be difficult for the managed care organization to know if a member has changed any of these exposures, except through a comprehensive, and certainly intrusive, monitoring system. Clinical indicators such as heart rate, blood pressure, or cholesterol level could be followed with clinic records. Biological markers for smoking, alcohol, or drug abuse are another possi-

bility. Most of the exposures categorized under physical activities, nutrition, and lifestyle and safety would be impossible to accurately track.

Adjusting Capitation Rates

If we are to avoid some of the perverse incentives regarding risk segmentation and selective enrollment, it may be necessary to risk-adjust capitation rates and design a methodology to charge community-rated premiums to enrollees by subsidizing higher-risk plans through some redistributive mechanism. If we assume that a community-rated premium is desirable, then the high-risk plans (i.e., those with sicker patients) will get more per member per month than the quoted premiums. In other words, they will have to be subsidized by the low-risk plans through some fund-distribution mechanism or fourth party. Thus, according to Giacomini, Luft, and Robinson (1995), risk adjustment will raise the "effective price" of the low-risk plans as it lowers the "effective price" of the high-risk plans.

The previous section discussed risk adjustment and described a number of potential risk adjusters. If the goal is to charge enrollees a similar community rate premium across healthcare plans, then it will be necessary to employ a risk-adjustment method to calculate the degree to which enrollee expected costs exceed or fall short of this premium. One method is to associate a marginal excess premium with each risk factor (e.g., smoking or a specific type of morbidity). The excess premium would represent the degree to which a high-risk enrollee is expected to incur costs in excess of the community-rated premium. These marginal excess premiums would be distributed to the high-risk plans from high-cost condition pools. Contributions to the high-cost condition pools would be derived from the "taxation" of low-risk plans, which would donate "marginal deficit premiums" to the pool. Alternatively, one could use general revenues, such as state or federal income taxes, to stock the high-cost pools with funds. The assumption with all of this, of course, is that social health insurance rather than actuarial fairness is the desirable objective (Giacomini, Luft, and Robinson 1995).

The question of whether or not capitation premiums should be risk-adjusted does not have a simple answer. Clearly, unadjusted capitation rates create incentives to attract low-risk enrollees and to disenroll the high-risk members. Adjustments to these rates would reduce the risk of enrolling an atypical population. This would be more attractive to providers of care (Manton, Tolley, and Vertrees 1989) and would perhaps prevent some health plans with higher-risk populations from leaving the market (Rogal and Gauthier 1998). On the other hand, capitation systems are supposed to create incentives different from those created by a fee-for-service system. If incentives are created only through risk, one might question how much risk adjustment would compromise managed care. As managed care markets mature, however,

TABLE 8.1
Hierarchical
Coexisting
Conditions
and
Incremental
Payment
Weights

| HCC | Example | Incremental Payment | |
		Diagnoses	With procedures
High-Cost Infectious Diseases	AIDS	$4,116	$3,045
High-Cost Cancers	lung cancer	4,226	3,457
High-Cost Nervous System	MS	1,556	1,436
Cardiac Arrest/Shock	—	1,759	1,271
Congestive Heart Failure	—	3,063	2,873
Coronary Artery Disease	angina pectoris	1,049	995
Respiratory Arrest	—	9,282	6,561
COPD	emphysema	1,555	1,448
Higher-Cost Pneumonia	pneumoccoal	2,943	2,673
Hip and verebral fractures	—	1,109	998

the relative profitability of improvements in efficiency may decrease. With no more "fat" left in the system, the relative profitability of risk selection would rise (Giacomini, Luft, and Robinson 1995). Risk-adjusted capitated rates would at least mitigate the process by which plans are forced to look for good risks in order to have a healthy bottom line.

Ellis and colleagues (1996) developed and tested a methodology using diagnosis and procedure information on claims data to risk-adjust the Medicare capitation payment known as the adjusted average per capita cost. Ellis and colleagues used total Medicare program expenditures for 1991 and 1992 on a 5 percent sample of Medicare beneficiaries. These expenses included hospital inpatient, outpatient, physician, home health, hospice, skilled nursing facility, laboratory, durable medical equipment, and other services. The basic approach used principal inpatient diagnoses from the preceding year as risk adjusters. One extension to this approach added secondary diagnoses from inpatient and outpatient claims, with the individual classified by the highest cost diagnosis. Another extension adjusted for the presence of multiple comorbidities by developing a hierarchy of coexisting conditions. A third extension included life-sustaining medical procedures. A final extension attempted to predict both concurrent (same year) and prospective (subsequent year) expenses. The hierarchy of coexisting conditions models actually aggregate the marginal predicted cost payments for each coexisting condition to get a total payment. Ellis and colleagues found that the inpatient diagnosis model explained about 5.53 percent of the total variance in expenditures, whereas the most robust model with hierarchical coexisting conditions and inpatient diagnoses, procedures, age, and sex explained 9.01 percent of the variance.

The Ellis methodology is particularly interesting because it suggests an epidemiological approach to adjusting capitation payments based on the prevalence of multiple comorbid conditions. The approach could essentially derive a type of marginal excess premium, described earlier: that high-risk plans could be reimbursed from a high-cost illness pool of some sort. Table 8.1 illustrates the incremental payments derived by Ellis and colleagues for ten illustrative conditions. Using a different methodology, Case Study 8.2 illustrates how incremental payments could be derived for two risk factors (smoking and obesity).

Case Study 8.2. Group Health East: Risk Factors and Capitation Rates

Group Health East (GHE) decides to incorporate two risk factors into the capitation rates that are charged to area employers. The risk factors are smoking and obesity (defined as a body mass index of at least 30). GHE wants to differentiate among obese members who are physically active versus those who are not. Each of these two risk factors has been linked to coronary heart disease (CHD), and each of these factors can be reduced in a population through behavioral and/or pharmaceutical intervention. Assume that the prevalence of smoking in GHE is 30 percent and that 25 percent of the members are considered obese (and only 20 percent of these are physically active). Assume that the ten-year incidence rate of CHD is 50 per 1,000 for both non smokers and those who are not obese, 100 per 1,000 for smokers, 175 per 1,000 for those who are obese and physically inactive, and 100 per 1,000 for those who are obese and physically active. Assume that the average cost of being hospitalized with CHD is about $7,500, and that patients with CHD have a 20 percent annual risk of being hospitalized. Further assume that each CHD member visits a physician once a year for CHD, with an average cost of $150 per visit.

QUESTIONS

1. Of the 100,000 members in GHE, how many smoke, are obese and physically active, and are obese and physically inactive?
2. For those who do not smoke or are not obese, what is the actual risk of developing CHD over the ten-year period?
3. For those who smoke or are obese, what is the actual risk of developing CHD over the ten-year period?
4. What is the additional risk of CHD (attributable risk, Chapter 11) of being either a smoker or obese?
5. By comparing the ten-year CHD incidence rates of either smokers or obese GHE members to those without either of those conditions (one rate divided by the other), how many times more likely is CHD among those who either smoke or are obese compared to members who do not smoke or are not obese (Chapter 12)?

6. Of the members who smoke, (1) how many should develop CHD over a ten-year period, (2) how many would have developed CHD even if they had not smoked, and (3) how much CHD among these members could be directly attributed to smoking?

7. Of the members who are obese and physically inactive, (1) how many should develop CHD over a ten-year period, (2) how many would have developed CHD even if they were not obese and physically inactive, and (3) how much CHD among these members could be directly attributed to being obese and physically inactive?

8. Of the members who are obese and physically active, (1) how many should develop CHD over a ten-year period, (2) how many would have developed CHD even if they were not obese, and (3) how much CHD among these members could be directly attributed to obesity?

9. With this simple example, what would be the additional costs incurred by members who develop CHD?

10. Use your answers from questions 8 and 9 to calculate (1) the total additional costs of CHD that can be directly attributed to either smoking or obesity and (2) the average additional costs of CHD to members in each of those risk categories.

11. With this simple example, how much more should GHE charge area employers for members who have either of these risk factors?

12. Why are the additional premiums for smokers (from question 11) less than you might expect?

13. What interventions could GHE implement to reduce the three risk factors?

14. The relationship between risk factors and disease is probabilistic. Only some people with these risk factors will develop disease. The time lag between exposure and disease onset is uncertain. The onset of a cost-related event, such as acute myocardial infarction, may (or may not) occur at some near (or distant) time in the future. Would this capitation system based on the prevalence of risk factors be "actuarially fair?"

ANSWERS

1. Of the 100,000 members, $0.30 \times 100,000 = 30,000$ are smokers, $0.25 \times 100,000 = 25,000$ are considered obese, and of the obese, $0.20 \times 25,000 = 5,000$ are physically active and 20,000 are physically inactive.

2. The actual risk of developing CHD among those who do not smoke or are not obese is $50/1,000 = 5\%$.

3. For smokers, $100/1,000 = 10\%$ will develop CHD over the ten years. Of the physically inactive obese, $175/1,000 = 17.5\%$ will develop CHD over the 10 years. Of the physically active obese, $100/1,000 = 10\%$ will develop CHD over the ten years.

4. The additional risk for a smoker is $10\% - 5\% = 5\%$. The additional risk for those who are obese and physically inactive is $17.5\% - 5\% = 12.5\%$. The additional risk for those who are obese but physically active is $10\% - 5\% = 5\%$.

5. Smokers are $[(100/1,000)/(50/1,000)] = 2$ times as likely to develop CHD over a ten-year period than those who don't smoke and are not obese. Obese members who are physically inactive are $[(175/1,000)/(50/1,000)] = 3.5$ times as likely to develop CHD than nonobese, nonsmoking members, while obese members who are physically active are $[(100/1,000)/(50/1,000)] = 2$ times as likely to develop CHD than nonobese nonsmokers.

6. Of the 30,000 smokers, $0.10 \times 30,000 = 3,000$ will develop CHD. Of these same smokers, $0.05 \times 30,000 = 1,500$ of them would have developed CHD even if they had not smoked. Therefore $3,000 - 1,500 = 1,500$ cases of CHD could be directly attributed to smoking.

7. Of the 20,000 physically inactive obese members, $0.175 \times 20,000 = 3,500$ will develop CHD. Of these same members, $0.05 \times 20,000 = 1,000$ of them would have developed CHD even if they were not obese. Therefore $3,500 - 1,000 = 2,500$ cases of CHD could be directly attributed to obesity among those who are physically inactive.

8. Of the 5,000 physically active obese members, $0.10 \times 5,000 = 500$ will develop CHD. Of these same members, $0.05 \times 5,000 = 250$ of them would have developed CHD even if they were not obese. Therefore $500 - 250 = 250$ cases of CHD could be directly attributed to obesity among the physically active.

9. Members who develop CHD will incur a cost of $150 for a CHD-related physician visit, and have a 20% risk of being hospitalized at a cost of $7,500. Therefore, for every five members with CHD each year, one will be hospitalized ($7,500), and all five will visit the physician ($5 \times \$150 = \$750$), for a total of $\$8,250/5 = \$1,650$ per person.

10. Among the 30,000 smokers, there would be 1,500 cases attributed to smoking, at a cost of $1,650 per case, $2,475,000 total costs, or $2,475,000/30,000 = \$82.50$ per smoker. Among the 20,000 physically inactive obese members, there would be 2,500 cases of CHD directly attributed to obesity among the physically inactive, at a cost of $1,650 per case, $4,125,000 total costs, or $4,125,000/20,000 = \$206.25$ per obese member who is physically inactive. Among the 5,000 physically active obese members, there would be 250 cases of CHD directly attributed to obesity among the physically active, at a cost of $1,650 per case, $412,500 total costs, or $412,500/5,000 = \$82.50$ per obese member who is physically active.

11. It would appear that employers of smokers should be charged an additional $82.50, while employers of the obese should be charged either an additional $82.50 or $206.25, depending on whether the member is physically active.

12. This analysis only considers the impact of smoking on the risks and costs of CHD. Smoking also affects the risks of lung cancer, pancreatic cancer, hypertension, and a number of other diseases, each of which would increase the risk of future costs due to morbidity.

13. Smoking cessation programs are the obvious solution to reduce the prevalence of smoking. The relative effectiveness of these programs is discussed in more detail in Chapter 14. Weight reduction programs can be targeted at

obese members in the plan; however, the relative effectiveness of these programs in terms of sustained weight loss is still under debate. Nevertheless, physical activity is desirable irrespective of sustained weight loss.

14. One of the problems with this approach is that future morbidity that can be attributed to these risk factors may occur years in the future, perhaps after members have switched to other plans. Current managed care plans would benefit from the additional premiums of these members, while other plans would have to endure the costs of this future morbidity.

Pay for Performance

Programs to improve the quality of healthcare have been around for decades (Chapter 5). The most recent innovation is pay for performance (P4P). These programs are well-entrenched in U.S. payment systems, including health maintenance organizations, Medicare, and Medicaid. With P4P, the quality of healthcare is measured and linked to payment, such that superior quality is rewarded and inferior quality is not. These programs come in a variety of "colors" and "flavors." A typical program would use the Healthcare Effectiveness Data and Information Set measures discussed in Chapter 5 to categorize providers as good, fair, or poor. The good providers enjoy a bonus in reimbursement (say, 1 percent or 2 percent), and the poor providers suffer a loss (e.g., 1 percent or 2 percent).

Rosenthal and Dudley (2007) describe five key design elements in these programs. The first element relates to whether the programs are aimed at individual physicians or a "group" of physicians. The authors argue for a mixed approach, with some incentives/penalties flowing to or from the individual, and some to or from the group. For example, rewards that are linked to behaviors that are directly under the control of the physician, such as smoking cessation, should flow directly to the physician.

The second design element relates to the "right amount" to pay, walking the fine line between spending as little money as possible and ineffectiveness. Economic theory, according to Rosenthal and Dudley (2007), suggests that the reward should equal the additional cost of the necessary quality improvement.

The third design element is the performance measures. They should be measures that have a "high impact" on patient care, rather than those that are just widely available. Since performance incentives may lead to quality improvement in the areas that are measured, it is important to determine whether such measures should relate to clinical quality, cost efficiency, information technology, or patient satisfaction (Rosenthal and Dudley 2007).

The fourth design element relates to the scope of the incentive program, that is, what proportion of "top performers" will be rewarded.

The final design element relates to how the P4P programs prioritize improvement in underserved populations, where the costs of improvement may be greater due to "patients' geographic, linguistic, educational, financial, or other barriers" (Rosenthal and Dudley 2007, 743).

Breakeven Analysis

Breakeven analysis is a common tool used by financial managers to demonstrate the volume of goods or services that must be sold in order for the organization to break even, that is, for revenues to equal expenses.

Boles and Fleming (1997) demonstrate that the concept of breakeven analysis within a capitation environment is complex, and that the incentives with regard to utilization rate in fee-for-services and capitation are diametrically opposed. The authors show that breakeven analysis in a normal fee-for-service environment is relatively stable and straightforward, with net income (revenues minus expenses) increasing as long as the number of patients or the utilization rate of existing patients increases. In a managed care environment, however, breakeven analysis is more dynamic, "driven by the utilization rate of existing enrollees and the cost per unit of utilization" (Boles and Fleming 1997).

With fee-for-service, breakeven analysis can be represented by a two-dimensional graph, with revenues/expenses on the y-axis and volume on the x-axis. Both revenues and expenses increase with volume, and the point at which the lines intersect—where the revenue line crosses the expenses line—represents the breakeven point. With capitation, breakeven is a three-dimensional concept, with revenues/expenses on one axis and number of enrollees and utilization on the other two. Total revenues increase as membership increases. Total costs increase with both membership and utilization rates. Thus, as utilization rates increase, the number of enrollees required for breakeven increases exponentially, rather than linearly. Furthermore, net income, or profit, increases with either increasing membership or decreasing utilization rate. The authors contend that it makes sense to view the three-dimensional breakeven analysis as a "trajectory over time" that relates profits to the future growth of the organization.

The breakeven formulations in either a fee-for-service or capitation environment make a number of assumptions regarding economics and epidemiology. With regard to economics, one must assume that the expenses incurred by the organization are determined by production, that is, how many patients are treated, what supplies are consumed, etc. The efficiency with which organizations and/or physicians choose, combine, and sequence resources, such as doctors, nurses, pharmaceuticals, and imaging technology, determines the costs that are incurred.

Insofar as epidemiology is concerned, the breakeven model makes no distinction among patients in terms of morbidity or disease severity. It may assume a nonlinear relationship between cost and volume of patients treated, so that it is proportionately more or less costly to increase volume. Presumably one could expand the three-dimensional breakeven model to include a fourth dimension, say, case mix. In this case, one could show that the breakeven point increases as case mix or disease severity increases.

Another approach would be to weigh volume (i.e., membership) by some measure of case mix or resource use. Giacomini, Luft, and Robinson (1995), for instance, suggest that one could associate a relative risk with each risk factor or risk-adjuster, such as those described earlier in this chapter. In this case, the relative risk has a financial rather than epidemiologic meaning. A relative risk of 1.2 would mean that the risk factor is likely to be associated with costs exceeding the "average" by 20 percent. This would be useful only for enrollees with one or no risk factors, in which case the volume for breakeven analysis would be the aggregated sum of the relative risks. For patients with multiple risk factors, one would have to combine this relative-risk concept with the hierarchical coexisting conditions method discussed in the last section and determine a way to assign a relative risk to each patient enrolled in the managed care organization. Breakeven analysis would simply aggregate these relative risks and represent the total as the volume of patients or membership.

Summary

We have described a changing, perhaps more colorful, and certainly expansive healthcare landscape, over which managed care has redirected the focus from sick patients to healthy populations. The fissures and faults of risk have been categorized as genetic, behavioral, environmental, and biological, with the burden placed on financial managers to recognize and measure the seismic potential of these exposures. We have described the basic principles of capitation, the problem of adverse selection, and the potential to incorporate risk into the process of setting capitation rates. The measurement of risk for the purpose of developing risk-adjusted capitation rates can include both upstream and midstream features. Upstream measures of risk include exposures of genetic, behavioral, environmental, and biological risk that make the insured more or less likely to develop disease and incur costs to the healthcare system. Midstream measures include measures of current morbidity burden. Even if we could develop these sophisticated systems to measure disease profiles, the more poignant question is, should we?

References

Boles, K. E., and S. T. Fleming. 1997. "Why Traditional Breakeven Analysis Doesn't Work with Managed Care." *Health Care Systems Economics Report* 1 (9): 7–12.

Cave, D. G., S. O. Schweitzer, and P. A. Lachenbruch. 1989. "Adjusting Employer Group Capitation Premiums by Community Rating by Class Factors." *Medical Care* 27 (9): 887–99.

Donabedian, A., J. R. C. Wheeler, and L. Wyszewianski. 1982. "Quality, Cost, and Health: An Integrative Model." *Medical Care* 20 (10): 975–92.

Ellis, R. P., G. C. Pope, L. I. Iezzoni, J. Z. Ayanian, D. W. Bates, H. Burstin, and A. S. Ash. 1996. "Diagnosis-Based Risk Adjustment for Medicare Capitation Payments." *Health Care Financing Review* 17 (3): 101–28.

Fleming, S. T. 1991. "The Relationship Between Quality and Cost: Pure and Simple?" *Inquiry* 28 (1): 29–38.

Fleming, S. T., and K. E. Boles. 1994. "Financial and Clinical Performance: Bridging the Gap." *Health Care Management Review* 19 (1): 11–17.

Fleming, S. T., and F. P. Kohrs. 1998. "Linking Claims and Registry Data: Is It Worth the Effort?" *Clinical Performance and Quality Health Care* 6 (2): 88–96.

Giacomini, M., H. S. Luft, and J. C. Robinson. 1995. "Risk Adjusting Community-Rated Health Plan Premiums: A Survey of Risk Assessment Literature and Policy Applications." *Annual Review of Public Health* 16: 401–30.

Hellinger, F. J. 1987. "Selection Bias in Health Maintenance Organizations: Analysis of the Evidence." *Health Care Financing Review* 9 (2): 55–63.

Hornbrook, M. C. 1999. "Commentary: Improving Risk-Adjustment Models for Capitation Payment and Global Budgeting." *Health Services Research* 33 (6): 1745–51.

Hornbrook, M. C., and M. J. Goodman. 1991. "Health Plan Case Mix: Definitions, Measurement, and Use." *Health Services Research* 26 (1): 111–48.

Kronick, R., Z. Zhou, and T. Dreyfus. 1995. "Making Risk Adjustment Work for Everyone." *Inquiry* 32 (1): 41–55.

Lamers, L. M. 1999. "Risk-Adjusted Capitation Based on the Diagnostic Cost Group Model: An Empirical Evaluation with Health Survey Information." *Health Services Research* 33 (6): 1727–44.

Lubitz, J. 1987. "Health Status Adjustments for Medicare Capitation." *Inquiry* 24 (4): 362–75.

Luft, H. S. 1995. "Potential Methods to Reduce Risk Selection and Its Effects." *Inquiry* 32 (1): 23–32.

Manton, K. G., H. D. Tolley, and J. C. Vertrees. 1989. "Controlling Risk in Capitation Payment: Multivariate Definitions of Risk Groups." *Medical Care* 27 (3): 259–71.

National Cancer Institute. 2008. "What Are Risk Factors?" [Online information; retrieved 3/19/08.] http://understandingrisk.cancer.gov/learn/whatareriskfactors.cfm.

Newhouse, J. P. 1982. "Is Competition the Answer?" *Journal of Health Economics* 1 (1): 109–15.

———. 1998. "Risk Adjustment: Where Are We Now?" *Inquiry* 35 (2): 122–31.

Newhouse, J. P., W. G. Manning, E. B. Keller, and E. M. Sloss. 1989. "Adjusting Capitation Rates Using Objective Health Measures and Prior Utilization." *Health Care Financing Review* 10 (3): 41–54.

RealAge.com. "The Real Age Test." [Online information; retrieved 2/7/08.] http://www.realage.com.

Robinson, J. C. 1993. "A Payment Method for Health Insurance Purchasing Cooperatives." *Health Affairs* (Suppl.): 66–75.

Rogal, D. L., and A. K. Gauthier. 1998. "Are Health-Based Payments a Feasible Tool for Addressing Risk Segmentation?" *Inquiry* 35 (2): 115–21.

Roizen, M. 2000. "What's Your Real Age?" *Reader's Digest* (January): 33–36.

Rosenthal, M. B., and R. A. Dudley. 2007. "Pay-for-Performance: Will the Latest Payment Trend Improve Care?" *Journal of the American Medical Association* 297 (7): 740–44.

Schauffler, H. H., J. Howland, and J. Cobb. 1992. "Using Chronic Disease Risk Factors to Adjust Medicare Capitation Payments." *Health Care Financing Review* 14 (1): 79–90.

Wennberg, J. E., and A. M. Gittelsohn. 1973. "Small Area Variations in Health Care Delivery." *Science* 182 (117): 1102–8.

COST-EFFECTIVENESS ANALYSIS

Steven T. Fleming

"There are risks and costs to a program of action. But they are far less than the long-range risks and costs of comfortable inaction."
John F. Kennedy

One of the fundamental principles of economics is that "there is no such thing as a free lunch." The meaning behind this phrase is that most things in life cost money, even though the trail of those costs may be obscure, diffuse, or apparently nonexistent.

In the United States, we have been spending an ever-increasing proportion of our gross national product on healthcare services, with no relief in sight, particularly as the baby boomers reach retirement age. Since resources are limited (another fundamental economic principle), choices must be made. A dollar spent on healthcare services is a dollar that cannot be spent on education, highway infrastructure, or national parks. A dollar spent on bone marrow transplantation for the terminally ill may be a dollar that cannot be spent on childhood immunization programs. It would be wise to spend healthcare dollars effectively, so as to maximize the return on the investment. This chapter examines a technique called cost-effectiveness analysis (CEA), the purpose of which is to formally evaluate the costs and effects (i.e., outcomes) of alternative programs, in order to make rational decisions. Hunink and Glasziou's (2001) chapter *Constrained Resources*, in their outstanding book on decision making, was instrumental in informing the discussion of cost-effectiveness that follows.

Figure 9.1 summarizes four options from Hunink and Glasziou that can be used to compare the costs and effects of a particular program in a world of constrained resources. *Positive health effects* are improvements in the health status of people for whom the program is intended. *Negative health effects* represent diminishing health status. *Positive costs* mean the program costs money, whereas *negative costs* imply that there is a cost saving with program implementation. A program that achieves positive health effects while saving money (upper left quadrant) is clearly a superior choice. For example, the movement of some medical services from the inpatient to outpatient setting might yield better outcomes (through fewer nosocomial infections), while costing less money. Such programs would always be desirable, from a cost-effectiveness standpoint, if logistically feasible. A program that costs money to achieve negative health effects (lower right quadrant) would be an inferior choice. It would not make sense to fund a program that leads to diminishing health status of the target population.

FIGURE 9.1
Trade–Off
Between
Costs and
Effects

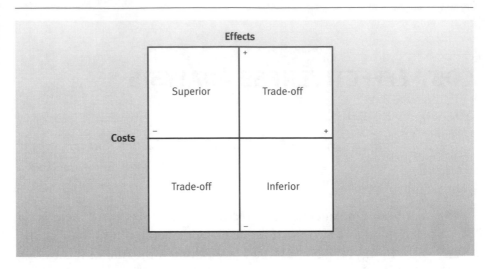

SOURCE: Hunink and Glasziou (2001). Reprinted with the permission of Cambridge University Press.

The remaining two options suggest trade-offs for which cost-effectiveness analysis may be useful, in a world of competing resources. Programs that cost money to achieve health improvements (lower right quadrant) must be systematically compared, so as to maximize health improvement per dollar spent. Programs that save money but lower health effects (lower left quadrant) must be evaluated also, since cost savings from these programs may be used to improve health effects through other, more cost-effective alternatives.

Cost-Effectiveness Ratios

Three kinds of cost-effectiveness ratios are important decision-making tools. The *average cost-effectiveness ratio* (ACER) is used to evaluate a single intervention or program against either no program at all or current practice, whatever that is. To obtain the ACER, one divides the net cost of the program by the net effects of the program (such as lives saved). For example, if the cost of a measles vaccination outreach program is $50,000 and the estimated effect is 100 cases prevented, then the ACER would be $50,000/100 = $500 per measles case prevented. The *incremental cost-effectiveness ratio* (ICER) compares the differences in both costs and outcomes for two interventions that compete with each other for resources. Thus, the ratio represents the "additional" cost of one program (compared to the next less-effective alternative), divided by the additional outcomes of that same program, compared to the next less-effective alternative.

The *marginal cost-effectiveness ratio* is for program expansion or contraction, and is therefore similar to the ICER, in that it measures "changes" in costs and outcomes. The remainder of this chapter focuses primarily on the ICER.

Cost-Effectiveness Model

The ICER is calculated as the net increase in costs divided by the net increase in effects (or outcomes) for one intervention, compared to an alternative, which is the next less-effective choice. According to Hunink and Glasziou (2001), costs would include: (1) those associated with the programs themselves (e.g., physicians, nurses, vaccines); (2) costs or savings that result from procedures that were induced or avoided (e.g., prostatectomies that resulted from a screening program, coronary artery bypass graft surgeries that were avoided); (3) costs or savings that resulted from morbidity that was averted (e.g., costs of caring for the cases of influenza that were avoided by a vaccination program); (4) costs of treating complications and side effects; and (5) costs of healthcare in additional years of life. The net increase in effects would include changes in some measure of healthcare outcomes, such as added years of life, cases of disease that were avoided, and quality-adjusted life years.

The ICER is calculated through a series of steps. One must: (1) describe the kind of program or intervention being considered, and the perspective from which the evaluation will take place; (2) identify the measure(s) of effect that will be used and calculate net effects; (3) identify the various components of costs and calculate net costs; and (4) calculate the cost-effectiveness ratio and use this ratio to make rational program choices.

Program Specification

Program specification involves formally delineating the scope of the intervention, or what some have referred to as "framing the analysis."

The first step in this process is to define the problem. For example, suppose that an examination of infant mortality data by county revealed serious racial disparities in a few adjacent counties. This may be the problem (racial disparities in infant mortality rates), or it may be part of a larger problem involving access to preventive healthcare services among the economically disadvantaged.

The second step in this process is to identify the types of interventions that will be formally compared with the CEA, in terms of delivery sites, personnel, technology, and so on. For example, to address the earlier program, we might want to consider a prenatal videotape educational intervention delivered by volunteer nurses in a local mall (home to several welfare agencies).

The third step is to frame the analysis in terms of perspective, reference, and target population. The healthcare "marketplace" is a complicated scene with many stakeholders. It is often difficult to determine where the costs and effects land once a program is implemented. For example, costs may be shifted across payers, or benefits may be enjoyed by others who have no part in the financial transaction. For example, the mother who refuses to have her child immunized against measles enjoys the benefit of the "herd immunity" (Chapter 2) financed by others.

The perspective of the analysis pertains to the range of people and stakeholders who will be included in the analysis. An *individual* perspective would attribute costs and effects to the people who are targeted by the intervention. The broader *organizational* perspective would factor in the costs and effects accrued to the organization, such as the increase in membership or profits to a managed care organization that adopts an innovative disease management program. The *payer* perspective would focus on the inflow and outflow of insurance payments as a result of changing morbidity patterns. The *societal* perspective is the most typical perspective used in CEA, because it includes costs and effects that spill over to others who are not part of the targeted population. The economists would call these externalities. A *positive externality* occurs when others enjoy a benefit without incurring a cost, such as the herd immunity example mentioned earlier. A *negative externality* occurs when others suffer a loss or harm through no fault of their own, such as those who develop morbidity as a result of passive smoke exposure.

Program specification also involves defining the reference program or intervention. To calculate the ICER for each alternative program choice, one must compare the costs and effects of each alternative with a reference. That reference will be the next less-effective choice. For most programs, the next less-effective choice will be another alternative program. For the least effective choice, the comparison group will be either no program at all or an existing program.

Program specification also entails defining who the target population is—that is, which people, patients, or population groups will enjoy benefits, or incur costs, as a result of the program intervention.

Finally, program specification requires defining the time horizon, or the period within which the evaluation will take place.

Measuring Effectiveness

A number of different measures of effect may be useful in the cost-effectiveness analysis. The challenge is to identify the best measure(s) that relates specifically to the operation of the program, and for which data are available. When several programs are being compared, one must select an outcome that has a common denominator across the programs. For example, we can compare two programs when the outcome is measured in disability-free years of life, or quality-adjusted life years (QALYs), but we cannot compare two programs if the outcome in one program is number of children immunized, while the outcome of the other is heart attacks avoided.

Often the critical outcomes of a program may not be manifested until years in the future, perhaps years beyond the time horizon of the study. For example, a diet modification program aimed at children in a managed care organization may seek to reduce the incidence of heart disease among these members. Such morbidity, however, may be 20 years beyond the time horizon of the study. In such cases, intermediate outcomes—such as a lowering of average cholesterol levels—may be suitable measures of effectiveness.

An important step in the process of identifying measures of effectiveness is to enumerate the harms and benefits associated with the problems for which the programs are intended, and then identify the harms and benefits associated with the programs being evaluated.

Suppose the problem is high infant mortality rates among teenaged mothers. Infant mortality would be among the list of harms, as would the present and future morbidity associated with low infant birth weight. The next step is to identify which harms and benefits can be specifically measured, which ones have proxy measures that are more readily available, and which ones cannot be measured at all. For example, infant mortality is a vital statistic routinely collected in most countries. While the literature may report the present and future morbidity of low infant birth weight, these data may be difficult to obtain. A sufficient measure may simply be the number of infants of low or very low birth weight. Present or future psychological distress caused by the death of an infant may be impossible to measure or gather.

The most common measures of effect in cost-effectiveness analysis are related either to changes in morbidity or survival. So, "number of cases of disease averted" is a common measure of effect, as is "lives saved," or "years of life added," or "disability-free years of life," or "quality-adjusted years of life." Epidemiologists are critical in securing such information, particularly morbidity, since programs designed to eliminate or reduce risk factors should lead to less disease in future years.

Consider the earlier example of teenage smoking, low infant birth weight, and infant mortality. Suppose that teenaged mothers who are smokers are twice as likely to give birth to a low birth weight infant than non-smokers are, and that 20 percent of teenaged mothers smoke. With these data, the attributable fraction (Chapter 11) would be $[0.2 (2 - 1)]/[0.2(2 - 1) + 1] \times 100 = 16.7$ percent, with the interpretation being that 16.7 percent of low birth weight infants among teenaged mothers can be attributed to smoking. Suppose we were evaluating a smoking cessation program aimed at teenaged mothers and decide that the number of low birth weight infants is an outcome we want to measure. We would estimate the effectiveness of our program in reducing the prevalence of smoking (say, 50 percent effective), estimate the number of low birth weight infants (say, 1,000), and use the attributable fraction to estimate changes in the number of low birth weight infants given our presumed effectiveness: $0.5 \times 0.167 \times 1,000 = 83.5$ infants who would be born at a normal, rather than low, birth weight, because of the smoking cessation program.

Quality-Adjusted Life Years

The measure of effect can be a single measure of health outcome, such as lives saved, morbidity avoided, or cancer detected, or it can be a multidimensional measure that captures various kinds of outcomes in a single index, such as longevity and quality of life.

The quality-adjusted life year is such a measure, since it incorporates both duration of life and quality of life. With the QALY, we add up the number of additional years of life a particular program is expected to generate, and weigh each year by the quality of life associated with a particular health state. It is because of this that the QALY has been called a "preference-based" or "utility-based" measure, because it assumes we can value different health states based on our preferences for good health and good functioning over poor health or functioning. In fact, the CEA that uses the QALY as the measure of effect is often referred to a *cost utility analysis*.

Several approaches can be used to assign a value, or weight, to each health state for the purpose of calculating QALYs, including the standard gamble, time trade-off, and rating scale.

With the *standard gamble*, you create disease "scenarios" and ask people how willing they would be to risk immediate, painless death for the chance of complete recovery from the given disease. For example, you ask them to envision disease scenario A, which features a 50 percent chance of immediate, painless death and a corresponding 50 percent chance of complete recovery. If they respond, "No, I would not be willing to take that risk!" you change the probabilities, say, to a 20 percent chance of immediate, painless death and an 80 percent chance of recovery. Eventually you reach a point where people agree to the gamble (say, at 13 percent death versus 87 percent recovery). The health state weight is assigned based on that point, in this case a value of 0.87. The theory behind this approach is that most people are willing to take a larger risk of death (and thus a lower health state weight) when the health state, or quality of life, is lower.

The time trade-off approach involves asking folks to give up years of life in a given state of disability in order to be disease-free. For example, suppose you are trying to evaluate the weight of a health state for a paraplegic. The question would be, "Given that you have 20 more years of life as a paraplegic, how many of those years would you be willing to give up in order to walk again?" If the answer was "five of those years," then the weight of the health state would be $(20 - 5)/20 = 0.75$.

The rating scale simply assigns weights to health states by asking people to assign a value of 1 to 100 to living in a particular health state, with the associated symptoms and disability.

The weights used in calculating the QALY can be derived using one of the methods discussed above via a survey, a questionnaire, or an interview. Regardless of the method used, the critical decision is who should determine the weights. One view is that the general public should assign these weights, not on the basis of actually having the disease or disability, but rather by evaluating "what it would be like" if they did. With this approach it would be necessary to educate, or inform, the public as to the symptoms, disabilities, and quality of life for particular diseases, perhaps through disease scenarios or vignettes. The alternative view is that those with the disease or disability should assign the weights using one of the three methods, on the basis of their actual experience. A middle position would be that a family member of those with disease or disability be involved in determining the weights. The concern is that these weights should accurately reflect the state of health or quality of life associated with a particular disease or disability. The general public, or even family members for that matter, may not be able to accurately judge such issues without going through the experience. On the other hand, patients may adapt to their disability over time, and even rate their state of health higher than the general public. One of my students who uses a wheelchair rated his state of health much higher than his colleagues, saying "I can do just about anything." Some would suggest that patients ought to assign the weights in the CEA if the frame of reference is the individual, but that the general public ought to be involved when the frame of reference is the community or society. Another approach would be to sample the general public to include some representative proportion of patients with the disease(s) being weighed.

The QALY is a weighted sum of the number of years of life remaining. The formula is $N(Y \times W)$, where N is the number of patients, Y is the number of years of extended life, and W is the quality weight of those years. If the quality weight changes as the patient ages, you simply account for that by creating more $(Y \times W)$ functions and adding them together, so the formula becomes $N[(Y_1 \times W_1) + (Y_2 \times W_2)...]$, where Y_1 is the number of years at the first quality weight, Y_2 is the number of years at the subsequent quality weight, etc.

Suppose you are conducting a CEA on angioplasty, and are calculating an ICER with the QALY as the measure of effectiveness. For every 100 symptomatic patients treated with angioplasty, you estimate a total of 20 remaining years of life per person, compared to 15 remaining years of life for those who are treated medically. The QALY would weigh each of those additional years of life by the quality of life in that health state. Assume that the angioplasty patients live ten years with a quality of life weight of 0.8, eight years with a weight of 0.7, and two years with a weight of 0.5, whereas the medically treated patients live ten years at a weight of 0.75 and five years at a weight of 0.5. The QALY for the angioplasty patients would be $100 \times [(10 \times 0.8) + (8 \times 0.7) + (2 \times 0.5)] = 1,460$, or 14.6 QALYs per person, and the QALY for the medically treated patients would be $100 \times [(10 \times 0.75) + (5 \times 0.5)] = 1,000$, or 10 QALYs per person, for a difference of 460 QALYs, or 4.6 QALYs per person. Case Study 9.1 reviews how the Oregon Health Services Commission originally used QALYs to rank healthcare services in its Medicaid program.

Case Study 9.1. The Oregon Medicaid Prioritization of Health Services Program

In 1991, the Oregon Health Services Commission submitted a report to the governor and legislature (Oregon Health Services Commission 1991), in which it recommended prioritization of health services based on cost-effectiveness. The program has been modified since then by eliminating CEA, since very inexpensive and effective treatments for trivial conditions (e.g., malocclusion due to thumb sucking) ranked higher than only moderately expensive and effective treatments for serious conditions. The approach, however, was bold, innovative, and illustrative of CEA using QALYs.

QUESTIONS

1. The Commission conducted a telephone survey in which it asked folks to assign a health state value (from 0 to 1.0) to a number of different symptoms and functional limitations, such as having chest pain (0.747) or having shortness of breath (0.682). How could these values be converted to "dysfunction" or "disutility" values so that health state values could be derived for diseases with "multiple" dysfunctions and symptoms?
2. Suppose that you want to evaluate treatment for acute myocardial infarction (AMI). Four health states are specified for those who *do not* get treatment: (1) died within five years; (2) experience frequent chest pain; (3) often experience shortness of breath; and (4) return to former level of health in five years. Four states of health are specified for those who *do* get treatment: (1) die despite treatment; (2) still experience chest pain; (3) have residual shortness of breath; and (4) return to former state of health. What weights would you assign to each of these states of health based on question 1?
3. What additional information is needed to calculate QALYs for those *with* and *without* treatment?

4. Suppose that the probabilities of being in each of the four health states listed above *without* treatment is 0.30, 0.30, 0.20, and 0.20, respectively; that the probabilities of being in each of the four health states listed above *with* treatment is 0.10, 0.30, 0.30, and 0.30, respectively; and that the average life expectancy of the median AMI patient (age 46) is 29 years. Calculate the difference in QALYs for those with and without treatment.
5. Suppose that the cost of treatment was estimated at $32,500. What is the cost per QALY associated with treatment for AMI?

ANSWERS

1. Subtract the numbers from 1.0. The dysfunction associated with chest pain would be $1.0 - 0.747 = 0.253$, and the dysfunction associated with shortness of breath would be $1.0 - 0.682 = 0.318$. If there were a disease state with both chest pain and shortness of breath, the health state weight would be $1.0 - 0.253 - 0.318 = 0.429$.
2. Assign death a value of 0 and restoration of health a value of 1.0. Chest pain would be assigned a value of 0.747 and shortness of breath a value of 0.682.
3. You need to know the probability of being in each of the four states for those *with* and *without* treatment. You also need to know the number of years the treatment is effective, in this case, the average life expectancy of patients with AMI.
4. Total QALYs without treatment would be $[(0.30 \times 0) + (0.30 \times 0.747) + (0.20 \times 0.682) + (0.20 \times 1.0)] \times 29 = 16.25$. Total QALYs with treatment would be $[(0.10 \times 0) + (0.30 \times 0.747) + (0.30 \times 0.682) + (0.30 \times 1.0)] \times 29 = 21.13$. The difference in QALYs would be $21.13 - 16.25 = 4.88$.
5. The cost/QALY would be $32,500/4.88 = $6,660 per QALY.

Biased Estimates

According to Last (2001, 14), *bias* is "any deviation of results or inferences from the truth." Bias is discussed in detail in chapters 11–13. At least two kinds of bias are problematic for CEA, particularly when screening programs are being evaluated: lead time and length bias.

Lead time bias refers to the length of time between when someone who is not showing symptoms is diagnosed with a disease through screening, and when that person would have been diagnosed had he or she not been screened. The reasoning is that screening usually detects cancer and other chronic diseases before symptoms occur, thus asymptomatic people who are screened are diagnosed sooner than symptomatic, unscreened individuals. If a study compares the survival of screened versus unscreened people without taking this bias into consideration, the data will inaccurately show that the screened people live longer.

Length bias relates to the mix of people with disease who are subject to a screening program. Subjects with a long preclinical phase of disease are: (1) more likely to be found by screening, because of the long asymptomatic, but detectable, phase of disease and (2) more likely to survive longer, since disease among them is typically less serious.

Measuring Costs

The measurement of costs is a difficult, but critical, task in any cost-effectiveness analysis. It involves multiple components and adjustments.

One of the most important components of cost is the money spent on healthcare resources needed to operate the program or intervention. This includes physical infrastructure (such as building or clinical space); physician, nursing, and other professional services; equipment (such as imaging technology); pharmaceuticals; and other supplies.

The other equally important cost component comprises non-healthcare expenditures. For example, there may be transportation costs borne by patients who travel from their homes to clinics or other treatment sites. Moreover, the wages lost to patients who seek treatment and do not get paid sick time are an additional cost. We all value leisure time, which, if reduced, represents a cost borne by program participants. The cost of caregiver time represents what the economists call an "opportunity cost," since these caregivers could be earning wages elsewhere, were it not for the fact that they were needed to provide care to their loved ones. There are lost productivity costs, to the extent that patients treated by the program being evaluated may produce fewer goods or services because of a reduced level of health. The costs associated with lost productivity can be included in either the numerator or the denominator of an ICER. To be in the numerator, these costs would represent the dollar value of goods and services not produced by program participants because of shortened life or disability. In the denominator, the cost of lost productivity is reflected by lower QALY levels. One should not measure the impact of lost productivity in both the numerator and denominator; the latter is preferred.

It is useful to conceptualize and measure costs as a sequence (or stream) of events that occurs over the time frame of the project. These costs may be associated with progressive stages of the project, and can be broadly categorized as (1) initial costs, (2) continuing costs, (3) induced costs, and (4) averted costs. The *initial costs* are those associated with the beginning of the program, such as new buildings, office space, the hiring of new staff, the purchasing of supplies, and so on. *Continuing costs* are expenses associated with the ongoing implementation of the program.

Induced costs refer to those that are spawned by the intervention. For example, a new screening program for breast cancer may result in both false positives and true positives. Additional testing or biopsies are necessary to repudiate the false positive diagnoses. Elmore and colleagues (1998) report on the ten-year risk of a false positive result for screening mammograms and clinical breast examinations in a retrospective cohort study of 2,400 women. The false positive tests led to 870 outpatient appointments, 539 diagnostic mammograms, 186 ultrasound examinations, 188 biopsies, and 1 hospitalization, all of which represent induced costs. Further treatment, such as surgery, chemotherapy, or radiation therapy, will be required for the true positive patients. These are all induced costs.

Averted costs are expenses that would have occurred if the intervention had not taken place, such as the costs associated with treating future morbidity. A screening program for breast cancer may generate costs associated with treating proportionately more early-stage cases than if the screening program didn't exist, but lack of such a program may result in the future costly treatment of late-stage disease. The former represents induced costs, the latter averted costs.

A final, somewhat controversial component of the costs is related to additional years of life. Presumably, a new program or intervention will result in additional years of life. Patients who enjoy the benefits of such an intervention will live longer, but with this longer life may suffer from morbidities that they would not have endured without the intervention. The care for such morbidities may be costly. Futhermore, these people will consume goods and services, but may also contribute to society in terms of additional productivity. Should this complex array of costs be included in the analysis? Some suggest that healthcare-related costs, such as the cost of treating future morbidities, may be estimated, but non-healthcare-related costs are probably too difficult to evaluate.

Table 9.1 summarizes some costs and effects from the four different perspectives discussed earlier.

All costs—initial, continuing, induced, and averted—should be estimated for each year of the program. Decisions need to be made regarding whether to include fixed costs (such as new buildings) in addition to variable costs (those that typically change with the level of output). The time-frame of the analysis is critical here, since even fixed costs are variable in the long term. One approach would be to include fixed costs only if there are long-term effects within the time frame of the program.

All costs need to be adjusted in two important ways: (1) inflation and (2) discounting to present value. Future prices will be higher than present prices, particularly in the area of healthcare. The purpose of adjusting for inflation is to make future dollars equal to present dollars in terms of buying power. When accumulating the cost "streams" over the time frame of the project, one must convert all present and future costs into "constant"

TABLE 9.1
Costs and
Effects from
Four Different
Perspectives

Perspective	Costs (Savings)	Effects

Individual	Out-of-pocket costs (savings)
	  a. for intervention
	  b. for induced treatments, etc.
	  c. savings from averted morbidity
	Travel costs
	Lost wages
	Cost of lost leisure time
	Cost of caregivers
		QALYs gained by
		  individuals

Organizational	Personnel costs Capital costs Cost of supplies Reimbursement from payer Fees from individuals	QALYs gained by individuals

Payer	Reimbursement to providers
	  a. for intervention
	  b. for induced treatment, etc.
	  c. savings from averted morbidity
	Costs shifting to/from other payers
		QALYs gained by
		  individuals

Society	All costs from individual, organization,
	  and payer
	Spillovers costs to other individuals
	Costs borne by society in other areas,
	  such as education, environment, etc.
		QALYs gained by
		  individuals
		Spillover QALYs to
		  other members
		  of society
		Productivity losses

dollars, typically by devaluing all future dollars based on projected inflation rates. The Consumer Price Index (CPI) (www.stats.bls.gov), or Medical CPI, is used in this process. Both indices estimate the cost of a market basket of goods and services. For example, assume that the CPI for 2007 and 2006 was 206.00 and 200.00, respectively, and that that you were doing a CEA with two years of cost streams, $130,000 for 2007 and $100,000 for 2006. You would want to convert all cost streams to constant dollars (using 2006 as the frame of reference) by "deflating" the $130,000 in 2007 dollars to 2006 dollars, using the CPI as follows: $(200.00/206.00) \times \$130,000 = \$126,214$.

The second important way that costs need to be adjusted when cost streams are accumulated over a multiple-year time frame is through discounting. *Discounting* refers to the process of determining how much future resource costs should be worth today, called the *present value*. You can think of discounting as the "reverse" of earning interest. The theory behind discounting is that future dollars are not worth as much as dollars today, because the latter can be invested and earn a return. For example, if I gave you one dollar right now, you could at least deposit it in the bank and earn, say, 5 percent interest, so that it would be worth $1.05 in one year. The *discount rate* is the rate by which future dollars are devalued, and is presumably related to some estimate of the projected return on investment, typically around 5 percent. The discount rate is net of inflation.

Both inflation adjustments and discounting allow us to evaluate future costs in present-day terms. The present value (PV) is the amount invested at the discount rate that will earn the future value (FV). The net present value (NPV) is the difference between the PV of income (or savings) and PV of costs.

Suppose that you are doing a CEA and project a total of $50,000 in costs, $10,000 initially and then $10,000 at the end of years 1, 2, 3, and 4. You would like to calculate the present value of these costs by discounting the value of future costs using a discount rate of 5 percent. To simplify, we will assume no inflation over the five-year period. The present value of all costs, initial plus subsequent, is calculated using the following formula:

$$PV = FV/(1 + r)^t$$

where PV = present value, FV = future value, r = discount rate, t = time in years

$PV(\text{initial}) = \$10,000/(1.05)^0 = \$10,000$
$PV(\text{year } 1) = \$10,000/(1.05)^1 = \$9,524$
$PV(\text{year } 2) = \$10,000/(1.05)^2 = \$9,070$
$PV(\text{year } 3) = \$10,000/(1.05)^3 = \$8,638$
$PV(\text{year } 4) = \$10,000/(1.05)^4 = \$8,227$
$$\text{Total} = \$45,459$$

The rationale behind using a discount rate for costs and savings is clear and intuitive. Current dollars can earn a return on the investment. Future dollars represent foregone investment income. Some would also argue that we should discount future health outcomes. Presumably most of us have a "time preference" for health. If given a choice, we would prefer five years of disability-free health today over five years of disability-free health in the future. In other words, future health status is worth less to us than current health status. To carry this argument further, a QALY in the future is worth less than a QALY today. With this argument, then, it makes sense to discount future outcomes in the same way that we discount future dollars.

Arguments against this approach are centered around a distaste for the implications. If we discount future health outcomes, then all programs with effects in the distant future, such as those aimed at children (e.g., reducing adolescent obesity), will be subject to a rather serious handicap. Many prevention programs would be at a great disadvantage in any CEA that compares them to other programs with proximal, rather than distant, outcomes.

Even if we accept the notion that outcomes should be discounted in addition to costs, we may still wrestle over the question of which discount rates to use for each. Discounting both costs and outcomes at the same rate is standard practice in CEA, even though it may be conceptually appealing to use different rates. A compelling argument against using different rates is the well-cited "Keeler-Cretin paradox," which states that discounting costs and health benefits at different rates will lead to the conclusion that it is always preferable to delay program implementation. For example, assume there is no discounting of health outcomes, and say you could spend $2 million on a cancer screening program now to save 100 lives, or $20,000 per life saved. The alternative would be to invest the money at, say, 5 percent interest, in which case you would have $2 million $\times$ 1.05 = $2.1 million at the end of one year. With this money you would be able to save $2.1 million/$20,000 = 105 lives, or invest the money for another year and save 110 lives, and so on. The "paradox" is that delay always improves the cost-effectiveness ratio, so it would never be rational to start a program.

Cost-Benefit Analysis

Cost-benefit analysis (CBA) is another methodology for comparing programs. The primary difference between the two methodologies is in how outcomes are measured. With CEA, there are many possible outcomes that can be measured, such as lives saved, cases of disease prevented, or QALYs, and it is imperative to compare programs using the same measure of outcome. With CBA, both costs and outcomes are converted to some monetary unit, for example, U.S. dollars, and the cost-benefit ratio is a number that can be directly interpreted. If the cost-to-benefit ratio is 1.2, then costs exceed benefits by 20 percent.

Earlier we discussed the challenges associated with measuring all components of costs for CEA, and the necessity of both adjusting for inflation and converting the cost streams into present value dollars. CBA poses an even greater challenge: the need to convert health outcomes into monetary units. How does one measure the value of a human life, or a case of disease prevented? Most theorists would recommend some kind of "human capital" approach, which envisions people as "production units" in society. Thus the loss of a life, or the burden of disability, represents a loss of productivity to society that can be evaluated. So, an individual life can be measured as future earnings that relate to its productivity over the years.

One approach would calculate the gross present value of earnings, and another the net present value of earnings, which subtracts the consumption of goods and services. Using the latter approach, the net present value of the early and later years of life would be negative, since children and retirees are net consumers of goods and services. The net present value of men and women during their productive employment years is likely to be positive.

While the human capital approach may seem appealing from an economic theory standpoint, we find it distasteful, because it evaluates life only on one dimension, and ignores the value that we have to our relatives or friends.

An alternative approach is to value outcomes according to our "willingness to pay" for these outcomes, using either a "revealed willingness to pay," for example, actual purchases, or a subjective willingness to pay. For example, some elective cosmetic surgery is not covered by most insurance, so we can estimate the value of such an outcome by how much consumers are willing to pay for these services. Alternatively, we can create various disease scenarios or vignettes, as mentioned earlier, and ask people to subjectively assign a dollar value to each: "How much would it be worth to you to be free of your paraplegia?" One particular problem with the willingness to pay approach is that the affluent place a higher value on health than the poor, and are therefore willing to pay more to remain healthy. We could justify these different preferences for health with economic theory, because the affluent have more to lose should they become disabled. The implications, however, of assigning different values to health outcomes for programs aimed at different economic groups are problematic, because the programs aimed at the poor would always be at a disadvantage due to a lower "benefit" yield.

Choosing Among Programs

Hunink and Glasziou (2001) describe two different kinds of CEA, where the alternatives are either: (1) competing choices or (2) noncompeting choices. A *competing choice analysis* is used when the choices are mutually exclusive. In other words, the alternatives are not independent, and one choice precludes the other. Two surgical alternatives are perhaps the best example. A *noncompeting choice analysis* is used when the choices are not mutually exclusive. In this scenario, the decision to implement one program does not preclude the implementation of another.

The CEA with noncompeting choices is the most simple. It entails calculating cost-effectiveness ratios for each program, and sorting the programs by increasing ratio. Presumably any combination of programs is

TABLE 9.2
Cost–
Effectiveness
of Four
Noncompeting
Health
Promotion
Campaigns

Program	QALYs	Cost ($)	C/E
A	10	50,000	50,000/10 = 5,000
B	20	−25,000	Superior choice—rule in
C	−10	40,000	Inferior choice—rule out
D	15	80,000	80,000/15 = 5,333

possible, and programs may be partially funded by dividing them into smaller units. Programs that cost money but have negative effects (lower right quadrant of Figure 9.1) are immediately "ruled out." Programs that save money and have positive effects (upper left quadrant of Figure 9.1) are immediately "ruled in." The savings from these programs are added to the available budget. Finally, programs are sequentially selected from the lowest to the highest cost-effectiveness ratio until the budget, including any savings from superior programs, runs out.

Table 9.2 illustrates this technique for four noncompeting health promotion campaigns and a budget of $50,000. Program B will always be implemented because it saves money and increases QALYs. Program C will never be implemented because it costs money while decreasing QALYs. The total budget of $75,000 ($50,000 + $25,000 savings from implementing program B) could fund all of program A, because it is more cost-effective than program D. The remaining $25,000 would be used to fund a scaled-down version of program D.

A CEA with competing choices is more difficult because it involves calculating ICERs. With this analysis, programs are mutually exclusive, and the objective is to maximize total incremental, or net, effectiveness with a limited budget. As stated earlier, the ICER involves comparing each program to the next most cost-effective alternative. Table 9.3 summarizes this strategy with four screening programs. Notice how the programs are sorted initially by increasing effectiveness (QALYs). Program G can be ruled out by what Hunink and Glasziou (2001) refer to as "simple dominance," since this program costs more, but with lower effects than program H.

The second step is to calculate the ICER for each program using the next effective alternative. Program E is compared to no program at all. Program F is compared to program E, and program H is compared to program F. The incremental cost (ΔC) and incremental effect (ΔE) are, in both cases, the difference between each program and the alternative. Programs F and H are ruled out by what Hunink and Glasziou (2001) refer to as "extended dominance," meaning that the ICER is higher for programs F and H than program E. The decision would be to fund program E. Case Study 9.2 describes a CEA using ICERs for treatment options for acute otitis media.

Program	QALYs	Cost ($)	ΔC/ΔE
E	10	50,000	$(50,000 - 0)/(10-0) = 5,000$
F	20	500,000	$(500,000 - 50,000)/(20 - 10) = 45,000$
G	30	1,200,000	Ruled out
H	50	1,000,000	$(1,000,000 - 500,000)/(50 - 20) = 16,667$

TABLE 9.3
Incremental Cost–Effectiveness of Four Competing Screening Programs

Case Study 9.2. Cost-Effectiveness Analysis of Treatment Options for Acute Otitis Media (Earache)

Coco (2007) conducts a CEA in which he compares four treatment options for the treatment of acute otitis media: (1) delayed prescription, (2) watchful waiting, (3) seven to ten days of amoxicillin, and (4) four days of amoxicillin. The time frame for the study was 30 days, and focused specifically on short-term outcomes. Mastoiditis refers to the hospitalization costs associated with acute

TABLE 9.4. COST-EFFECTIVENESS ANALYSIS OF FOUR TREATMENT OPTIONS FOR TREATMENT OF ACUTE OTITIS MEDIA

Variable	Delayed Prescription	Watchful Waiting	7–10 Days of Amoxicillin	5 Days of Amoxicillin
Cost, $				
Nonhealthcare	12.78	14.52	15.10	15.47
Work loss	95.31	98.43	94.70	97.34
Office consultation	22.52	31.47	33.83	34.61
Antibiotic	1.68	1.47	11.61	9.42
Mastoiditis	0.11	0.11	0.06	0.06
Total	132.40	146.00	155.30	156.90
Effectiveness (QALYs)	0.99460	0.99472	0.99501	0.99487

SOURCE: Coco (2007). Used with permission of the American Academy of Family Physicians.

mastoiditis. Nonmedical costs include an average of 5.6 hours of work lost, and other nonhealthcare costs such as the cost of babysitting, day care, travel, and parking. Table 9.4 summarizes the results of this study.

QUESTIONS

1. From which perspective is this study being conducted?
2. Calculate incremental costs and effectiveness for each option by comparing it to the less effective alternative (to the left).
3. Can any of the alternatives be eliminated based on simple dominance, that is, it costs more and yields less effectiveness?
4. Calculate the incremental cost-effectiveness ratios for watchful waiting and seven to ten days of amoxicillin. Which has the highest ICER? What is the next step?
5. Calculate the final ICER for the best option.

ANSWERS

TABLE 9.5. INCREMENTAL COST-EFFECTIVENESS ANALYSIS OF FOUR TREATMENT OPTIONS FOR TREATMENT OF ACUTE OTITIS MEDIA

Variable	Delayed Prescription	Watchful Waiting	7–10 Days of Amoxicillin	5 Days of Amoxicillin
Incremental cost	—	13.6	9.3	1.60
Incremental effectiveness	—	0.00012	0.00029	−0.00014

SOURCE: Coco (2007). Used with permission of the American Academy of Family Physicians.

1. The author argues that the study is being conducted from a societal perspective because it includes "non-healthcare costs of parental work loss and transportation" (Coco 2007, 30).
2. Table 9.5 summarizes these calculations.
3. The "5-days of amoxicillin" option can be eliminated because it costs more than "7-10 days of amoxicillin" ($156.90 vs. $155.30) and yields less effectiveness (0.99487 vs. 0.99501).
4. The ICER for "watchful waiting" is 13.6/0.00012 = $113,333 per QALY and for "7-10 days of amoxicillin" it is 9.3/0.00029 = $32,069 per QALY. Watchful waiting has a higher ICER, which means that it can be eliminated based on "extended dominance." The next step would be to calculate the ICER com-

paring "7–10 days of amoxicillin" to "delayed prescription."

5. The final ICER for "7–10 days of amoxicillin" is ($155.30 – $132.40)/
   (0.99501 – 0.99460) = $55,854 per QALY.

Uncertainty

Throughout this chapter, we have seen the need to obtain estimates for numerous components of a cost-effectiveness analysis. The measurement of effectiveness requires that we estimate the effect of various program interventions on health status. For example, smoking cessation will have an impact on the risk of various types of future morbidity, such as lung cancer, pancreatic cancer, and heart disease, just to mention a few. We need to obtain estimates of the degree to which a program will have an impact on this risk. Other kinds of treatment, such as angioplasty, will affect the risk of future morbidity as well.

There is uncertainty with each of these estimates, which means that we do not know for sure the magnitude of the risk reduction. Even estimates obtained from the literature will typically include confidence intervals, which quantify, at least to some degree, the magnitude of the uncertainty. The cost estimates are also subject to uncertainty, as is the choice of projected inflation rates and the choice of a discount rate. What should be done to deal with this uncertainty, and how will this uncertainty affect the results of the cost-effectiveness analysis?

A common approach to encapsulating this uncertainty is with a process called *sensitivity analysis*. With sensitivity analysis, you provide a range of values around each uncertain estimate. The cost-effectiveness ratio is calculated multiple times, using the upper and lower estimates for each uncertain parameter. This reveals any changes in decisions. If the upper and lower bound estimate of a parameter—say, the risk of disease associated with a particular risk factor—leads to different program choices, we seek more refined estimates. Case Study 9.3 illustrates the use of a sensitivity analysis for the cost-effectiveness of health insurance.

Case Study 9.3. Cost-Effectiveness of Health Insurance

Muennig, Franks, and Gold (2005) conducted a cost-effectiveness analysis of health insurance in the United States using the 1993 National Health Interview Survey linked to the National Death Index (through 1995). A regression analysis on a sample of the privately insured 25–65-year-olds estimated the effects of sociodemographic and clinical variables on expenditures, quality of life, and mortality. Parameter estimates from the regression were then used to predict the expenditures, quality of life, and mortality for the uninsured, assuming that they could secure health insurance. Finally, a decision-analysis model was used to predict both costs and benefits of insuring the average 25-year-old through age 65, with societal costs discounted at a rate of 3 percent.

Table 9.6 reports observed expenditures, quality of life, and mortality, by age group, for the insured and uninsured, as well as predicted values for each of these three measures for the uninsured, assuming that they could obtain insurance. Note, the authors of the study report slightly different results due to rounding.

QUESTIONS

1. What is the relationship between expenditures and age for both the insured and uninsured groups?
2. What is the relationship between quality of life, mortality, and age for both the insured and uninsured groups?
3. For the average 25-year-old, assume that the discounted societal costs are $47,000 for those with insurance and $17,000 for those without insurance. Further, assume that effectiveness, measured in QALYs, would be 22.5 for those with insurance and 21.7 for those without. Effectiveness measured in life years (LYs) would be 27.1 for those with insurance and 26.5 for those without. Calculate the incremental cost and incremental effectiveness (in both QALYs and LYs).
4. Calculate the incremental ICER using both measures of effectiveness, and interpret these results.
5. The authors conducted a sensitivity analysis to see how the ICER (using QALYs) would change with low and high limits for administrative costs, annual expenditures for both the insured and uninsured, and quality of life measures for the insured, among other factors. What effect on the ICER should a higher limit on each of these values have?
6. The authors report that ICERs decrease for each five-year age increment up until age 65. For example, ICER for 45-year-olds is approximately $21,000, and for 60-year olds, approximately $14,000. Why do the ICERs decrease with increasing age, and how might this affect policy recommendations?
7. What effect would these two opposing biases have on the ICERs? (1) Suppose that people with health insurance are healthier and more health-conscious, and that such an orientation has an impact on health outcomes. (2) Suppose that people choose health insurance because they are at a higher health risk than is captured in the model.

ANSWERS

1. Expenditures increase with age for the insured and uninsured. The disparities by insurance status are particularly noticeable in the younger age groups.

TABLE 9.6. OBSERVED AND PREDICTED EXPENDITURES AND HEALTH OUTCOMES

	Age Group	Insured	Uninsured	Predicted[a]
Expenditures	25–34	$1,169	$326	$1,193
	35–44	$1,543	$519	$1,613
	45–54	$1,935	$742	$2,219
	55–64	$2,820	$2,280	$3,385
HRQL score	25–34	0.92	0.88	0.88
	35–44	0.90	0.84	0.86
	45–54	0.87	0.79	0.83
	55–64	0.84	0.73	0.78
Mortality[b]	25–34	0.001	0.002	0.001
	35–44	0.002	0.003	0.002
	45 54	0.006	0.009	0.006
	55–64	0.012	0.020	0.013

SOURCE: Muennig, Franks, and Gold (2005). Copyright © 2005 American Journal of Preventive Medicine. Published by Elsevier Inc. Used with permission.

NOTE: a: Values for insuring the presently uninsured using predictive regression models. b: Proportion dying within 24 months. HRQL, health-related quality of life.

For example, 25–34-year-olds spend 3.6 times as much if they have insurance compared to those who do not.

2. Quality of life decreases, while mortality rates increase, with age for both insured and uninsured groups. Uninsured persons in each age group have lower quality of life and higher mortality.

3. The incremental cost would be $47,000 – $17,000 = $30,000. The incremental effectiveness, measured in QALYs, would be 22.5 – 21.7 = 0.8. The incremental effectiveness, measured in LYs, would be 27.1 – 26.5 = 0.6.

4. The ICER using QALYs would be $30,000/0.8 = $37,500. The ICER using LYs would be $30,000/0.6 = $50,000. This means providing health insurance to the uninsured would cost society $37,500 for every quality-adjusted life year gained, and $50,000 for every life year gained.

5. Higher administrative costs result in a higher ICER. Higher annual expenditures for the uninsured mean that the gap between insured and uninsured is smaller; the ICER decreases. Higher annual expenses for the insured mean that the gap between insured and uninsured is larger; the ICER increases. If the quality of life score for the insured is higher, then the gap between insured and uninsured is larger, thus the effect of insurance on this group increases, as does the ICER.

6. The authors argue that the increase in benefits associated with advancing age outweighs the increase in health expenditures, so the ICERs are lower with advancing age. In terms of policy recommendations, lowering the eli-

gibility age for Medicare would be more cost-effective than providing insurance to those in the younger age groups.

7. If the health orientation of the insured group was the reason behind better health outcomes, then the incremental effectiveness is higher than it should be, resulting in a lower ICER; that is, the ICER is underestimated. If people at higher risk tend to purchase insurance, then the incremental effectiveness is lower than it should be, resulting in a higher ICER; that is, the ICER is overestimated.

Summary

Former President John F. Kennedy warned of the complacency of the status quo, or what he called "comfortable inaction." Innovation requires a willingness to bear costs and take risks. This chapter described a methodology called cost-effectiveness analysis (CEA) that is used to evaluate alternatives in a systematic, rational manner. We showed how such a method can be applied in the healthcare field to many diverse options, such as (1) ranking healthcare services for the purpose of Medicaid reimbursement; (2) selecting the appropriate treatment option for acute otitis media (earache); and (3) deciding whether health insurance is cost-effective. The chapter discussed various metrics for evaluating effectiveness, including the popular quality-adjusted life year (QALY), and described the different components of costs, such as the averted costs of future morbidity avoided and the induced costs of follow-up or treatment for morbidity that is discovered. CEA requires that all costs and effects be "collapsed" over the time frame of the project into "present day" costs and effects, by adjusting for future inflation and taking into consideration that both costs and effects in the future are "worth less" today. Sensitivity analysis was proposed as a way of dealing with the uncertainty of estimates, and two different CEA techniques were presented to select among various alternatives. One technique is designed for programs that do not compete with each other; programs are selected based on the average cost-effectiveness and the budgetary constraint. The other technique, based on an incremental cost-effectiveness ratio, is for programs that are mutually exclusive; only one program can be selected, and we want that program to be the most cost-effective. By way of review, Case Study 9.4 uses cost-effectiveness analysis to evaluate whether universal or targeted screening for prostate cancer is the best approach.

Case Study 9.4. CEA for Targeted or Universal Prostate Cancer Testing

Testing for prostate cancer has been the subject of considerable controversy because of the relatively poor performance of the prostate-specific antigen

(PSA) test in discriminating between those with and without prostate cancer. Suppose you were charged with deciding whether to recommend universal or targeted screening for prostate cancer, with the targeted group being African American men. Assume that the sensitivity and specificity for the PSA test with a 4.0 ng/ml cutoff level for men at least 50 years old are 71.3 percent and 85.2 percent, respectively, as reported by Sun and colleagues (2007). A new blood test for prostate cancer has recently been developed with better discriminating characteristics. Assume that the early prostate cancer antigen-2 (EPCA-2) test has a sensitivity and specificity of 94 percent and 97 percent, respectively, for all ages. Further assume the prevalence of undiagnosed prostate cancer among whites and African Americans 50–69 years old is 15 percent and 25 percent, respectively. Calculate the ICER for each test on an entire population of 100,000 men and a targeted population of 15,000 African American men. (Note: The numbers used in this case study were made up for illustrative purposes; they are not actual statistics.)

QUESTIONS

1. How are sensitivity and specificity used to provide estimates of induced costs?
2. Calculate the frequency of true and false positives for both the PSA and EPCA-2 tests if the test is targeted to the 15,000 African American men with a prevalence of prostate cancer of 25 percent.
3. Calculate the frequency of true and false positives for both the PSA and EPCA-2 tests if the tests are given to the entire population of 100,000 men. Assume that 15 percent of the population is African American, and that the prevalence of prostate cancer is 15 percent and 25 percent among whites and African Americans, respectively.
4. Assume that 50- to 69-year-old whites and African Americans who do not have cancer have an average life expectancy of 25 and 23 years, respectively. Assume that all those who test positive are treated. White and black men who test positive for cancer and are treated live an average of 23 years and 21 years, respectively. Assume the false positives (those who do not have cancer but test positive) are biopsied or otherwise retested and shown to be negative, and thus seek no treatment. False negatives (those who have cancer but test negative) fall into two categories: (1) 40 percent develop serious symptoms and seek treatment—whites and African Americans in this category live 20 years and 18 years, respectively; (2) 60 percent do not develop symptoms severe enough to seek treatment—whites and African Americans in this category live 21 and 19 years, respectively. The baseline health states of whites and African Americans in that age group are 1.0 and 0.9, respectively, and 40 percent of those who undergo treatment suffer complications that reduce the average health state to 0.7. Calculate the average QALY per person for whites, African Americans, and all subjects.

5. Assume that the cost per person of PSA and EPCA-2 testing is $40 and $80, respectively; that the cumulative costs of radical prostatectomy, radiation therapy, and conservative therapy are $36,888, $59,455, and $32,135, respectively (Wilson et al. 2007); and that the cost of a prostate biopsy is about $1,200. Assume that the percentage of white men who choose prostatectomy, radiation therapy, and conservative therapy is 55.5 percent, 28.6 percent, and 15.9 percent, respectively (Hoffman et al. 2003), and that the same rates for African Americans are 54.3 percent, 20.0 percent, and 25.7 percent, respectively. Assume that 50 percent of men who test positive will get a prostate biopsy, 40 percent (all) of the false negatives who seek treatment will get a prostate biopsy, and all of those who seek treatment without testing will be biopsied. What is the cost per person for whites, African Americans, and all subjects using the PSA test, the EPCA-2 test, or no testing at all? Why are the costs higher with the EPCA-2 test despite the superior test characteristics?

6. Calculate ICERs for the targeted and universal screening strategies. Assume that the QALYs for the no testing groups are 23.84 and 19.03 for whites and African Americans, respectively. Note that these QALYs are less than the life expectancy for these two groups (25 and 23, respectively, question 4), because some men in each group will actually have prostate cancer, which will reduce their life expectancy, and in some cases, their quality of life. Interpret the ICERs.

7. Why was the targeted screening of African Americans with the PSA the preferred strategy?

ANSWERS

1. The specificity is used to calculate the number of false positives. The induced cost of verifying a false positive diagnosis involves other testing, such as transurethral ultrasound, or biopsy. The sensitivity is used to calculate the number of true positives. The costs associated with various treatment modalities would apply to the true positive cases.

2. Among the African American men, $15,000 \times 0.25 = 3,750$ of them will actually have prostate cancer and $15,000 - 3,750 = 11,250$ of them will not. With the PSA test, $0.713 \times 3,750 = 2,674$ of the men will be correctly diagnosed (true positives), and $(1 - 0.852) \times 11,250 = 1,665$ of the men will be incorrectly diagnosed (false positives). With the EPCA-2 test, $0.94 \times 3,750 = 3,525$ of the men will be correctly diagnosed (true positives) and $(1 - 0.97) \times 11,250 = 338$ of the men will be incorrectly diagnosed.

3. Among the African American men, 3,750 of them will actually have cancer and 11,250 will not (answer 2). Among the white men, $85,000 \times 0.15 = 12,750$ of them will have cancer, and $85,000 - 12,750 = 72,250$ of them will not. From answer 2, true positives with the PSA and EPCA-2 tests are, respectively, 2,674 and 3,525 for African American men. False positives are 1,665 and 338, respectively, for African American men. With the PSA test applied to white men,

0.713 × 12,750 = 9,091 of them will be correctly diagnosed (true positives), and (1 – 0.852) × 72,250 = 10,693 of the men will be incorrectly diagnosed (false positives). With the EPCA-2 test applied to white men, 0.94 × 12,750 = 11,985 of the men will be correctly diagnosed (true positives) and (1 – 0.97) × 72,250 = 2,168 of the men will be incorrectly diagnosed.

4. Refer to Table 9.7 for calculation of the QALYs. Using the PSA false negative ratio (1 – sensitivity), there will be (1 – 0.713) × 12,750 = 3,659 false negatives among white men, of whom 40 percent (1,464) will seek treatment. Of those, 40 percent (586) will have complications. The QALY/person among white men screened using PSA is calculated as follows: [(72,250 × 25) + (3,636 × 0.7 × 23) + (9,091 – 3,636) × 23 + (586 × 0.7 × 20) + (1,464 – 586) × 20 + (2,196 × 21)]/85,000 = 24.26. Notice the similarities in QALYs between both tests despite the much higher sensitivity and specificity of the EPCA-2 test.

TABLE 9.7. CALCULATION OF QALYS FOR PSA AND EPCA-2 TESTS

	Whites		African Americans		All	
	PSA	EPCA-2	PSA	EPCA-2	PSA	EPCA-2
Positives	9,091	11,985	2,674	3,525	11,765	15,510
True positive w/comp	3,636	4,794	1,070	1,410	4,706	6,204
False negatives 40%	1,464	306	430	90	1,894	396
False negatives 40% w/comp	586	122	172	36	758	158
True negatives (including false positives)	72,250	72,250	11,251	11,251	83,500	83,500
False negatives 60% (untreated)	2,195	459	646	135	2,840	594
QALYs/person	24.26	24.28	21.82	21.86	23.89	23.92

5. Refer to Table 9.8 for calculation of costs. Costs are probably higher for the EPCA-2 test because more cancer cases are found and treated. Sample calculations are as follows: (1) the number of white men tested with PSA who get a prostatectomy is true positives + false negatives × 0.40 (proportion who seek treatment) = 9,091 (true positives) + 1,464 (false negatives × 0.4, the proportion who seek treatment) = 10,555 × 0.555 = 5,858; (2) with no testing,

85,000 × 0.15 = 12,750 white men will actually have prostate cancer and 12,750 × 0.40 = 5,100 of them will seek treatment; 15,000 × 0.25 = 3,750 African American men will actually have prostate cancer, and 3,750 × 0.40 = 1,500 of them will seek treatment; and (3) the number of prostate biopsies for white men with the PSA test would be half of the men who test positive (including the false positives, which is 14.8 percent of the men without cancer) plus 40 percent of the false negatives = (9,091 + 10,693) × 0.5 + 1,464 = 11,356.

TABLE 9.8. CALCULATION OF COSTS FOR PSA AND EPCA-2 TESTS

	Whites		African Americans		All Subjects	
PSA Test	Freq.	Cost	Freq.	Cost	Freq.	Cost
Prostatectomy	5,858	216,089,904	1,685	62,156,280	7,543	278,246,184
Radiation	3,019	179,494,645	621	36,921,555	3,640	216,416,200
Conservative	1,678	53,922,530	798	25,643,730	2,476	79,566,260
Prostate biopsy	11,356	13,627,200	2,600	3,120,000	13,956	16,747,200
PSA test	85,000	3,400,000	15,000	600,000	100,000	4,000,000
Cost/person		5,489		8,563		5,950
EPCA-2 Test	Freq.	Cost	Freq.	Cost	Freq.	Cost
Prostatectomy	6,822	251,649,936	1,963	72,411,144	8,785	324,061,080
Radiation	3,515	208,984,325	723	42,985,965	4,238	251,970,290
Conservative	1,954	62,791,790	929	29,853,415	2,883	92,645,205
Prostate biopsy	7,383	8,859,600	2,022	2,426,400	9,405	11,286,000
EPCA-2 test	85,000	6,800,000	15,000	1,200,000	100,000	8,000,000
Cost/person		6,342		9,925		6,880
No testing (assume 40% with cancer get treatment)	5,100		1,500		6,600	
Prostatectomy	2,831	104,429,928	815	30,063,720	3,646	134,493,648
Radiation	1,459	86,744,845	300	17,836,500	1,759	104,581,345
Conservative	811	26,061,485	386	12,404,110	1,197	38,465,595
Prostate biopsy	5,100	6,120,000	1,500	1,800,000	6,600	7,920,000
Cost/person		2,628		4,140		2,855

6. Refer to Table 9.9 for calculating ICERs. The ICER for targeted screening of African Americans with the PSA test was the preferred strategy at an incremental cost of $1,970 per QALY. Universal screening was nearly 20 times as high, but still below the conservative $100,000 cost/QALY threshold for cost-effectiveness.
7. African Americans have a higher incidence of prostate cancer, thus benefit the most from screening. The PSA test had the lowest ICER.

TABLE 9.9. ICER TARGETED OR UNIVERSAL SCREENING FOR PROSTATE CANCER

	Cost/Person	QALY/Person	ΔCosts	ΔQALY	ICER
No Screening	2,868	24.2 × 0.85 (whites) + 19.57 × 0.15 (African Americans) = 23.51	—	—	—
Targeted Screening African Americans only (PSA)	8,563 × 0.15 (African Americans) + 2,628 × 0.85 (whites) = 3,518	21.82 × 0.15 (African Americans) + 24.2 × 0.85 (whites) = 23.84	650	0.33	1,970
Targeted Screening (EPCA-2)	9,925 × 0.15 (African Americans) + 2,628 × 0.85 (whites) = 3,723	21.86 × 0.15 (African Americans) + 24.2 × 0.85 (whites) = 23.85	205	0.01	20,500
Universal Screening (PSA)	5,950	23.89	2,227	0.04	55,675
Universal Screening (ECPA-2)	6,880	23.92	930	0.03	31,000

References

Centers for Disease Control and Prevention. "Cost Effectiveness Analysis." [Online information; retrieved 2/7/08.] http://www.cdc.gov/owcd/EET/CostEffect2/fixed/4.html.

Coco, A. S. 2007. "Cost-Effectiveness Analysis of Treatment Options for Acute Otitis Media." *Annals of Family Medicine* 5 (1): 29–38.

Elmore, J. G., M. B. Barton, V. M. Moceri, S. Polk, P. J. Arena, and S. W. Fletcher. 1998. "Ten-Year Risk of False Positive Screening Mammograms and Clinical Breast Examinations." *New England Journal of Medicine* 338 (16): 1089–96.

Hoffman, R. M., L. C. Harlan, C. N. Klabunde, F. D. Gilliland, R. A. Stephenson, W. C. Hunt, and A. L. Potosky. 2003. "Racial Differences in Initial Treatment for Clinically Localized Prostate Cancer: Results from the Prostate Cancer Outcomes Study." *Journal of General Internal Medicine* 18: 845–53.

Hunink, M., and P. Glasziou. 2001. *Decision Making in Health and Medicine: Integrating Evidence and Values.* New York: Cambridge University Press.

Last, J. M. 2001. *A Dictionary of Epidemiology.* New York: Oxford University Press.

Muennig, P., P. Franks, and M. Gold. 2005. "The Cost Effectiveness of Health Insurance." *American Journal of Preventive Medicine* 28 (1): 59–64.

Oregon Health Services Commission. 1991. *Prioritization of Health Services: A Report to the Governor and Legislature, 1991.* Salem, OR: Oregon Health Services Commission.

Sun, L., J. W. Moul, J. M. Hotaling, E. Rampersaud, P. Dahm, C. Robertson, N. Fitzsimons, D. Albala, and T. J. Polascik. 2007. "Prostate-Specific Antigen (PSA) and PSA Velocity for Prostate Cancer Detection in Men Aged <50 Years." *BJU International* 99 (4): 753–57.

Wilson, L. S., R. Tesoro, E. P. Elkin, N. Sadetsky, J. M. Broering, D. M. Latini, J. DuChane, R. R. Mody, and P. R. Carroll. 2007. "Cumulative Cost Pattern Comparison of Prostate Cancer Treatments." *Cancer* 109 (3): 518–27.

EVIDENCE-BASED MANAGEMENT AND MEDICINE

Evidence-based medicine refers to clinicians' use of the best available scientific evidence, rather than tradition or hunches, to make decisions regarding the diagnosis, treatment, or prognosis of the patients under their care. Evidence-based management is rooted in this practice in the medical realm, and similarly involves using the best available scientific evidence to make managerial decisions. Such evidence may be based on clinical studies and trials, other epidemiologic research, or research from other disciplines such as management or behavioral science. Presumably managers who are equipped with the facts make better decisions than those who rely only on experience, tradition, or hunches. In fact, this entire text is aimed at convincing present and future managers that they would be wise to integrate epidemiologic theory and reasoning into their everyday decision making.

This section consists of five chapters. Chapter 10 is a review of basic statistical tools, including both descriptive and inferential statistics. Chapters 11 through 13 deal primarily with three important study designs that are used regularly in epidemiologic research: the case-control study, the cohort study, and the randomized clinical trial. Each of these three designs has its own characteristics, strengths, and weaknesses. Some of the designs are prospective, or forward-looking. The prospective cohort study and randomized clinical trial enroll subjects in the present and track their progress for years into the future. The case-control study and retrospective cohort study are backward-looking, in the sense that while the study is conducted in the present, information from the past must be retrieved. Finally, Chapter 14 deals with clinical epidemiology, a term that is similar to, if not identical to, evidence-based medicine. Here the authors compare clinical decision making with and without a solid grounding in the scientific literature. A case study in this chapter provides a set of decision-making tools to aid in clinical judgment. The purpose of this chapter is not to transform managers into "armchair" clinicians. That would be both risky and unproductive. Rather the purpose is to expose future managers to how clinicians reason and make decisions with and without the use of the best available scientific evidence.

One of the main thrusts of epidemiologic research is trying to establish a causal relationship between a particular exposure, risk factor, or intervention, and an outcome or disease. It is one thing to demonstrate an association between an exposure and disease—exercise and heart disease, for instance. It is quite another, however, to demonstrate that the relationship is causal. Exercise may be associated with heart disease in such a way that it would seem that exercise is "protective," i.e., exercise seems to be associated with lower rates of heart disease. On the other hand, heart disease may prevent people from exercising regularly, or at least as vigorously, due to pain or risk of infarction. The challenge of epidemiologic research is to demonstrate causal relationship (low exercise → heart disease), not simply an association.

On a practical level, the physician or manager is faced with at least two tasks. One task involves trying to interpret a particular study from a practice standpoint, which means deciding what the results of the study mean in terms of the practice of medicine or management. Second, the physician or manager must decide whether the results of the study can be trusted, which involves an evaluation of the characteristics of the study design, including whether such characteristics support any causal relationship(s) reported in the study.

Perhaps the most basic principle in deciding whether the exposure, risk factor, or intervention is a true "cause" of disease or outcome is whether the cause is necessary and/or sufficient. A *necessary* cause is a factor whose presence is required for disease to occur. In other words, disease occurs "only if" that factor is present. For example, if HIV is a necessary factor for AIDS, it means that HIV must be present for AIDS to develop. The disease cannot occur without the presence of this agent. A *sufficient* factor is one that inevitably produces disease. The ebola virus would be considered a sufficient factor for ebola if the people who are exposed to the virus always develop this disease. The link between cause and effect is strongest for factors that are proven to be both necessary and sufficient causes of disease because there may be a one-to-one relationship between agent and disease. The agent is necessary for the disease to occur, and always leads to the development of disease. Most chronic disease risk factors are neither necessary nor sufficient causes of disease. For example, cigarette smoking is not a necessary cause of lung cancer because nonsmokers get lung cancer from other causes. Neither is smoking a sufficient risk factor for lung cancer because smoking will not inevitably lead to lung cancer. Some long-term smokers escape the ravages of lung cancer, despite research that demonstrates that they are about 10–20 times as likely to develop the disease as people who do not smoke.

Chapter 14 summarizes a number of criteria that strengthen our confidence that the results of a particular study demonstrate a causal relationship. This involves determining whether the study has "internal validity," i.e., whether it is designed in such as way as to truly isolate the relationship between a cause and an effect. A "strong" relationship between an exposure and a disease, or a treatment and an outcome, is supportive of causality, as is a consistent finding across different populations or using different methods. High specificity as demonstrated by the necessary and sufficient conditions discussed earlier—a one-to-one link between cause and effect—is supportive of causality. Studies with a correct time relationship, such that we know that the cause precedes the effect (and not vice-versa) are supportive of causality, as are studies that demonstrate a dose-response relationship, or biological gradient, where a higher dose or longer exposure leads to increased risk. Finally, studies that are plausible from a scientific standpoint, in terms of theory, and coherent with other known facts about the disease, are more likely to demonstrate causality.

In summary, the physician or manager should not only be aware of the scientific literature, but be able to determine whether such literature is trustworthy, and if so, be able to distill important results and apply such results to the practice of medicine or management. This involves determining the presence or absence of the various criteria for causality, and eliminating any other alternative explanations for the significant research findings reported in the literature.

STATISTICAL TOOLS

Mary Kay Rayens and Thomas C. Tucker

Epidemiology can be viewed as the set of tools used to measure the need for and impact of healthcare interventions. This chapter describes the basic statistical tools used by epidemiologists that can be employed by health service managers to guide the decision-making process. The chapter is intended to serve as an overview of these concepts; more detailed information may be found in the included references.

There are two basic sets of statistical tools, *descriptive epidemiology* and *inferential epidemiology*.

Descriptive and Inferential Epidemiology

Descriptive epidemiology describes a characteristic or characteristics of a defined population, including health needs, health events, and health outcomes. Descriptive epidemiology typically consists of summarizing the quantitative attributes of a sample from the population of observations (when the population is too large to assess completely) or a known characteristic of the entire population of interest. For example, if you as a health manager need to assess the compliance of the hospital staff with the standard protocol for chart documentation, one way to assess this would be to review a randomly selected sample of charts to determine the number of charts from the sample that are in compliance (see Table 10.1 in the appendix at the end of this chapter for a table of random numbers). Another example of the use of descriptive statistics would be to record all the reported cases of a particular disease and then summarize the incidence of this illness in the population during a specific period. In other words, the tools of epidemiology can be used to describe characteristics of a population or estimate these characteristics from a sample.

Inferential epidemiology is used to compare two or more populations for differences or similarities. For example, one could use inferential epidemiology to ascertain whether males differed from females in the risk of developing hepatitis after exposure. In this situation, we could examine the frequency of cases in each gender, and use that information to infer whether the risk of disease is the same for both groups. Inferential methods allow epidemiologists to use randomly chosen samples to compare the underlying populations.

Levels of Measurement

There are two basic classes of data, *continuous* and *categorical*. Variables that are measured on an *interval scale*—which indicates that for these variables the distance between points is meaningful and the variable can take any value within a continuous range—are continuous. Examples of continuous variables are age, height, weight, and systolic blood pressure. Categorical variables can take values in only a fixed number of categories. These types of variables may be either *ordinal*, meaning the categories can be ordered in some meaningful way, or *nominal*, meaning the categories are qualitative rather than quantitative. An example of an ordinal variable would be the assessment of patient satisfaction graded on a four-point scale from "very satisfied" to "very dissatisfied," or the extent of cancer at diagnosis coded as stage I, II, III, or IV. Examples of nominal variables include race and gender.

Sampling

When it is not possible or practical to collect data from an entire population, a subset of that population, a *sample*, is used to provide an estimate of the characteristic being studied. The purpose of sampling is typically to estimate population characteristics, but usually the sample is drawn from a *sampling frame* rather than from the population itself. The sampling frame is a compilation of the members of the population who are available to be chosen in the sample, and should include as many of the population members as possible. An example of a sampling frame is a telephone book. If the goal of a survey is to estimate the percentage of citizens in a certain town who wear seatbelts, it may be impossible to have an exhaustive list of citizens, but the phone book may be used as a reasonable sampling frame from which to randomly choose participants. Random-digit-dialing techniques would increase the sampling frame to include citizens with unlisted numbers; this may improve the ability of the survey to provide a realistic estimate of the underlying population percentage of seatbelt users.

The two basic ways to choose a set of elements from a sampling frame are *convenience sampling* and *probability sampling*. Convenience sampling is a nonrandom selection of elements from the population. An example of data collected using a convenience sampling scheme would be an assessment of a relevant disease state (e.g., diabetic status) of the next 50 patients to enter a particular clinic.

A probability sample is drawn using the concept of randomness. The simplest example of a probability sample is a *simple random sample* in which a random mechanism is used to select patients or records from an exhaustive list of the population. Using this sampling scheme, each member of the population is equally likely to be chosen. This type of sampling is considered the optimal type to use when planning an experiment, but it can be difficult to implement in practice. Rather than just taking the next 50 patients visiting a clinic, as we did in the convenience sampling example, in a simple random sampling the surveyors would randomly select 50 patients from the entire list of patients seen at that clinic. While this may be a relatively straightforward task in this example (since the population is well-defined and can be listed), it becomes difficult or even impossible in settings where the population defies enumeration.

Other types of probability sampling include *systematic sampling, cluster sampling,* and *stratified random sampling.* Each of these types of sampling involves schemes in which the sample of subjects is chosen in a more patterned way than is done with simple random sampling. An example of systematic sampling would be to randomly choose one of a clinic's first 20 patient charts, and then pull every 20th chart from the clinic's entire population. This would give the researcher a 5 percent sample of the population, which could be used to describe the entire population of clinic patients.

The goal of probability sampling is to garner samples that are representative of the populations from which they come, so that conclusions can be extended from the sample comparisons to the populations. Convenience sampling, while easier to implement, may lead to estimates that are not representative, since the specific population the sample members represent is not clear. If a convenience sample is drawn from a population of clinic patients seen during cold and flu season, for example, the sample may represent the subpopulation of patients who are most likely to succumb to these illnesses, rather than the larger population of all clinic patients.

Descriptive Statistics for Continuous Variables

Once a sample has been chosen and the relevant characteristics measured, the first step in describing a continuous variable is typically to assess the *mean* and *standard deviation* of that measure in the sample. The mean is the average value of that measure, and the standard deviation is a measure of the variability of the observations.

The formula for the sample mean, $\overline{X}$, is given below. With n subjects in the sample,

$$\overline{X} = \frac{\sum_{i=1}^{n} X_i}{n}$$

In plain English, the mean equals the sum of all the measures, divided by the number of subjects. For example, let's say a nurse weighed five toddlers, and their weights were 25 pounds, 32 pounds, 27 pounds, 24 pounds, and 22 pounds. To find the mean weight, the nurse would add 25, 32, 27, 24, and 22 (which equals 130) and divide by 5, getting 26. Thus, the mean weight of the five toddlers is 26 pounds.

Standard deviation is the average distance the variables fall from the mean. Statistical data are often viewed in a bell curve, where the top of the curve is the mean and the values above and below the mean form the sides of the bell. The lower the standard deviation, the steeper the bell, because more of the values are close to the mean.

When you want to know the standard deviation of a sample of a population, this is the formula:

$$s = \sqrt{\frac{\sum_{i=1}^{n}(X_i - \overline{X})^2}{n-1}} = \sqrt{\frac{n\sum_{i=1}^{n} X_i^2 - (\sum_{i=1}^{n} X_i)^2}{n(n-1)}}$$

This formula can broken into four simple steps:

1. Subtract the mean, $\overline{X}$, from each value, X.
2. Square the resulting number for each value.
3. Add up those squares, and divide that sum by the number of values minus one.
4. Take the square root of that result.

Notice the first formula given for the standard deviation illustrates how this statistic is a function of the distance of each of the sample values from the mean value, while the second formula provides a shortcut for computation.

The *variance* is simply the square of the standard deviation, and thus also is a gauge of variability of the measurements. In the case of simple random sampling, the *standard error of the mean* is the sample standard deviation divided by the square root of the sample size. While the standard deviation is a measure of the variability of observations about the sample mean, the standard error of the mean is a measure of how accurate the sample mean is likely to be in estimating the true population mean.

An additional summary measure for sample data is the *median*, or 50th percentile. Half of the observations lie above this value and half below (in the case of an even number of observations, the median is the average of the middle two values).

An additional method for describing the variability of the sample data would be to assess the *range*, or the difference between the highest and lowest observed value.

The mean and median are measures of *central tendency*, while the standard deviation, variance, and range are measures of *dispersion* or variation.

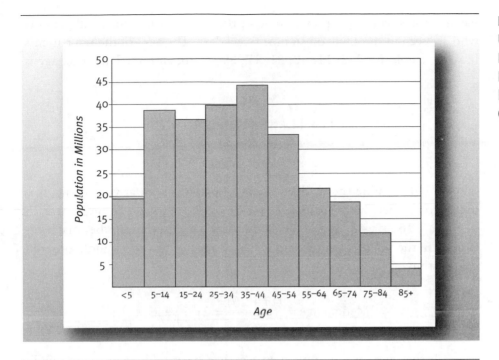

FIGURE 10.1
U.S. Resident Population by Age Group, 1997

SOURCE: National Center for Health Statistics (1999).

A graphical method for summarizing continuous data is a *histogram*, which is a display of bars whose size is determined by the number or percentage of the sample that falls within the range of values prescribed for that bar. Two distinguishing features of a histogram are bars that touch and equally spaced ranges for each bar. This graphical method allows one to discern patterns in the distribution of values, such as age of the population (Figure 10.1).

Example 1

The example helps illustrate how descriptive measures for continuous variables are calculated. As the manager of a health clinic, you want to describe the age of patients who come to your clinic on weekdays in the summer. Age is a continuous variable, so you decide to calculate the mean age, the median age, the standard deviation of ages observed, and the range of ages.

You have selected a random sample of ten patients seen at the clinic between Monday and Friday during the first week in July. (In practice, your sample may be considerably larger, but this limited sample size is used here to calculate the measures of central tendency and variability without being too computationally cumbersome.) The presumption is that this sampling frame (i.e., patients who come on the weekdays during the first week in July) has members who are representative of the population, namely all patients who are seen in the clinic on summer weekdays. The ages of the ten patients in your sample are 9, 3, 11, 42, 81, 17, 59, 7, 26, and 32. The mean age is

$$\bar{X} = \frac{\sum_{i=1}^{10} X_i}{10} = \frac{(9 + 3 + 11 + 42 + 81 + 17 + 59 + 7 + 26 + 32)}{10} = 28.7 \text{ years}$$

To determine the median age of all patients seen at your clinic, it is useful to reorder the ten sample observations from lowest to highest: 3, 7, 9, 11, 17, 26, 32, 42, 59, 81. Because there are an even number of observations in the sample, the median is the average of the two middle ordered values, thus

$$\text{Median age} = \frac{(17 + 26)}{2} = 21.5 \text{ years}$$

If the number of sample members had been odd, the median would have been simply the middle value from the ordered list of ages.

To determine the sample standard deviation using the shortcut formula, it is necessary to calculate both $\sum X_i$ and $\sum X_i^2$.

$$\sum_{i=1}^{10} X_i = 9 + 3 + 11 + 42 + 81 + 17 + 59 + 7 + 26 + 32 = 287$$

$$\sum_{i=1}^{10} X_i^2 = 9^2 + 3^2 + 11^2 + 42^2 + 81^2 + 17^2 + 59^2 + 7^2 + 26^2 + 32^2 = 14{,}055$$

Using the shortcut formula for the standard deviation,

$$s = \sqrt{\frac{n\sum_{i=1}^{n} X_i^2 (\sum_{i=1}^{n} X_i)^2}{n(n-1)}} = \sqrt{\frac{(10 \times 14{,}055) - (287 \times 287)}{(10 \times 9)}} = 25.4 \text{ years}$$

The standard error of the mean for this sample is $\frac{25.4}{\sqrt{10}} = 8.0$ years. Finally, the age range of this sample of ten patients is the difference between the oldest and youngest patients, or 78 years.

Descriptive Statistics for Categorical Variables

The descriptive summary for categorical data usually consists of a *frequency distribution*, which is a tabular or graphical way of summarizing

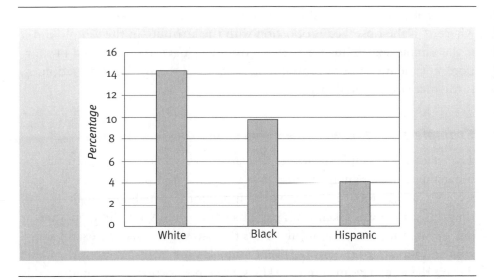

FIGURE 10.2
Mothers Who
Smoked
Cigarettes
During
Pregnancy,
1997

SOURCE: National Center for Health Statistics (1999).

the percentage or number of responses in each category. In its graphical form, the frequency distribution can be summarized in a *bar chart*. The bar chart is differentiated from the histogram by the fact that the bars should have spaces between them. This is to underscore the fact that one should resist the temptation to look for trends indicated by the bars, particularly in the case of nominal data when the ordering of the bars is arbitrary (Figure 10.2). Another summary measure that may be used for categorical data is the *mode*, the most commonly occurring value for the variable of interest. It is possible for sample data to have multiple modes or no mode.

It is common in epidemiology to study *binary variables*, categorical variables with only two outcomes. Examples of binary variables include survival status (alive or dead), disease status (present or absent), and gender (male or female). In this context, it is often useful to summarize binary data as either a *proportion* or a *rate*.

A proportion is calculated by dividing the number of observations with an attribute (i.e., characteristic of interest) by the total number of observations. The *percentage* is the proportion multiplied by 100.

A rate is a proportion that has been multiplied by a factor to make the order of magnitude of the proportion more meaningful. For example, in the case of a rare health event, it is more meaningful to present incidence, prevalence, or mortality rates as per 1,000 or per 100,000 population than as a percentage. For example, if the proportion of people in the United States who have a particular rare disease in the current year is equal to 0.000042, the rate of this disease in the U.S. population would then be 4.2 cases per 100,000 people. Rates are typically used only to describe populations, while proportions may be used to summarize populations or samples.

The sample standard deviation in this context is $s_{\hat{p}} = \sqrt{[\hat{p}_1(1-\hat{p}_1) / n]}$ where $\hat{p}$ is the observed proportion with the attribute in the sample and n is the sample size. Thus for the case of binary data, the observed proportion $\hat{p}$ is the measure of central tendency, while the standard deviation, s_p, is the measure of variability.

Example 2

The following example illustrates the calculation of descriptive statistics for binary measures. When the previous sample of ten patient ages was collected, you also recorded whether each patient was male or female. Recall that this sample was taken from patients who visited your clinic on a weekday during the first week in July. Thus this sample can also be used to provide an estimate of the proportion of females (or males) seen in the clinic during the weekdays in summer. The sample proportion is denoted $\hat{p}$; this statistic is an estimate of the population proportion, **p**. In your sample, seven patients were males and three were females. The proportion of the sample who are female is 3/10 or 0.3. The proportion of the sample who are male is 7/10 or 0.7. Thus 70 percent of the sample are males and 30 percent are females. The sample standard deviation is

$$s_{\hat{p}} = \sqrt{\frac{\hat{p}(1-\hat{p})}{n}} = \sqrt{\frac{(.03) \times (1-0.3)}{10}} = \sqrt{0.021} = 0.14$$

Notice that because this is a binary variable, it does not matter if you calculate the standard deviation based on the male proportion or the female proportion, since the proportion of males is equal to one minus the proportion of females and vice versa.

Inferential Statistics

Overview

The statistical comparison of two or more samples representing distinct underlying populations can be accomplished in a variety of ways, depending on the goals of the study and whether the variables are continuous or categorical.

Many inferential techniques are designed to test specific *hypotheses*, or statements that compare populations in a quantitative way. A simple example is the comparison of two population means. The *null hypothesis*, or the statement to be tested, would be that the two populations have the same mean. The *alternative hypothesis*, which will be assumed to be true if the null hypothesis is rejected, would be that the two population means are different. This is an example of a *two-sided hypothesis*—that is, a hypothesis in which the null hypothesis can be disproved by significant differences on either side (up or down, hotter or colder) of the null hypothesis—since there is not a presumption that one mean should necessarily be greater than the other one. As an example of a *one-sided hypothesis*, we may want to test whether a new drug is *more effective* than the current standard, and thus are only interested in obtaining a significant difference in mean response in a particular direction. In practice, two-sided hypothesis tests are more widely used. In the context of hypothesis testing, the *test statistic*, which is a function of the sample data, is used to reject the null hypothesis or fail to reject it. The conclusion in the former case is that the groups are not equal, while the conclusion in the latter case is that there is not enough evidence to suggest that the groups are significantly different. Note that hypotheses are never "proved"; they can only be disproved or not disproved.

A key element of hypothesis testing is the concept of the **p** *value*. The p value is the probability of the observed differences being due to random chance. Stated another way, the **p** value is the probability of a test statistic as extreme as the one obtained if the null hypothesis of equality is actually true. Intuitively, then, the smaller the **p** value, the more evidence there is to suggest that the null hypothesis is false. The general rule of thumb is that p values less than 0.05 are considered *significant*, thus giving ample evidence to reject the null. *P* values larger than 0.05 but less than 0.1 are typically considered *marginally significant*, perhaps indicative of a trend that did not quite reach strict statistical significance. **p** values below 0.01, or in some contexts below 0.005, may be considered *highly significant*.

When conducting a hypothesis test, one of four possible outcomes will occur. Two positive outcomes would be either to reject the null hypothesis when in fact it is false or to fail to reject it when it is actually true. If the null hypothesis is rejected even though it is true, this is considered making a *type I error*. Conversely, if the null hypothesis is not rejected even though it is false, a *type II error* has been committed. The probability of making a type I error is denoted α, and the probability of making a type II error is commonly referred to as β. While it would be ideal to make both α and β as small as possible so that the likelihood of reaching a wrong conclusion is minuscule, there is an inverse relationship between β and α, such that it is impossible to minimize one without increasing the other. The conventions for α and β are typically 0.05 and 0.20, respectively. That is, we are willing to wrongly reject the null hypothesis 5 percent of the time and fail to reject the null when it is false 20 percent of the time.

The probability that we will *correctly* discern that the null hypothesis is false is the *power* of the test. The power and the type II error rate sum to one; a type II error rate of 0.2 is equivalent to a power of 80 percent. The convention of setting α to 0.05 is what drives the comparison of p values to this level. The α level, also referred to as the *level of significance*, is a general guideline set in the planning stage of hypothesis testing, while the p value is associated with a specific test statistic. If the p value is less than the α level, the conclusion is that the test statistic is significant. In other words, if the p value is less than the α level, we would reject the null hypothesis.

Two-Sample t Test

The most common type of hypothesis testing involves the comparison of the mean values for two groups on some continuous attribute. The null hypothesis in this situation is

$$H_o: M_1 = M_2$$

The parameters M_1 and M_2 are the true population means for the continuous variable of interest. These population means are estimated using the sample means (i.e., $\overline{X}_1$ and $\overline{X}_2$) from each of the two groups. In order to test this hypothesis, a two-sample t test can be used. The formula for the test statistic is

$$t = \frac{\overline{X}_1 - \overline{X}_2}{\sqrt{(s_1^2 / n) + (s_2^2 / n_2)}}$$

The sample sizes from each group are n_1 and n_2, respectively. This is the general form of the t test. For the special case in which the standard deviations of the two groups are not statistically different (which may be ascertained via another hypothesis test, this one for equality of variances; see below for details), the t test formula simplifies to

$$t = \frac{\overline{X}_1 - \overline{X}_2}{\sqrt{(s_1^2 / n) + (s_2^2 / n_2)}} \text{ with } s^2 = \frac{(n_1 - 1)s_1^2 + (n_2 - 1)s_2^2}{(n_1 + n_2 - 2)}$$

The formula given above for s^2 provides a *pooled* estimate of the variance for this case, in which the two variances are not significantly different. The null hypothesis of no difference between the group means is rejected when the observed value of the t test statistic is "large" in absolute value. To determine the significance level, the test statistic is compared to a t distribution, which has a bell-shaped form that is approximately normal, particularly for large sample sizes. Assuming a sample size of at least 30 per group and an alpha level of 0.05, the *critical value* for the test statistic is approximately 2. The critical value associated with a particular hypothesis test gives a cutoff beyond which the observed test statistic (in absolute value) is deemed to be significant. The interpretation is that with this sample size, if the absolute value of the test statistic obtained is at least as large as the critical value, the null hypothesis is rejected since the **p** value is at most 0.05. The critical value is a function of both the α level and the *degrees of freedom*. The sample size does play a role in determining the critical value since the degrees of freedom are a function of the sample size. In particular, the degrees of freedom (ν) for the *t* test based on pooled variances are equal to $n_1 + n_2 - 2$. For the *t* test based on unpooled variances, the degrees of freedom are determined by

$$\nu = \frac{\left\{ \dfrac{s_1^2}{n_1} + \dfrac{s_2^2}{n_2} \right\}^2}{\dfrac{s_1^4}{n_1^2(n_1 - 1)} + \dfrac{s_2^4}{n_2^2(n_2 - 1)}}$$

If the above formula leads to a fractional value for the degrees of freedom, this may be rounded to the nearest degree. Once the degrees of freedom are known and the test statistic has been calculated, the observed test statistic may be compared to the appropriate critical value displayed in Table 10.2, located in the appendix at the end of this chapter.

To determine which form of the *t* test is appropriate, a test for the equality of variances is needed. The null and alternative hypotheses in this case are

$$H_o : \sigma_1^2 = \sigma_2^2$$

$$H_o : \sigma_1^2 \neq \sigma_2^2$$

The population variance for each group, σ_i^2, is estimated using the sample variance, s_i^2, to test the null hypothesis. To test this hypothesis, label the larger sample variance as s_1^2 and the smaller as s_2^2. The corresponding sample sizes for each are labeled n_1 and n_2, respectively. The form of the test statistic is simply s_1^2 / s_2^2. This observed test statistic is then compared to an *F* distribution with $\nu_1 = n_1 - 1$ numerator degrees of freedom and $\nu_2 = n_2 - 1$ denominator degrees of freedom. Tables 10.3 and 10.4 in the appendix of this chapter present the critical values of the *F* distribution for one-sided tests with $\alpha = 0.05$, and 0.01. These tabled critical values are equivalent to the critical values for two-sided tests with significance levels of 0.10 and 0.02, respectively.

Example 3

The following is an example of the use of the *t* test in comparing a continuous measure between two populations.

As the manager of a clinic, you want to compare the average age of the previous sample of ten patients seen during weekdays in the summer with that of a sample of ten patients seen during weekdays in the winter. The hypothesis you would like to test is whether there is a significant age difference between the two patient groups, given the possibility that there may be more injuries in summer involving young patients and more viral infections in winter involving older patients. Given this hypothesis, you would expect the average age in summer to be significantly different from the average patient age in winter. The null and alternative hypotheses are

$$H_o: \mu_s = \mu_w$$
$$H_A: \mu_s \neq \mu_w$$

It has already been shown in Example 1 that the average age of the summer weekday patients (denoted $\overline{X}_1$) was 28.7 years with a standard deviation (s_1) of 25.4 years. In order to test the hypothesis of equal age in the two groups of patients, you select a random sample of ten patients treated at the clinic on a weekday during the first week of February. The average age of the second sample ($\overline{X}_2$) is 47.1 years with a standard deviation (s_2) of 21.0 years. We first test the null hypothesis of equality of variances using the sample standard deviations,

$$\frac{s_1^2}{s_2^2} = \frac{25.4^2}{21.0^2} = 1.5$$

Notice the critical value for the two-sided test from Table 10.2 with $\alpha = 0.1$ and 9 degrees of freedom for both the numerator and denominator is equal to 1.833. Since our test statistic is less than the tabled value, the conclusion is that the *p* value for this test exceeds 0.1, so the null hypothesis is not rejected. Since the variances are not significantly different, the correct form of the *t* test is

$$t = \frac{\overline{X}_1 - \overline{X}_2}{\sqrt{s^2 / n_1 + (s^2 / n_2)}} \text{ with } s^2 = \frac{(n_1 - 1)s_1^2 + (n_2 - 1)s_2^2}{(n_1 + n_2 - 2)}$$

In this case, $s^2 = \dfrac{(9 \times 25.4) + (9 \times 21.09 \times 21.0)}{18} = 543.1$ so that

$$t = \frac{(28.7 - 47.1)}{\sqrt{(543.1/10) + (543.1/10)}} = -1.8 \text{ and } |t| = 1.8$$

The critical value for a two-sided test with $\alpha = 0.05$ and 18 degrees of freedom is 2.101 (see Table 10.2). Thus, we conclude that the *p* value for this observed test statistic exceeds 0.05, so we fail to reject the null hypothesis and conclude that there is insufficient evidence to suggest that the two patient groups differ significantly on age. This conclusion may seem counterintuitive given the apparent large difference in means between the two samples. However, the standard deviations are relatively large and the sample sizes are modest, both of which impact the *p* value of the test statistic.

z Test for Differences in Proportions

The *z* test for differences in proportions between two groups is similar in form to the *t* test for two group means. The null and alternative hypotheses in this case are

$$H_o: p_1 = p_2$$
$$H_A: p_1 \neq p_2$$

The statistics $\hat{p}_1$ and $\hat{p}_2$ are the sample proportions of subjects with the attribute of interest from each of the groups. These are estimates of the population parameters, p_1 and p_2. As before, n_1 and n_2 are the sample sizes obtained from the two groups. The critical value for the *z* test is determined using the standard normal distribution (also denoted the *z* distribution). A table of critical values from this distribution (Table 10.5) is found in the chapter appendix.

The *z* test has the form

$$z = \frac{\hat{p}_1 - \hat{p}_2}{\sqrt{[\hat{p}_1(1 - \hat{p}_1)/n_1] = [\hat{p}_2(1 - \hat{p}_2)/n_2}}$$

In general, the *z* distribution provides accurate critical values for the *z* test statistic. However, if the sample sizes are limited, the *z* test tends to underestimate the true *p* value, which may lead to an increased type I error rate. To correct for this, a slight adjustment to the test statistic is suggested. The correction is referred to as the *Yates correction*, and is a subtraction from the numerator of the test statistic; this modification decreases the test statistic, which in turn increases the *p* value. As the sample sizes get large, the impact of the Yates correction is negligible. The form of the test statistic with this correction is

$$z = \frac{\left|\hat{p}_1 - \hat{p}_2\right| - \frac{1}{2}(1/n_1 + 1/n_2)}{\sqrt{[\hat{p}_1(1-\hat{p}_1)/n_1] + [\hat{p}_2(1-\hat{p}_2)/n_2]}}$$

The observed test statistic is compared to the standard normal (z) distribution; critical values are displayed in Table 10.5 found in the appendix of this chapter. The body of the table contains the probabilities, or area under the curve, for each possible value of the test statistic. For example, 95 percent of the z distribution is contained between –1.96 and 1.96, so choosing 1.96 as a critical value for a z test would result in a test with an α level of 0.05.

Example 4

As the manager of a clinic, you want to know if there is a significant difference between the proportion of males or females seen during the summer and the gender distribution of patients seen in winter. You have already determined (in Example 2) that the proportion of males seen in summer is 0.7. If the sample of ten patients seen during the first week of February has four males, the test statistic for the comparison of these two proportions is

$$z = \frac{(0.7 - 0.4) - \frac{1}{2}(1/10 + 1/10)}{\sqrt{[(0.7 \times 0.3)/10] + [0.4 \times 0.6)/10]}}$$

It is important to use the Yates correction since the sample sizes are small. Comparing this observed value to Table 10.5 in the chapter appendix reveals that the probability associated with observing 0.94 under the null hypothesis of equal proportions is equal to $(1 - [.3264 \times 2])$ or 0.34. This is the proportion of area under the standard normal curve that is in the two tails with a critical value of 0.94. With a *p* value of 0.34, there is no evidence to reject the null hypothesis, so we conclude the two proportions are not significantly different.

Confidence Intervals

The construction of a confidence interval around a sample estimate provides an alternative to the hypothesis test. The general form of the confidence interval is the test statistic plus or minus a particular quantity; this quantity is a function of the variability and the sample size. This method provides a range of values within which the true population parameter is likely to lie. Test statistics with relatively high variability and/or small sample sizes will have wider confidence intervals than those based on smaller standard deviations and/or more robust sample sizes. While confidence intervals can be constructed for virtually any test statistic, the confidence interval for the difference in means is

$$(\overline{X}_1 - \overline{X}_2) - t_\alpha \times s < \mu_2 < (\overline{X}_1 - \overline{X}_2) + t_\alpha \times s$$

The sample means $\overline{X}_1$ and $\overline{X}_2$ are used in this calculation, as is the appropriate form of the sample standard deviation, s. This standard deviation is either the pooled or unpooled version discussed in the previous section on the two-sample t test, depending on whether the variances are significantly different or not. The quantity t_α is a function of the alpha level and sample size and may be determined using Table 10.2 in the chapter appendix. For example, if there are 16 subjects in each group, the significance level is chosen to be 0.05, and the two population variances are not different, the correct t_α would be 2.042 and s is the pooled standard deviation. If the α level is 0.05, the resulting confidence interval is referred to as a *95 percent confidence interval*. For alternative levels of significance, different t_α values would be specified to increase or decrease the width of the interval according to whether the percent confidence is increased or decreased. As the percent confidence increases, the size of t_α also increases so that the width of the interval is larger. Conversely, t_α is smaller for smaller levels of confidence so that the width of the confidence interval shrinks.

The interpretation of a 95 percent confidence interval is that we are 95 percent confident of the method used to generate it. In other words, we don't know for certain whether the obtained confidence interval contains the true population parameter of interest, but we do know that 95 percent of the time the obtained confidence interval will contain the population parameter. We summarize this interpretation by stating that we are 95 percent confident that the difference between the two population means is between a and b, where a and b are the lower and upper limits of the obtained 95 percent confidence interval.

The relationship between hypothesis testing and confidence intervals is direct. In the example of the confidence interval for the difference in means, if the obtained $(1 - \alpha)100$ percent confidence interval does not contain 0, this is analogous to the conclusion that the two means are significantly different at a significance level α. The appeal of the confidence interval over the hypothesis test is that it provides what is perhaps a more concrete representation of the "typical" range of values the sample statistics are likely to take. The appeal of hypothesis testing compared to confidence intervals is that the former provides a **p** value that may be compared with various α levels to determine significance, while the latter is calculated for a preset α level.

Example 5

This example will indicate the differences and similarities between hypothesis testing and confidence intervals. Recall in Example 3 the comparison of mean ages between summer and winter patients. The 95 percent confidence interval for the difference in mean ages is

$$(47.1 - 28.7) - (2.1 \times 23.3) < \mu_1 - \mu_2 < (47.1 - 28.7) + (2.1 \times 23.3)$$

Thus the 95 percent confidence interval for the difference in means is from −30.5 to 67.3. Since the interval contains zero, this is confirmation of the fact that the two means are not statistically different at the $\alpha = 0.05$ level. Notice how the width of the interval is influenced both by the variability (i.e., the pooled standard deviation) as well as the sample size (through the degrees of freedom associated with the t value, which determines the magnitude of the t value used).

Summary

The material in this chapter and the examples provided introduce the statistical tools used in epidemiology. These basic tools can be useful to health services managers by providing more objective ways of making decisions. The chapter has provided a brief overview of the univariate (i.e., descriptive) and bivariate (i.e., inferential methods for two groups) statistics commonly used in epidemiology. Multivariate methods, such as multiple regression, multiple logistic regression, and analysis of variance, are beyond the scope of this overview. For more detailed information on the methods presented here or on multivariate analysis strategies, note the suggested references. Health services managers are encouraged to consult practicing statisticians or epidemiologists for assistance in planning the studies, making the important decisions, or answering the complex questions that may come up in the pursuit of epidemiologic problem solving.

A Bibliography of Epidemiologic Tools for Healthcare Managers

Glantz, S. A. 1997. *Primer of Biostatistics.* New York: McGraw-Hill.

Hamilton, L. C. 1990. *Modern Data Analysis: A First Course in Applied Statistics.* Belmont, CA: Brooks/Cole.

Kanji, G. K. 1999. *100 Statistical Tests.* London: Sage.

Motulsky, H. 1995. *Intuitive Biostatistics.* New York: Oxford University Press.

National Center for Health Statistics. 1999. "Health, United States, 1999, with Health and Aging Chartbook." Hyattsville, MD: National Center for Health Statistics.

Selvin, S. 1996. *Statistical Analysis of Epidemiologic Data*. New York: Oxford University Press.

Snedecor, G. W., and W. G. Cochran. 1980. *Statistical Methods*. Ames, IA: The Iowa State University Press.

Vogt, W. P. 1999. *Dictionary of Statistics & Methodology: A Nontechnical Guide for the Social Sciences*. London: Sage.

TABLE 10.1

Ten Thousand Randomly Assorted Digits

Appendix

	00–04	05–09	10–14	15–19	20–24	25–29	30–34	35–39	40–44	45–49
00	54463	22662	65905	70639	79365	67382	29085	69831	47058	08186
01	15389	85205	18850	39226	42249	90669	96325	23248	60933	26927
02	85941	40756	82414	02015	13858	78030	16269	65978	01385	15345
03	61149	69440	11286	88218	58925	03638	52862	62733	33451	77455
04	05219	81619	10651	67079	92511	59888	84502	72095	83463	75577
05	41417	98326	87719	92294	46614	50948	64886	20002	97365	30976
06	28357	94070	20652	35774	16249	75019	21145	05217	47286	76305
07	17783	00015	10806	83091	91530	36466	39981	62481	49177	75779
08	40950	84820	29881	85966	62800	70326	84740	62660	77379	90279
09	82995	64157	66164	41180	10089	41757	78258	96488	88629	37231
10	96754	17676	55659	44105	47361	34833	86679	23930	53249	27093
11	34357	88040	53364	71726	45690	66334	60332	22554	90600	71113
12	06318	37403	49927	57715	50423	67372	63116	48888	21505	80182
13	62111	52820	07243	79931	89292	84767	85693	73947	22278	11551
14	47534	09243	67879	00544	23410	12740	02540	54440	32949	13491
15	98614	75993	84460	62846	59844	14922	48730	73443	48167	34770
16	24856	03648	44898	09351	98795	18644	39765	71058	90368	44104
17	96887	12479	80621	66223	86085	78285	02432	53342	42846	94771
18	90801	21472	42815	77408	37390	76766	52615	32141	30268	18106
19	55165	77312	83666	36028	28420	70219	81369	41943	47366	41067
20	75884	12952	84318	95108	72305	64620	91318	89872	45375	85436
21	16777	37116	58550	42958	21460	43910	01175	87894	81378	10620
22	46230	43877	80207	88877	89380	32992	91380	03164	98656	59337
23	42902	66892	46134	01432	94710	23474	20423	60137	60609	13119
24	81007	00333	39693	28039	10154	95425	39220	19774	31782	49037
25	68089	01122	51111	72373	06902	74373	96199	97017	41273	21546
26	20411	67081	99950	16944	93054	87687	96693	87236	77054	33848
27	58212	13160	06468	15718	82627	76999	05999	58680	96739	63700
28	70577	42866	24969	61210	76046	67699	42054	12696	93758	03283
29	94522	74358	71659	62038	79643	79169	44741	05437	39038	13163
30	42626	86819	85651	88678	17401	03252	99547	32404	17918	62880
31	16051	33763	57194	16752	54450	19031	58580	47629	54132	60631
32	08244	27647	33851	44705	94211	46716	11738	55784	95374	72655
33	59497	04392	09419	99964	51211	04894	72882	17805	21896	83864
34	97155	13428	40293	09985	58434	01412	69124	82171	59058	82859
35	98409	66162	95763	47420	20792	61527	20441	39435	11859	41567
36	45476	84882	65109	96597	25930	66790	65706	61203	53634	22557
37	89300	69700	50741	30329	11658	23166	05400	66669	48708	03887
38	50051	95137	91631	66315	91428	12275	24816	68091	71710	33258
39	31753	85178	31310	89642	98364	02306	24617	09609	83942	22716
40	79152	53829	77250	20190	56535	18760	69942	77448	33278	48805
41	44560	38750	83635	56540	64900	42912	13953	79149	18710	68618
42	68328	83378	63369	71381	39564	05615	42451	64559	97501	65747
43	46939	38689	58625	08342	30459	85863	20781	09284	26333	91777
44	83544	86141	15707	96256	23068	13782	08467	89469	93942	55349
45	91621	00881	04900	54224	46177	55309	17852	27491	89415	23466
46	91896	67126	04151	03795	59077	11848	12630	98375	52068	60142
47	55751	62515	21108	80830	02263	29303	37204	96926	30506	09808
48	85156	87689	95493	88842	00664	55017	55539	17771	69448	87530
49	07521	56898	12236	60277	39102	62315	12239	07105	11844	01117

	50–54	55–59	60–64	65–69	70–74	75–79	80–84	85–89	90–94	95–99
00	59391	58030	52098	82718	87024	82848	04190	96574	90464	29065
01	99567	76364	77204	04615	27062	96621	43918	01896	83991	51141
02	10363	97518	51400	25670	98342	61891	27101	37855	06235	33316
03	86859	19558	64432	16706	99612	59798	32803	67708	15297	28612
04	11258	24591	36863	55368	31721	94335	34936	02566	80972	08188
05	95068	88628	35911	14530	33020	80428	39936	31855	34334	64865
06	54463	47237	73800	91017	36239	71824	83671	39892	60518	37092
07	16874	62677	57412	13215	31389	62233	80827	73917	82802	84420
08	92494	63157	76593	91316	03505	72389	96363	52887	01087	66091
09	15669	56689	35682	40844	53256	81872	35213	09840	34471	74441
10	99116	75486	84989	23476	52967	67104	39495	39100	17217	74073
11	15696	10703	65178	90637	63110	17622	53988	71087	84148	11670
12	97720	15369	51269	69620	03388	13699	33423	67453	43269	56720
13	11666	13841	71681	98000	35979	39719	81899	07449	47985	46967
14	71628	73130	78783	75691	41632	09847	61547	18707	85489	69944
15	40501	51089	99943	91843	41995	88931	73631	69361	05375	15417
16	22518	55576	98215	82068	10798	86211	36584	67466	69373	40054
17	75112	30485	62173	02132	14878	92879	22281	16783	86352	00077
18	80327	02671	98191	84342	90813	49268	95441	15496	20168	09271
19	60251	45548	02146	05597	48228	81366	34598	72856	66762	17002
20	57430	82270	10421	00540	43648	75888	66049	21511	47676	33444
21	73528	39559	34434	88596	54086	71693	43132	14414	79949	85193
22	25991	65959	70769	64721	86413	33475	42740	06175	82758	66248
23	78388	16638	09134	59980	63806	48472	39318	35434	24057	74739
24	12477	09965	96657	57994	59439	76330	24596	77515	09577	91871
25	83266	32883	42451	15579	38155	29793	40914	65990	16255	17777
26	76970	80876	10237	39515	79152	74798	39357	09054	73579	92359
27	37074	65198	44785	68624	98336	84481	97610	78735	46703	98265
28	83712	06514	30101	78295	54656	85417	43189	60048	72781	72606
29	20287	56862	69727	94443	64936	08366	27227	05158	50326	59566
30	74261	32592	86538	27041	65172	85532	07571	80609	39285	65340
31	64081	49863	08478	96001	18888	14810	70545	89755	59064	07210
32	05617	75818	47750	67814	29575	10526	66192	44464	27058	40467
33	26793	74951	95466	74307	13330	42664	85515	20632	05497	33625
34	65988	72850	48737	54719	52056	01596	03845	35067	03134	70322
35	27366	42271	44300	73399	21105	03280	73457	43093	05192	48657
36	56760	10909	98147	34736	33863	95256	12731	66598	50771	83665
37	72880	43338	93643	58904	59543	23943	11231	83268	65938	81581
38	77888	38100	03062	58103	47961	83841	25878	23746	55903	44115
39	28440	07819	21580	51459	47971	29882	13990	29226	23608	15873
40	63525	94441	77033	12147	51054	49955	58312	76923	96071	05813
41	47606	93410	16359	89033	89696	47231	64498	31776	05383	39902
42	52669	45030	96279	14709	52372	87832	02735	50803	72744	88208
43	16738	60159	07425	62369	07515	82721	37875	71153	21315	00132
44	59348	11695	45751	15865	74739	05572	32688	20271	65128	14551
45	12900	71775	29845	60774	94924	21810	38636	33717	67598	82521
46	75086	23537	49939	33595	13484	97588	28617	17979	70749	35234
47	99495	51434	29181	09993	38190	42553	68922	52125	91077	40197
48	26075	31671	45386	36583	93459	48599	52022	41330	60651	91321
49	13636	93596	23377	51133	95126	61496	42474	45141	46660	42338

Continued

TABLE 10.1
(Continued)

	00–04	05–09	10–14	15–19	20–24	25–29	30–34	35–39	40–44	45–49
50	64249	63664	39652	40646	97306	31741	07294	84149	46797	82487
51	26538	44249	04050	48174	65570	44072	40192	51153	11397	58212
52	05845	00512	78630	55328	18116	69296	91705	86224	29503	57071
53	74897	68373	67359	51014	33510	83048	17056	72506	82949	54600
54	20872	54570	35017	88132	25730	22626	86723	91691	13191	77212
55	31432	96156	89177	75541	81355	24480	77243	76690	42507	84362
56	66890	61505	01240	00660	05873	13568	76082	79172	57913	93448
57	41894	57790	79970	33106	86904	48119	52503	24130	72824	21627
58	11303	87118	81471	52936	08555	28420	49416	44448	04269	27029
59	54374	57325	16947	45356	78371	10563	97191	53798	12693	27928
60	64852	34421	61046	90849	13966	39810	42699	21753	76192	10508
61	16309	20384	09491	91588	97720	89846	30376	76970	23063	35894
62	42587	37065	24526	72602	57589	98131	37292	05967	26002	51945
63	40177	98590	97161	41682	84533	67588	62036	49967	01990	72308
64	82309	76128	93965	26743	24141	04838	40254	26065	07938	76236
65	79788	68243	59732	04257	27084	14743	17520	95401	55811	76099
66	40538	79000	89559	25026	42274	23489	34502	75508	06059	86682
67	64016	73598	18609	73150	62463	33102	45205	87440	96767	67042
68	49767	12691	17903	93871	99721	79109	09425	26904	07419	76013
69	76974	55108	29795	08404	82684	00497	51126	79935	57450	55671
70	23854	08480	85983	96025	50117	64610	99425	62291	86943	21541
71	68973	70551	25098	78033	98573	79848	31778	29555	61446	23037
72	36444	93600	65350	14971	25325	00427	52073	64280	18847	24768
73	03003	87800	07391	11594	21196	00781	32550	57158	58887	73041
74	17540	26188	36647	78386	04558	61463	57842	90382	77019	24210
75	38916	55809	47982	41968	69760	79422	80154	91486	19180	15100
76	64288	19843	69122	42502	48508	28820	59933	72998	99942	10515
77	86809	51564	38040	39418	49915	19000	58050	16899	79952	57849
78	99800	99566	14742	05028	30033	94889	53381	23656	75787	59223
79	92345	31890	95712	08279	91794	94068	49337	88674	35355	12267
80	90363	65162	32245	82279	79256	80834	06088	99462	56705	06118
81	64437	32242	48431	04835	39070	59702	31508	60935	22390	52246
82	91714	53662	28373	34333	55791	74758	51144	18827	10704	76803
83	20902	17646	31391	31459	33315	03444	55743	74701	58851	27427
84	12217	86007	70371	52281	14510	76094	96579	54853	78339	20839
85	45177	02863	42307	53571	22532	74921	17735	42201	80540	54721
86	28325	90814	08804	52746	47913	54577	47525	77705	95330	21866
87	29019	28776	56116	54791	64604	08815	46049	71186	34650	14994
88	84979	81353	56219	67062	26146	82567	33122	14124	46240	92973
89	50371	26347	48513	63915	11158	25563	91915	18431	92978	11591
90	53422	06825	69711	67950	64716	18003	49581	45378	99878	61130
91	67453	35651	89316	41620	32048	70225	47597	33137	31443	51445
92	07294	85353	74819	23445	68237	07202	99515	62282	53809	26685
93	79544	00302	45338	16015	66613	88968	14595	63836	77716	79596
94	64144	85442	82060	46471	24162	39500	87351	36637	42833	71875
95	90919	11883	58318	00042	52402	28210	34075	33272	00840	73268
96	06670	57353	86275	92276	77591	46924	60839	55437	03183	13191
97	36634	93976	52062	83678	41256	60948	18685	48992	19462	96062
98	75101	72891	85745	67106	26010	62107	60885	37503	55461	71213
99	05112	71222	72654	51583	05228	62056	57390	42746	39272	96659

	50–54	55–59	60–64	65–69	70–74	75–79	80–84	85–89	90–94	95–99
50	32847	31282	03345	89593	69214	70381	78285	20054	91018	16742
51	16916	00041	30236	55023	14253	76582	12092	86533	92426	37655
52	66176	34037	21005	27137	03193	48970	64625	22394	39622	79085
53	46299	13335	12180	16861	38043	59292	62675	63631	37020	78195
54	22847	47839	45385	23289	47526	54098	45683	55849	51575	64689
55	41851	54160	92320	69936	34803	92479	33399	71160	64777	83378
56	28444	59497	91586	95917	68553	28639	06455	34174	11130	91994
57	47520	62378	98855	83174	13088	16561	68559	26679	06238	51254
58	34978	63271	13142	82681	05271	08822	06490	44984	49307	61717
59	37404	80416	69035	92980	49486	74378	75610	74976	70056	15478
60	32400	65482	52099	53676	74648	94148	65095	69597	52771	71551
61	89262	86332	51718	70663	11623	29834	79820	73002	84886	03591
62	86866	09127	98021	03871	27789	58444	44832	36505	40672	30180
63	90814	14833	08759	74645	05046	94056	99094	65091	32663	73040
64	19192	82756	20553	58446	55376	88914	75096	26119	83898	43816
65	77585	52593	56612	95766	10019	29531	73064	20953	53523	58136
66	23757	16364	05096	03192	62386	45389	85332	18877	55710	96459
67	45989	96257	23850	26216	23309	21526	07425	50254	19455	29315
68	92970	94243	07316	41467	64837	52406	25225	51553	31220	14032
69	74346	59596	40088	98176	17896	86900	20249	77753	19099	48885
70	87646	41309	27636	45153	29988	94770	07255	70908	05340	99751
71	50099	71038	45146	06146	55211	99429	43169	66259	97786	59180
72	10127	46900	64984	75348	04115	33624	68774	60013	35515	62556
73	67995	81977	18984	64091	02785	27762	42529	97144	80407	64524
74	26304	80217	84934	82657	69291	35397	98714	35104	08187	48109
75	81994	41070	56642	64091	31229	02595	13513	45148	78722	30144
76	59537	34662	79631	89403	65212	09975	06118	86197	58208	16162
77	51228	10937	62396	81460	47331	91403	95007	06047	16846	64809
78	31089	37995	29577	07828	42272	54016	21950	86192	99046	84864
79	38207	97938	93459	75174	79460	55436	57206	87644	21296	43393
80	88666	31142	09474	89712	63153	62333	42212	06140	42594	43671
81	53365	56134	67582	92557	89520	33452	05134	70628	27612	33738
82	89807	74530	38004	90102	11693	90257	05500	79920	62700	43325
83	18682	81038	85662	90915	91631	22223	91588	80774	07716	12548
84	63571	32579	63942	25371	09234	94592	98475	76884	37635	33608
85	68927	56492	67799	95398	77642	54913	91583	08421	81450	76229
86	56401	63186	39389	88798	31356	89235	97036	32341	33292	73757
87	24333	95603	02359	72942	46287	95382	08452	62862	97869	71775
88	17025	84202	95199	62272	06366	16175	97577	99304	41587	03686
89	02804	08253	52133	20224	68034	50865	57868	22343	55111	03607
90	08298	03879	20995	19850	73090	13191	18963	82244	78479	99121
91	59883	01785	82403	96062	03785	03488	12970	64896	38336	30030
92	46982	06682	62864	91837	74021	89094	39952	64158	79614	78235
93	31121	47266	07661	02051	67599	24471	69843	83696	71402	76287
94	97867	56641	63416	17577	30161	87320	37752	73276	48969	41915
95	57364	86746	08415	14621	49430	22311	15836	72492	49372	44103
96	09559	26263	69511	28064	75999	44540	13337	10918	79846	54809
97	53873	55571	00608	42661	91332	63956	74087	59008	47493	99581
98	35531	19162	86406	05299	77511	24311	57257	22826	77555	05941
99	28229	88629	25695	94932	30721	16197	78742	34974	97528	45447

SOURCE: Snedecor, G. W., and W.G. Cochran. 1967. *Statistical Methods*, 6th ed. Ames, IA: Iowa State University Press.

TABLE 10.2
The
Distribution
of *t* (Two–
Tailed Tests)

Degrees of Freedom	Probability of a Larger Value, Sign Ignored								
	0.500	0.400	0.200	0.100	0.050	0.025	0.010	0.005	0.001
1	1.000	1.376	3.078	6.314	12.706	25.452	63.657		
2	0.816	1.061	1.886	2.920	4.303	6.205	9.925	14.089	31.598
3	.765	0.978	1.638	2.353	3.182	4.176	5.841	7.453	12.941
4	.741	.941	1.533	2.132	2.776	3.495	4.604	5.598	8.610
5	.727	.920	1.476	2.015	2.571	3.163	4.032	4.773	6.859
6	.718	.906	1.440	1.943	2.447	2.969	3.707	4.317	5.959
7	.711	.896	1.415	1.895	2.365	2.841	3.499	4.029	5.405
8	.706	.889	1.397	1.860	2.306	2.752	3.355	3.832	5.041
9	.703	.883	1.383	1.833	2.262	2.685	3.250	3.690	4.781
10	.700	.879	1.372	1.812	2.228	2.634	3.169	3.581	4.587
11	.697	.876	1.363	1.796	2.201	2.593	3.106	3.497	4.437
12	.695	.873	1.356	1.782	2.179	2.560	3.055	3.428	4.318
13	.694	.870	1.350	1.771	2.160	2.533	3.012	3.372	4.221
14	.692	.868	1.345	1.761	2.145	2.510	2.977	3.326	4.140
15	.691	.866	1.341	1.753	2.131	2.490	2.947	3.286	4.073
16	.690	.865	1.337	1.746	2.120	2.473	2.921	3.252	4.015
17	.689	.863	1.333	1.740	2.110	2.458	2.898	3.222	3.965
18	.688	.862	1.330	1.734	2.101	2.445	2.878	3.197	3.922
19	.688	.861	1.328	1.729	2.093	2.433	2.861	3.174	3.883
20	.687	.860	1.325	1.725	2.086	2.423	2.845	3.153	3.850
21	.686	.859	1.323	1.721	2.080	2.414	2.831	3.135	3.819
22	.686	.858	1.321	1.717	2.074	2.406	2.819	3.119	3.792
23	.685	.858	1.319	1.714	2.069	2.398	2.807	3.104	3.767
24	.685	.857	1.318	1.711	2.064	2.391	2.797	3.090	3.745
25	.684	.856	1.316	1.708	2.060	2.385	2.787	3.078	3.725
26	.684	.856	1.315	1.706	2.056	2.379	2.779	3.067	3.707
27	.684	.855	1.314	1.703	2.052	2.373	2.771	3.056	3.690
28	.683	.855	1.313	1.701	2.048	2.368	2.763	3.047	3.674
29	.683	.854	1.311	1.699	2.045	2.364	2.756	3.038	3.659
30	.683	.854	1.310	1.697	2.042	2.360	2.750	3.030	3.646
35	.682	.852	1.306	1.690	2.030	2.342	2.724	2.996	3.591
40	.681	.851	1.303	1.684	2.021	2.329	2.704	2.971	3.551
45	.680	.850	1.301	1.680	2.014	2.319	2.690	2.952	3.520
50	.680	.849	1.299	1.676	2.008	2.310	2.678	2.937	3.496
55	.679	.849	1.297	1.673	2.004	2.304	2.669	2.925	3.476
60	.679	.848	1.296	1.671	2.000	2.299	2.660	2.915	3.460
70	.678	.847	1.294	1.667	1.994	2.290	2.648	2.899	3.435
80	.678	.847	1.293	1.665	1.989	2.284	2.638	2.887	3.416
90	.678	.846	1.291	1.662	1.986	2.279	2.631	2.878	3.402
100	.677	.846	1.290	1.661	1.982	2.276	2.625	2.871	3.390
120	.677	.845	1.289	1.658	1.980	2.270	2.617	2.860	3.373
∞	.6745	.8416	1.2816	1.6448	1.9600	2.2414	2.5758	2.8070	3.2905

Parts of this table are reprinted by permission from R. A. Fisher's Statistical Methods for Research Workers, published by Oliver and Boyd, Edinburgh (1925–1950); from Maxine Merrington's "Table of Percentage Points of the t-Distribution," Biometrika, 32:300 (1942); and from Bernard Ostle's Statistics in Research, Iowa State Univeristy Press (1954).
Source: Snedecor, G. W. and W. G. Cochran. 1967. *Statistical Methods, 6th ed.* Ames: The Iowa State University Press.

TABLE 10.3 5% and 1% (Bold) Points for the Distribution of F

f_1 Degrees of Freedom (for greater mean square)

Each cell shows the 5% point (regular) / 1% point (**bold**).

f_2	1	2	3	4	5	6	7	8	9	10	11	12	14	16	20	24	30	40	50	75	100	200	500	∞
1	161 / **4,052**	200 / **4,999**	216 / **5,403**	225 / **5,625**	230 / **5,764**	234 / **5,859**	237 / **5,928**	239 / **5,981**	241 / **6,022**	242 / **6,056**	243 / **6,082**	244 / **6,106**	245 / **6,142**	246 / **6,169**	248 / **6,208**	249 / **6,234**	250 / **6,261**	251 / **6,286**	252 / **6,302**	253 / **6,323**	253 / **6,334**	254 / **6,352**	254 / **6,361**	254 / **6,366**
2	18.51 / **98.49**	19.00 / **99.00**	19.16 / **99.17**	19.25 / **99.25**	19.30 / **99.30**	19.33 / **99.33**	19.36 / **99.36**	19.37 / **99.37**	19.38 / **99.39**	19.39 / **99.40**	19.40 / **99.41**	19.41 / **99.42**	19.42 / **99.43**	19.43 / **99.44**	19.44 / **99.45**	19.45 / **99.46**	19.46 / **99.47**	19.47 / **99.48**	19.47 / **99.48**	19.48 / **99.49**	19.49 / **99.49**	19.49 / **99.49**	19.50 / **99.50**	19.50 / **99.50**
3	10.13 / **34.12**	9.55 / **30.82**	9.28 / **29.46**	9.12 / **28.71**	9.01 / **28.24**	8.94 / **27.91**	8.88 / **27.67**	8.84 / **27.49**	8.81 / **27.34**	8.78 / **27.23**	8.76 / **27.13**	8.74 / **27.05**	8.71 / **26.92**	8.69 / **26.83**	8.66 / **26.69**	8.64 / **26.60**	8.62 / **26.50**	8.60 / **26.41**	8.58 / **26.35**	8.57 / **26.27**	8.56 / **26.23**	8.54 / **26.18**	8.54 / **26.14**	8.53 / **26.12**
4	7.71 / **21.20**	6.94 / **18.00**	6.59 / **16.69**	6.39 / **15.98**	6.26 / **15.52**	6.16 / **15.21**	6.09 / **14.98**	6.04 / **14.80**	6.00 / **14.66**	5.96 / **14.54**	5.93 / **14.45**	5.91 / **14.37**	5.87 / **14.24**	5.84 / **14.15**	5.80 / **14.02**	5.77 / **13.93**	5.74 / **13.83**	5.71 / **13.74**	5.70 / **13.69**	5.68 / **13.61**	5.66 / **13.57**	5.65 / **13.52**	5.64 / **13.48**	5.63 / **13.46**
5	6.61 / **16.26**	5.79 / **13.27**	5.41 / **12.06**	5.19 / **11.39**	5.05 / **10.97**	4.95 / **10.67**	4.88 / **10.45**	4.82 / **10.29**	4.78 / **10.15**	4.74 / **10.05**	4.70 / **9.96**	4.68 / **9.89**	4.64 / **9.77**	4.60 / **9.68**	4.56 / **9.55**	4.53 / **9.47**	4.50 / **9.38**	4.46 / **9.29**	4.44 / **9.24**	4.42 / **9.17**	4.40 / **9.13**	4.38 / **9.07**	4.37 / **9.04**	4.36 / **9.02**
6	5.99 / **13.74**	5.14 / **10.92**	4.76 / **9.78**	4.53 / **9.15**	4.39 / **8.75**	4.28 / **8.47**	4.21 / **8.26**	4.15 / **8.10**	4.10 / **7.98**	4.06 / **7.87**	4.03 / **7.79**	4.00 / **7.72**	3.96 / **7.60**	3.92 / **7.52**	3.87 / **7.39**	3.84 / **7.31**	3.81 / **7.23**	3.77 / **7.14**	3.75 / **7.09**	3.72 / **7.02**	3.71 / **6.99**	3.69 / **6.94**	3.68 / **6.90**	3.67 / **6.88**
7	5.59 / **12.25**	4.74 / **9.55**	4.35 / **8.45**	4.12 / **7.85**	3.97 / **7.46**	3.87 / **7.19**	3.79 / **7.00**	3.73 / **6.84**	3.68 / **6.71**	3.63 / **6.62**	3.60 / **6.54**	3.57 / **6.47**	3.52 / **6.35**	3.49 / **6.27**	3.44 / **6.15**	3.41 / **6.07**	3.38 / **5.98**	3.34 / **5.90**	3.32 / **5.85**	3.29 / **5.78**	3.28 / **5.75**	3.25 / **5.70**	3.24 / **5.67**	3.23 / **5.65**
8	5.32 / **11.26**	4.46 / **8.65**	4.07 / **7.59**	3.84 / **7.01**	3.69 / **6.63**	3.58 / **6.37**	3.50 / **6.19**	3.44 / **6.03**	3.39 / **5.91**	3.34 / **5.82**	3.31 / **5.74**	3.28 / **5.67**	3.23 / **5.56**	3.20 / **5.48**	3.15 / **5.36**	3.12 / **5.28**	3.08 / **5.20**	3.05 / **5.11**	3.03 / **5.06**	3.00 / **5.00**	2.98 / **4.96**	2.96 / **4.91**	2.94 / **4.88**	2.93 / **4.86**
9	5.12 / **10.56**	4.26 / **8.02**	3.86 / **6.99**	3.63 / **6.42**	3.48 / **6.06**	3.37 / **5.80**	3.29 / **5.62**	3.23 / **5.47**	3.18 / **5.35**	3.13 / **5.26**	3.10 / **5.18**	3.07 / **5.11**	3.02 / **5.00**	2.98 / **4.92**	2.93 / **4.80**	2.90 / **4.73**	2.86 / **4.64**	2.82 / **4.56**	2.80 / **4.51**	2.77 / **4.45**	2.76 / **4.41**	2.73 / **4.36**	2.72 / **4.33**	2.71 / **4.31**
10	4.96 / **10.04**	4.10 / **7.56**	3.71 / **6.55**	3.48 / **5.99**	3.33 / **5.64**	3.22 / **5.39**	3.14 / **5.21**	3.07 / **5.06**	3.02 / **4.95**	2.97 / **4.85**	2.94 / **4.78**	2.91 / **4.71**	2.86 / **4.60**	2.82 / **4.52**	2.77 / **4.41**	2.74 / **4.33**	2.70 / **4.25**	2.67 / **4.17**	2.64 / **4.12**	2.61 / **4.05**	2.59 / **4.01**	2.56 / **3.96**	2.55 / **3.93**	2.54 / **3.91**
11	4.84 / **9.65**	3.98 / **7.20**	3.59 / **6.22**	3.36 / **5.67**	3.20 / **5.32**	3.09 / **5.07**	3.01 / **4.88**	2.95 / **4.74**	2.90 / **4.63**	2.86 / **4.54**	2.82 / **4.46**	2.79 / **4.40**	2.74 / **4.29**	2.70 / **4.21**	2.65 / **4.10**	2.61 / **4.02**	2.57 / **3.94**	2.53 / **3.86**	2.50 / **3.80**	2.47 / **3.74**	2.45 / **3.70**	2.42 / **3.66**	2.41 / **3.62**	2.40 / **3.60**
12	4.75 / **9.33**	3.88 / **6.93**	3.49 / **5.95**	3.26 / **5.41**	3.11 / **5.06**	3.00 / **4.82**	2.92 / **4.65**	2.85 / **4.50**	2.80 / **4.39**	2.76 / **4.30**	2.72 / **4.22**	2.69 / **4.16**	2.64 / **4.05**	2.60 / **3.98**	2.54 / **3.86**	2.50 / **3.78**	2.46 / **3.70**	2.42 / **3.61**	2.40 / **3.56**	2.36 / **3.49**	2.35 / **3.46**	2.32 / **3.41**	2.31 / **3.38**	2.30 / **3.36**
13	4.67 / **9.07**	3.80 / **6.70**	3.41 / **5.74**	3.18 / **5.20**	3.02 / **4.86**	2.92 / **4.62**	2.84 / **4.44**	2.77 / **4.30**	2.72 / **4.19**	2.67 / **4.10**	2.63 / **4.02**	2.60 / **3.96**	2.55 / **3.85**	2.51 / **3.78**	2.46 / **3.67**	2.42 / **3.59**	2.38 / **3.51**	2.34 / **3.42**	2.32 / **3.37**	2.28 / **3.30**	2.26 / **3.27**	2.24 / **3.21**	2.22 / **3.18**	2.21 / **3.16**
14	4.60 / **8.86**	3.74 / **6.51**	3.34 / **5.56**	3.11 / **5.03**	2.96 / **4.69**	2.85 / **4.46**	2.77 / **4.28**	2.70 / **4.14**	2.65 / **4.03**	2.60 / **3.94**	2.56 / **3.86**	2.53 / **3.80**	2.48 / **3.70**	2.44 / **3.62**	2.39 / **3.51**	2.35 / **3.43**	2.31 / **3.34**	2.27 / **3.26**	2.24 / **3.21**	2.21 / **3.14**	2.19 / **3.11**	2.16 / **3.06**	2.14 / **3.02**	2.13 / **3.00**
15	4.54 / **8.68**	3.68 / **6.36**	3.29 / **5.42**	3.06 / **4.89**	2.90 / **4.56**	2.79 / **4.32**	2.70 / **4.14**	2.64 / **4.00**	2.59 / **3.89**	2.55 / **3.80**	2.51 / **3.73**	2.48 / **3.67**	2.43 / **3.56**	2.39 / **3.48**	2.33 / **3.36**	2.29 / **3.29**	2.25 / **3.20**	2.21 / **3.12**	2.18 / **3.07**	2.15 / **3.00**	2.12 / **2.97**	2.10 / **2.92**	2.08 / **2.89**	2.07 / **2.87**
16	4.49 / **8.53**	3.63 / **6.23**	3.24 / **5.29**	3.01 / **4.77**	2.85 / **4.44**	2.74 / **4.20**	2.66 / **4.03**	2.59 / **3.89**	2.54 / **3.78**	2.49 / **3.69**	2.45 / **3.61**	2.42 / **3.55**	2.37 / **3.45**	2.33 / **3.37**	2.28 / **3.25**	2.24 / **3.18**	2.20 / **3.10**	2.16 / **3.01**	2.13 / **2.96**	2.09 / **2.89**	2.07 / **2.86**	2.04 / **2.80**	2.02 / **2.77**	2.01 / **2.75**
17	4.45 / **8.40**	3.59 / **6.11**	3.20 / **5.18**	2.96 / **4.67**	2.81 / **4.34**	2.70 / **4.10**	2.62 / **3.93**	2.55 / **3.79**	2.50 / **3.68**	2.45 / **3.59**	2.41 / **3.52**	2.38 / **3.45**	2.33 / **3.35**	2.29 / **3.27**	2.23 / **3.16**	2.19 / **3.08**	2.15 / **3.00**	2.11 / **2.92**	2.08 / **2.86**	2.04 / **2.79**	2.02 / **2.76**	1.99 / **2.70**	1.97 / **2.67**	1.96 / **2.65**
18	4.41 / **8.28**	3.55 / **6.01**	3.16 / **5.09**	2.93 / **4.58**	2.77 / **4.25**	2.66 / **4.01**	2.58 / **3.85**	2.51 / **3.71**	2.46 / **3.60**	2.41 / **3.51**	2.37 / **3.44**	2.34 / **3.37**	2.29 / **3.27**	2.25 / **3.19**	2.19 / **3.07**	2.15 / **3.00**	2.11 / **2.91**	2.07 / **2.83**	2.04 / **2.78**	2.00 / **2.71**	1.98 / **2.68**	1.95 / **2.62**	1.93 / **2.59**	1.92 / **2.57**
19	4.38 / **8.18**	3.52 / **5.93**	3.13 / **5.01**	2.90 / **4.50**	2.74 / **4.17**	2.63 / **3.94**	2.55 / **3.77**	2.48 / **3.63**	2.43 / **3.52**	2.38 / **3.43**	2.34 / **3.36**	2.31 / **3.30**	2.26 / **3.19**	2.21 / **3.12**	2.15 / **3.00**	2.11 / **2.92**	2.07 / **2.84**	2.02 / **2.76**	2.00 / **2.70**	1.96 / **2.63**	1.94 / **2.60**	1.91 / **2.54**	1.90 / **2.51**	1.88 / **2.49**
20	4.35 / **8.10**	3.49 / **5.85**	3.10 / **4.94**	2.87 / **4.43**	2.71 / **4.10**	2.60 / **3.87**	2.52 / **3.71**	2.45 / **3.56**	2.40 / **3.45**	2.35 / **3.37**	2.31 / **3.30**	2.28 / **3.23**	2.23 / **3.13**	2.18 / **3.05**	2.12 / **2.94**	2.08 / **2.86**	2.04 / **2.77**	1.99 / **2.69**	1.96 / **2.63**	1.92 / **2.56**	1.90 / **2.53**	1.87 / **2.47**	1.85 / **2.44**	1.84 / **2.42**
21	4.32 / **8.02**	3.47 / **5.78**	3.07 / **4.87**	2.84 / **4.37**	2.68 / **4.04**	2.57 / **3.81**	2.49 / **3.65**	2.42 / **3.51**	2.37 / **3.40**	2.32 / **3.31**	2.28 / **3.24**	2.25 / **3.17**	2.20 / **3.07**	2.15 / **2.99**	2.09 / **2.88**	2.05 / **2.80**	2.00 / **2.72**	1.96 / **2.63**	1.93 / **2.58**	1.89 / **2.51**	1.87 / **2.47**	1.84 / **2.42**	1.82 / **2.38**	1.81 / **2.36**

continued

TABLE 10.3 (Continued)

	22	23	24	25	26	27	28	29	30	32	34	36	38	40	42	44	46	48	50	55	60	65	70	80
22	4.30 / 7.94	3.44 / 5.72	3.05 / 4.82	2.82 / 4.31	2.66 / 3.99	2.55 / 3.76	2.47 / 3.59	2.40 / 3.45	2.35 / 3.35	2.30 / 3.26	2.26 / 3.18	2.23 / 3.12	2.18 / 3.02	2.13 / 2.94	2.07 / 2.83	2.03 / 2.75	1.98 / 2.67	1.93 / 2.55	1.91 / 2.53	1.87 / 2.46	1.84 / 2.42	1.81 / 2.37	1.80 / 2.33	1.78 / 2.31
23	4.28 / 7.88	3.42 / 5.66	3.03 / 4.76	2.80 / 4.26	2.64 / 3.94	2.53 / 3.71	2.45 / 3.54	2.38 / 3.41	2.32 / 3.30	2.28 / 3.21	2.24 / 3.14	2.20 / 3.07	2.14 / 2.97	2.10 / 2.89	2.04 / 2.78	2.00 / 2.70	1.96 / 2.62	1.91 / 2.53	1.88 / 2.48	1.84 / 2.41	1.82 / 2.37	1.79 / 2.32	1.77 / 2.28	1.76 / 2.26
24	4.26 / 7.82	3.40 / 5.61	3.01 / 4.72	2.78 / 4.22	2.62 / 3.90	2.51 / 3.67	2.43 / 3.50	2.36 / 3.36	2.30 / 3.25	2.26 / 3.17	2.22 / 3.09	2.18 / 3.03	2.13 / 2.93	2.09 / 2.85	2.02 / 2.74	1.98 / 2.66	1.94 / 2.58	1.89 / 2.49	1.86 / 2.44	1.82 / 2.36	1.80 / 2.33	1.76 / 2.27	1.74 / 2.23	1.73 / 2.21
25	4.24 / 7.77	3.38 / 5.57	2.99 / 4.68	2.76 / 4.18	2.60 / 3.86	2.49 / 3.63	2.41 / 3.46	2.34 / 3.32	2.28 / 3.21	2.24 / 3.13	2.20 / 3.05	2.16 / 2.99	2.11 / 2.89	2.06 / 2.81	2.00 / 2.70	1.96 / 2.62	1.92 / 2.54	1.87 / 2.45	1.84 / 2.40	1.80 / 2.32	1.77 / 2.29	1.74 / 2.23	1.72 / 2.19	1.71 / 2.17
26	4.22 / 7.72	3.37 / 5.53	2.98 / 4.64	2.74 / 4.14	2.59 / 3.82	2.47 / 3.59	2.39 / 3.42	2.32 / 3.29	2.27 / 3.17	2.22 / 3.09	2.18 / 3.02	2.15 / 2.96	2.10 / 2.86	2.05 / 2.77	1.99 / 2.66	1.95 / 2.58	1.90 / 2.50	1.85 / 2.41	1.82 / 2.36	1.78 / 2.28	1.76 / 2.25	1.72 / 2.19	1.70 / 2.15	1.69 / 2.13
27	4.21 / 7.68	3.35 / 5.49	2.96 / 4.60	2.73 / 4.11	2.57 / 3.79	2.46 / 3.56	2.37 / 3.39	2.30 / 3.26	2.25 / 3.14	2.20 / 3.06	2.16 / 2.98	2.13 / 2.93	2.08 / 2.83	2.03 / 2.74	1.97 / 2.63	1.93 / 2.55	1.88 / 2.47	1.84 / 2.38	1.80 / 2.33	1.76 / 2.25	1.74 / 2.21	1.71 / 2.16	1.68 / 2.12	1.67 / 2.10
28	4.20 / 7.64	3.34 / 5.45	2.95 / 4.57	2.71 / 4.07	2.56 / 3.76	2.44 / 3.53	2.36 / 3.36	2.29 / 3.23	2.24 / 3.11	2.19 / 3.03	2.15 / 2.95	2.12 / 2.90	2.06 / 2.80	2.02 / 2.71	1.96 / 2.60	1.91 / 2.52	1.87 / 2.44	1.81 / 2.35	1.78 / 2.30	1.75 / 2.22	1.72 / 2.18	1.69 / 2.13	1.67 / 2.09	1.65 / 2.06
29	4.18 / 7.60	3.33 / 5.42	2.93 / 4.54	2.70 / 4.04	2.54 / 3.73	2.43 / 3.50	2.35 / 3.33	2.28 / 3.20	2.22 / 3.08	2.18 / 3.00	2.14 / 2.92	2.10 / 2.87	2.05 / 2.77	2.00 / 2.68	1.94 / 2.57	1.90 / 2.49	1.85 / 2.41	1.80 / 2.32	1.77 / 2.27	1.73 / 2.19	1.71 / 2.15	1.68 / 2.10	1.65 / 2.06	1.64 / 2.03
30	4.17 / 7.56	3.32 / 5.39	2.92 / 4.51	2.69 / 4.02	2.53 / 3.70	2.42 / 3.47	2.34 / 3.30	2.27 / 3.17	2.21 / 3.06	2.16 / 2.98	2.12 / 2.90	2.09 / 2.84	2.04 / 2.74	1.99 / 2.66	1.93 / 2.55	1.89 / 2.47	1.84 / 2.38	1.79 / 2.29	1.76 / 2.24	1.72 / 2.16	1.69 / 2.13	1.66 / 2.07	1.64 / 2.03	1.62 / 2.01
32	4.15 / 7.50	3.30 / 5.34	2.90 / 4.46	2.67 / 3.97	2.51 / 3.66	2.40 / 3.42	2.32 / 3.25	2.25 / 3.12	2.19 / 3.01	2.14 / 2.94	2.10 / 2.86	2.07 / 2.80	2.02 / 2.70	1.97 / 2.62	1.91 / 2.51	1.86 / 2.42	1.82 / 2.34	1.76 / 2.25	1.74 / 2.20	1.69 / 2.12	1.67 / 2.08	1.64 / 2.02	1.61 / 1.98	1.59 / 1.96
34	4.13 / 7.44	3.28 / 5.29	2.88 / 4.42	2.65 / 3.93	2.49 / 3.61	2.38 / 3.38	2.30 / 3.21	2.23 / 3.08	2.17 / 2.97	2.12 / 2.89	2.08 / 2.82	2.05 / 2.76	2.00 / 2.66	1.95 / 2.58	1.89 / 2.47	1.84 / 2.38	1.80 / 2.30	1.74 / 2.21	1.71 / 2.15	1.67 / 2.08	1.64 / 2.04	1.61 / 1.98	1.59 / 1.94	1.57 / 1.91
36	4.11 / 7.39	3.26 / 5.25	2.86 / 4.38	2.63 / 3.89	2.48 / 3.58	2.36 / 3.35	2.28 / 3.18	2.21 / 3.04	2.15 / 2.94	2.10 / 2.86	2.06 / 2.78	2.03 / 2.72	1.98 / 2.62	1.93 / 2.54	1.87 / 2.43	1.82 / 2.35	1.78 / 2.26	1.72 / 2.17	1.69 / 2.12	1.65 / 2.04	1.62 / 2.00	1.59 / 1.94	1.56 / 1.90	1.55 / 1.87
38	4.10 / 7.35	3.25 / 5.21	2.85 / 4.34	2.62 / 3.86	2.46 / 3.54	2.35 / 3.32	2.26 / 3.15	2.19 / 3.02	2.14 / 2.91	2.09 / 2.82	2.05 / 2.75	2.02 / 2.69	1.96 / 2.59	1.92 / 2.51	1.85 / 2.40	1.80 / 2.32	1.76 / 2.22	1.70 / 2.14	1.67 / 2.08	1.63 / 2.00	1.60 / 1.97	1.57 / 1.90	1.54 / 1.86	1.53 / 1.84
40	4.08 / 7.31	3.23 / 5.18	2.84 / 4.31	2.61 / 3.83	2.45 / 3.51	2.34 / 3.29	2.25 / 3.12	2.18 / 2.99	2.12 / 2.88	2.07 / 2.80	2.04 / 2.73	2.00 / 2.66	1.95 / 2.56	1.90 / 2.49	1.84 / 2.37	1.79 / 2.29	1.74 / 2.20	1.69 / 2.11	1.66 / 2.05	1.61 / 1.97	1.59 / 1.94	1.55 / 1.88	1.53 / 1.84	1.51 / 1.81
42	4.07 / 7.27	3.22 / 5.15	2.83 / 4.29	2.59 / 3.80	2.44 / 3.49	2.32 / 3.26	2.24 / 3.10	2.17 / 2.96	2.11 / 2.86	2.06 / 2.77	2.02 / 2.70	1.99 / 2.64	1.94 / 2.54	1.89 / 2.46	1.82 / 2.35	1.78 / 2.26	1.73 / 2.17	1.68 / 2.08	1.64 / 2.02	1.60 / 1.94	1.57 / 1.91	1.54 / 1.85	1.51 / 1.81	1.49 / 1.78
44	4.06 / 7.24	3.21 / 5.12	2.82 / 4.26	2.58 / 3.78	2.43 / 3.46	2.31 / 3.24	2.23 / 3.07	2.16 / 2.94	2.10 / 2.84	2.05 / 2.75	2.01 / 2.68	1.98 / 2.62	1.92 / 2.52	1.88 / 2.44	1.81 / 2.32	1.76 / 2.24	1.72 / 2.15	1.67 / 2.06	1.63 / 2.00	1.58 / 1.92	1.56 / 1.88	1.52 / 1.82	1.50 / 1.78	1.48 / 1.75
46	4.05 / 7.21	3.20 / 5.10	2.81 / 4.24	2.57 / 3.76	2.42 / 3.44	2.30 / 3.22	2.22 / 3.05	2.14 / 2.92	2.09 / 2.82	2.04 / 2.73	2.00 / 2.66	1.97 / 2.60	1.91 / 2.50	1.87 / 2.42	1.80 / 2.30	1.75 / 2.22	1.71 / 2.13	1.65 / 2.04	1.62 / 1.98	1.57 / 1.90	1.54 / 1.86	1.51 / 1.80	1.48 / 1.76	1.46 / 1.72
48	4.04 / 7.19	3.19 / 5.08	2.80 / 4.22	2.56 / 3.74	2.41 / 3.42	2.30 / 3.20	2.21 / 3.04	2.14 / 2.90	2.08 / 2.80	2.03 / 2.71	1.99 / 2.64	1.96 / 2.58	1.90 / 2.48	1.86 / 2.40	1.79 / 2.29	1.74 / 2.20	1.70 / 2.11	1.64 / 2.02	1.61 / 1.96	1.56 / 1.88	1.53 / 1.84	1.50 / 1.78	1.47 / 1.73	1.45 / 1.70
50	4.03 / 7.17	3.18 / 5.06	2.79 / 4.20	2.56 / 3.72	2.40 / 3.41	2.29 / 3.18	2.20 / 3.02	2.13 / 2.88	2.07 / 2.78	2.02 / 2.70	1.98 / 2.62	1.95 / 2.56	1.90 / 2.46	1.85 / 2.39	1.78 / 2.26	1.74 / 2.18	1.69 / 2.10	1.63 / 2.00	1.60 / 1.94	1.55 / 1.86	1.52 / 1.82	1.48 / 1.76	1.46 / 1.71	1.44 / 1.68
55	4.02 / 7.12	3.17 / 5.01	2.78 / 4.16	2.54 / 3.68	2.38 / 3.37	2.27 / 3.15	2.18 / 2.98	2.11 / 2.85	2.05 / 2.75	2.00 / 2.66	1.97 / 2.59	1.93 / 2.53	1.88 / 2.43	1.83 / 2.35	1.76 / 2.23	1.72 / 2.15	1.67 / 2.06	1.61 / 1.96	1.58 / 1.90	1.52 / 1.82	1.50 / 1.78	1.46 / 1.71	1.43 / 1.66	1.41 / 1.64
60	4.00 / 7.08	3.15 / 4.98	2.76 / 4.13	2.52 / 3.65	2.37 / 3.34	2.25 / 3.12	2.17 / 2.95	2.10 / 2.82	2.04 / 2.72	1.99 / 2.63	1.95 / 2.56	1.92 / 2.50	1.86 / 2.40	1.81 / 2.32	1.75 / 2.20	1.70 / 2.12	1.65 / 2.03	1.59 / 1.93	1.56 / 1.87	1.50 / 1.79	1.48 / 1.74	1.44 / 1.68	1.41 / 1.63	1.39 / 1.60
65	3.99 / 7.04	3.14 / 4.95	2.75 / 4.10	2.51 / 3.62	2.36 / 3.31	2.24 / 3.09	2.15 / 2.93	2.08 / 2.79	2.02 / 2.70	1.98 / 2.61	1.94 / 2.54	1.90 / 2.47	1.85 / 2.37	1.80 / 2.30	1.73 / 2.18	1.68 / 2.09	1.63 / 2.00	1.57 / 1.90	1.54 / 1.84	1.49 / 1.76	1.46 / 1.71	1.42 / 1.64	1.39 / 1.60	1.37 / 1.56
70	3.98 / 7.01	3.13 / 4.92	2.74 / 4.08	2.50 / 3.60	2.35 / 3.29	2.23 / 3.07	2.14 / 2.91	2.07 / 2.77	2.01 / 2.67	1.97 / 2.59	1.93 / 2.51	1.89 / 2.45	1.84 / 2.35	1.79 / 2.28	1.72 / 2.15	1.67 / 2.07	1.62 / 1.98	1.56 / 1.88	1.53 / 1.82	1.47 / 1.74	1.45 / 1.69	1.40 / 1.62	1.37 / 1.56	1.35 / 1.53
80	3.96 / 6.96	3.11 / 4.88	2.72 / 4.04	2.48 / 3.56	2.33 / 3.25	2.21 / 3.04	2.12 / 2.87	2.05 / 2.74	1.99 / 2.64	1.95 / 2.55	1.91 / 2.48	1.88 / 2.41	1.82 / 2.32	1.77 / 2.24	1.70 / 2.11	1.65 / 2.03	1.60 / 1.94	1.54 / 1.84	1.51 / 1.78	1.45 / 1.70	1.42 / 1.65	1.38 / 1.57	1.35 / 1.52	1.32 / 1.49

TABLE 10.3

f_1 Degrees of Freedom (for greater mean square)

f_2	1	2	3	4	5	6	7	8	9	10	11	12	14	16	20	24	30	40	50	75	100	200	500	∞	f_2
100	3.94 / 6.90	3.09 / 4.82	2.70 / 3.98	2.46 / 3.51	2.30 / 3.20	2.19 / 2.99	2.10 / 2.82	2.03 / 2.69	1.97 / 2.55	1.92 / 2.51	1.88 / 2.43	1.85 / 2.36	1.79 / 2.26	1.75 / 2.19	1.68 / 2.06	1.63 / 1.98	1.57 / 1.89	1.51 / 1.79	1.48 / 1.73	1.42 / 1.54	1.39 / 1.59	1.34 / 1.51	1.30 / 1.46	1.28 / 1.43	100
125	3.92 / 6.84	3.07 / 4.78	2.68 / 3.94	2.44 / 3.47	2.29 / 3.17	2.17 / 2.95	2.08 / 2.79	2.01 / 2.65	1.95 / 2.56	1.90 / 2.47	1.86 / 2.40	1.83 / 2.33	1.77 / 2.23	1.72 / 2.15	1.65 / 2.03	1.60 / 1.94	1.55 / 1.85	1.49 / 1.75	1.45 / 1.68	1.39 / 1.59	1.36 / 1.54	1.31 / 1.46	1.27 / 1.40	1.25 / 1.37	125
150	3.91 / 6.81	3.06 / 4.75	2.67 / 3.91	2.43 / 3.44	2.27 / 3.14	2.16 / 2.92	2.07 / 2.76	2.00 / 2.62	1.94 / 2.53	1.89 / 2.44	1.85 / 2.37	1.82 / 2.30	1.76 / 2.20	1.71 / 2.12	1.64 / 2.00	1.59 / 1.91	1.54 / 1.83	1.47 / 1.72	1.44 / 1.66	1.37 / 1.56	1.34 / 1.51	1.29 / 1.43	1.25 / 1.37	1.22 / 1.33	150
200	3.89 / 6.76	3.04 / 4.71	2.65 / 3.88	2.41 / 3.41	2.26 / 3.11	2.14 / 2.90	2.05 / 2.73	1.98 / 2.60	1.92 / 2.50	1.87 / 2.41	1.83 / 2.34	1.80 / 2.28	1.74 / 2.17	1.69 / 2.09	1.62 / 1.97	1.57 / 1.88	1.52 / 1.79	1.45 / 1.69	1.42 / 1.62	1.35 / 1.53	1.32 / 1.48	1.26 / 1.39	1.22 / 1.33	1.19 / 1.28	200
400	3.86 / 6.70	3.02 / 4.66	2.62 / 3.83	2.39 / 3.36	2.23 / 3.06	2.12 / 2.85	2.03 / 2.69	1.96 / 2.55	1.90 / 2.46	1.85 / 2.37	1.81 / 2.29	1.79 / 2.23	1.72 / 2.12	1.67 / 2.04	1.60 / 1.92	1.54 / 1.84	1.49 / 1.74	1.42 / 1.64	1.38 / 1.57	1.32 / 1.47	1.28 / 1.42	1.22 / 1.32	1.16 / 1.24	1.13 / 1.19	400
1000	3.85 / 6.66	3.00 / 4.62	2.61 / 3.80	2.38 / 3.34	2.22 / 3.04	2.10 / 2.82	2.02 / 2.66	1.95 / 2.53	1.89 / 2.43	1.84 / 2.34	1.80 / 2.26	1.76 / 2.20	1.70 / 2.09	1.65 / 2.01	1.58 / 1.89	1.53 / 1.81	1.47 / 1.71	1.41 / 1.61	1.36 / 1.54	1.30 / 1.44	1.26 / 1.38	1.19 / 1.28	1.13 / 1.19	1.09 / 1.11	1000
∞	3.84 / 6.63	2.99 / 4.60	2.60 / 3.78	2.37 / 3.32	2.21 / 3.02	2.09 / 2.80	2.01 / 2.64	1.94 / 2.51	1.88 / 2.41	1.83 / 2.32	1.79 / 2.24	1.75 / 2.18	1.69 / 2.07	1.64 / 1.99	1.57 / 1.87	1.52 / 1.79	1.46 / 1.69	1.40 / 1.59	1.35 / 1.52	1.28 / 1.41	1.24 / 1.36	1.17 / 1.25	1.11 / 1.15	1.00 / 1.00	∞

The function, F = i with exponent 2z, is computed in part from Fisher's table VI (7). Additional entries are by interpolation, mostly graphical.

TABLE 10.4 25%, 10%, 2.5%, and 0.5% Points for the Distribution of F*

f_1 Degrees of Freedom (for greater mean square)

f_2	P	1	2	3	4	5	6	7	8	9	10	12	15	20	24	30	40	60	120	∞
1	.250	5.83	7.50	8.20	8.58	8.82	8.98	9.10	9.19	9.26	9.32	9.41	9.49	9.59	9.63	9.67	9.71	9.76	9.80	9.85
	.100	39.86	49.50	53.59	55.83	57.2	58.20	58.91	59.44	59.86	60.2	60.70	61.22	61.74	62.00	62.26	62.53	62.79	63.06	63.33
	.025	648	800	864	900	924	937	948	957	963	969	977	985	993	997	1,001	1,006	1,010	1,014	1,018
	.005	16,211	20,000	21,615	22,500	23,056	23,437	23,715	23,925	24,091	24,224	24,426	24,630	24,836	24,940	25,044	25,148	25,253	25,359	25,465
2	.250	2.57	3.00	3.15	3.23	3.28	3.31	3.34	3.35	3.37	3.38	3.39	3.41	3.43	3.43	3.44	3.45	3.46	3.47	3.48
	.100	8.53	9.00	9.16	9.24	9.29	9.33	9.35	9.37	9.38	9.39	9.41	9.42	9.44	9.45	9.46	9.47	9.47	9.48	9.49
	.025	38.51	39.00	39.16	39.25	39.30	39.33	39.35	39.37	39.39	39.40	39.41	39.43	39.45	39.46	39.46	39.47	39.48	39.49	39.50
	.005	198	199	199	199	199	199	199	199	99	99	199	199	199	199	199	199	199	199	200
3	.250	2.02	2.28	2.36	2.39	2.41	2.42	2.43	2.44	2.44	2.44	2.45	2.46	2.46	2.46	2.46	2.47	2.47	2.47	2.47
	.100	5.54	5.46	5.39	5.34	5.31	5.28	5.27	5.25	5.24	5.23	5.22	5.20	5.18	5.18	5.17	5.16	5.15	5.14	5.13
	.025	17.44	16.04	15.44	15.10	14.88	14.74	14.62	14.54	14.47	14.42	14.34	14.25	14.17	14.12	14.08	14.04	13.99	13.95	13.90
	.005	55.55	49.80	47.47	46.20	45.39	44.84	44.43	44.13	43.88	43.69	43.39	43.08	42.78	42.62	42.47	42.31	42.15	41.99	41.83
4	.250	1.81	2.00	2.05	2.06	2.07	2.08	2.08	2.08	2.08	2.08	2.08	2.08	2.08	2.08	2.08	2.08	2.08	2.08	2.08
	.100	4.54	4.32	4.19	4.11	4.05	4.01	3.98	3.95	3.94	3.92	3.90	3.87	3.84	3.83	3.82	3.80	3.79	3.78	3.76
	.025	12.22	10.65	9.98	9.60	9.36	9.20	9.07	8.98	8.90	8.84	8.75	8.66	8.56	8.51	8.46	8.41	8.36	8.31	8.26
	.005	31.33	26.28	24.26	23.16	22.46	21.98	21.62	21.35	21.14	20.97	20.70	20.44	20.17	20.03	19.89	19.75	19.61	19.47	19.32
5	.250	1.69	1.85	1.88	1.89	1.89	1.89	1.89	1.89	1.89	1.89	1.89	1.89	1.88	1.88	1.88	1.88	1.87	1.87	1.87
	.100	4.06	3.78	3.62	3.52	3.45	3.40	3.37	3.34	3.32	3.30	3.27	3.24	3.21	3.19	3.17	3.16	3.14	3.12	3.10
	.025	10.01	8.43	7.76	7.39	7.15	6.98	6.85	6.76	6.68	6.62	6.52	6.43	6.33	6.28	6.23	6.18	6.12	6.07	6.02
	.005	22.78	18.31	16.53	15.56	14.94	14.51	14.20	13.96	13.77	13.62	13.38	13.15	12.90	12.78	12.66	12.53	12.40	12.27	12.14
6	.250	1.62	1.76	1.78	1.79	1.79	1.78	1.78	1.78	1.77	1.77	1.77	1.76	1.76	1.75	1.75	1.75	1.74	1.74	1.74
	.100	3.78	3.46	3.29	3.18	3.11	3.05	3.01	2.98	2.96	2.94	2.90	2.87	2.84	2.82	2.80	2.78	2.76	2.74	2.72
	.025	8.81	7.26	6.60	6.23	5.99	5.82	5.70	5.60	5.52	5.46	5.37	5.27	5.17	5.12	5.07	5.01	4.96	4.90	4.85
	.005	18.64	14.54	12.92	12.03	11.46	11.07	10.79	10.57	10.39	10.25	10.03	9.81	9.59	9.47	9.36	9.24	9.12	9.00	8.88
7	.250	1.57	1.70	1.72	1.72	1.71	1.71	1.70	1.70	1.69	1.69	1.68	1.67	1.67	1.67	1.66	1.66	1.65	1.65	1.65
	.100	3.59	3.26	3.07	2.96	2.88	2.83	2.78	2.75	2.72	2.70	2.67	2.63	2.59	2.58	2.56	2.54	2.51	2.49	2.47
	.025	8.07	6.54	5.89	5.52	5.29	5.12	4.99	4.90	4.82	4.76	4.67	4.57	4.47	4.42	4.36	4.31	4.25	4.20	4.14
	.005	16.24	12.40	10.88	10.05	9.52	9.16	8.89	8.68	8.51	8.38	8.18	7.97	7.75	7.64	7.53	7.42	7.31	7.19	7.08
8	.250	1.54	1.66	1.67	1.66	1.66	1.65	1.64	1.64	1.64	1.63	1.62	1.62	1.62	1.60	1.60	1.59	1.59	1.58	1.58
	.100	3.46	3.11	2.92	2.81	2.73	2.67	2.62	2.59	2.56	2.54	2.50	2.46	2.42	2.40	2.38	2.36	2.34	2.32	2.29
	.025	7.57	6.06	5.42	5.05	4.82	4.65	4.53	4.43	4.36	4.30	4.20	4.10	4.00	3.95	3.89	3.84	3.78	3.73	3.67
	.005	14.69	11.04	9.60	8.81	8.30	7.95	7.69	7.50	7.34	7.21	7.01	6.81	6.61	6.50	6.40	6.29	6.18	6.06	5.95
9	0.250	1.51	1.62	1.63	1.63	1.62	1.61	1.60	1.60	1.59	1.59	1.58	1.57	1.56	1.56	1.55	1.54	1.54	1.53	1.53
	.100	3.36	3.01	2.81	2.69	2.61	2.55	2.51	2.47	2.44	2.42	2.38	2.34	2.30	2.28	2.25	2.23	2.21	2.18	2.16
	.025	7.21	5.71	5.08	4.72	4.48	4.32	4.20	4.10	4.03	3.96	3.87	3.77	3.67	3.61	3.56	3.51	3.45	3.39	3.33
	.005	13.61	10.11	8.72	7.96	7.47	7.13	6.88	6.69	6.54	6.42	6.23	6.03	5.83	5.73	5.62	5.52	5.41	5.30	5.19
10	.250	1.49	1.60	1.60	1.59	1.59	1.58	1.57	1.56	1.56	1.55	1.54	1.53	1.52	1.52	1.51	1.51	1.50	1.49	1.48
	.100	3.28	2.92	2.73	2.61	2.52	2.46	2.41	2.38	2.35	2.32	2.28	2.24	2.20	2.18	2.16	2.13	2.11	2.08	2.06
	.025	6.94	5.46	4.83	4.47	4.24	4.07	3.95	3.85	3.78	3.72	3.62	3.52	3.42	3.37	3.31	3.26	3.20	3.14	3.08
	.005	12.83	9.43	8.08	7.34	6.87	6.54	6.30	6.12	5.97	5.85	5.66	5.47	5.27	5.17	5.07	4.97	4.86	4.75	4.64
11	.250	1.47	1.58	1.58	1.57	1.56	1.55	1.54	1.53	1.53	1.52	1.51	1.50	1.49	1.49	1.48	1.47	1.47	1.46	1.45
	.100	3.23	2.86	2.66	2.54	2.45	2.39	2.34	2.30	2.27	2.25	2.21	2.17	2.12	2.10	2.08	2.05	2.03	2.00	1.97
	.025	6.72	5.26	4.63	4.28	4.04	3.88	3.76	3.66	3.59	3.53	3.43	3.33	3.23	3.17	3.12	3.06	3.00	2.94	2.83
	.005	12.23	8.91	7.60	6.88	6.42	6.10	5.86	5.68	5.54	5.42	5.24	5.05	4.86	4.76	4.65	4.55	4.44	4.34	4.23
12	.250	1.46	1.56	1.56	1.55	1.54	1.53	1.52	1.51	1.51	1.50	1.49	1.48	1.47	1.46	1.45	1.45	1.44	1.43	1.42
	.100	3.18	2.81	2.61	2.48	2.39	2.33	2.28	2.24	2.21	2.19	2.15	2.10	2.06	2.04	2.01	1.99	1.96	1.93	1.90
	.025	6.55	5.10	4.47	4.12	3.89	3.73	3.61	3.51	3.44	3.37	3.28	3.18	3.07	3.02	2.96	2.91	2.85	2.79	2.72
	.005	11.75	8.51	7.23	6.52	6.07	5.76	5.52	5.35	5.20	5.09	4.91	4.72	4.53	4.43	4.33	4.23	4.12	4.01	3.90

TABLE 10.4

f_1 Degrees of Freedom (for greater mean square)

f_2	P	1	2	3	4	5	6	7	8	9	10	12	15	20	24	30	40	60	120	∞
13	.250	1.45	1.55	1.55	1.53	1.52	1.51	1.50	1.49	1.49	1.43	1.47	1.46	1.45	1.44	1.43	1.42	1.42	1.41	1.40
	.100	3.14	2.76	2.56	2.43	2.35	2.28	2.23	2.20	2.16	2.14	2.10	2.05	2.01	1.98	1.96	1.93	1.90	1.88	1.85
	.025	6.41	4.97	4.35	4.00	3.77	3.60	3.48	3.39	3.31	3.25	3.15	3.05	2.95	2.89	2.84	2.78	2.72	2.66	2.60
	.005	11.37	8.19	6.93	6.23	5.79	5.48	5.25	5.08	4.94	4.82	4.64	4.26	4.27	4.17	4.07	3.97	3.87	3.76	3.65
14	.250	1.44	1.53	1.53	1.52	1.51	1.50	1.49	1.48	1.47	1.45	1.45	1.44	1.43	1.42	1.41	1.41	1.40	1.39	1.38
	.100	3.10	2.73	2.52	2.39	2.31	2.24	2.19	2.15	2.12	2.10	2.05	2.01	1.96	1.94	1.91	1.89	1.86	1.83	1.80
	.025	6.30	4.86	4.24	3.89	3.66	3.50	3.38	3.29	3.21	3.15	3.05	2.95	2.84	2.79	2.73	2.67	2.61	2.55	2.49
	.005	11.06	7.92	6.68	6.00	5.56	5.26	5.03	4.86	4.72	4.60	4.43	4.25	4.06	3.96	3.86	3.76	3.66	3.55	4.44
15	.250	1.43	1.52	1.52	1.51	1.49	1.48	1.47	1.46	1.46	1.45	1.44	1.43	1.41	1.41	1.40	1.39	1.38	1.37	1.36
	.100	3.07	2.70	2.49	2.36	2.27	2.21	2.16	2.12	2.09	2.06	2.02	1.97	1.92	1.90	1.87	1.85	1.82	1.79	1.76
	.025	6.20	4.76	4.15	3.80	3.58	3.41	3.29	3.20	3.12	3.06	2.96	2.86	2.76	2.70	2.64	2.58	2.52	2.46	2.40
	.005	10.80	7.70	6.48	5.80	5.37	5.07	4.85	4.67	4.54	4.42	4.25	4.07	3.88	3.79	3.69	3.58	3.48	3.37	3.26
16	.250	1.42	1.51	1.51	1.50	1.48	1.47	1.46	1.45	1.44	1.44	1.43	1.41	1.40	1.39	1.38	1.37	1.36	1.35	1.34
	.100	3.05	2.67	2.46	2.33	2.24	2.18	2.13	2.09	2.06	2.03	1.99	1.94	1.89	1.87	1.84	1.81	1.78	1.75	1.72
	.025	6.12	4.69	4.08	3.73	3.50	3.34	3.22	3.12	3.05	2.99	2.89	2.79	2.68	2.63	2.57	2.51	2.45	2.38	2.32
	.005	10.58	7.51	6.30	5.64	5.21	4.91	4.69	4.52	4.38	4.27	4.10	3.92	3.73	3.64	3.54	3.44	3.33	3.22	3.11
17	.250	1.42	1.51	1.50	1.49	1.47	1.46	1.45	1.44	1.43	1.43	1.41	1.40	1.39	1.38	1.37	1.36	1.35	1.34	1.13
	.100	3.03	2.64	2.44	2.31	2.22	2.15	2.10	2.06	2.03	2.00	1.96	1.91	1.86	1.84	1.81	1.78	1.75	1.72	1.69
	.025	6.04	4.62	4.01	3.66	3.44	3.28	3.16	3.06	2.98	2.92	2.82	2.72	2.62	2.56	2.50	2.44	2.38	2.32	2.25
	.005	10.38	7.35	6.16	5.50	5.07	4.78	4.56	4.39	4.25	4.14	3.97	3.79	3.61	3.51	3.41	3.31	3.21	3.10	2.98
18	.250	1.41	1.50	1.49	1.48	1.46	1.45	1.44	1.43	1.42	1.42	1.40	1.39	1.38	1.37	1.36	1.35	1.34	1.33	1.32
	.100	3.01	2.62	2.42	2.29	2.20	2.13	2.08	2.04	2.00	1.98	1.93	1.89	1.84	1.81	1.78	1.75	1.72	1.69	1.66
	.025	5.98	4.56	3.95	3.61	3.38	3.22	3.10	3.01	2.93	2.87	2.77	2.67	2.56	2.50	2.44	2.38	2.32	2.26	2.19
	.005	10.22	7.21	6.03	5.37	4.96	4.66	4.44	4.28	4.14	4.03	3.86	3.68	3.50	3.40	3.30	3.20	3.10	2.99	2.70
19	.250	1.41	1.49	1.49	1.47	1.46	1.44	1.43	1.42	1.41	1.41	1.40	1.38	1.37	1.36	1.35	1.34	1.33	1.32	1.30
	.100	2.99	2.61	2.40	2.27	2.18	2.11	2.06	2.02	1.98	1.96	1.91	1.86	1.81	1.79	1.76	1.73	1.70	1.67	1.63
	.025	5.92	4.51	3.90	3.56	3.33	3.17	3.05	2.96	2.88	2.82	2.72	2.62	2.51	2.45	2.39	2.33	2.27	2.20	2.13
	.005	10.07	7.09	5.92	5.27	4.85	4.56	4.34	4.18	4.04	3.93	3.76	3.59	3.40	3.31	3.21	3.11	3.00	2.89	2.78
20	.250	1.40	1.49	1.48	1.47	1.45	1.44	1.43	1.42	1.41	1.40	1.39	1.37	1.36	1.35	1.34	1.33	1.32	1.31	1.29
	.100	2.97	2.59	2.38	2.25	2.16	2.09	2.04	2.00	1.96	1.94	1.89	1.84	1.79	1.77	1.74	1.71	1.68	1.64	1.61
	.025	5.87	4.46	3.86	3.51	3.29	3.13	3.01	2.91	2.84	2.77	2.68	2.57	2.46	2.41	2.35	2.29	2.22	2.16	2.09
	.005	9.94	6.99	5.82	5.17	4.76	4.47	4.26	4.09	3.96	3.85	3.68	3.50	3.32	3.22	3.12	3.02	2.92	2.81	2.69
21	.250	1.40	1.48	1.48	1.46	1.44	1.43	1.42	1.41	1.40	1.39	1.38	1.37	1.35	1.34	1.33	1.32	1.31	1.30	1.28
	.100	2.96	2.57	2.36	2.23	2.14	2.08	2.02	1.98	1.95	1.92	1.88	1.83	1.78	1.75	1.72	1.69	1.66	1.62	1.59
	.025	5.83	4.42	3.82	3.48	3.25	3.09	2.97	2.87	2.80	2.73	2.64	2.53	2.42	2.37	2.31	2.25	2.18	2.11	2.04
	.005	9.83	6.89	5.73	5.09	4.68	4.39	4.18	4.01	3.88	3.77	3.60	3.43	3.24	3.15	3.05	2.95	2.84	2.73	2.61
22	.250	1.40	1.48	1.47	1.45	1.44	1.42	1.41	1.40	1.39	1.39	1.37	1.36	1.34	1.33	1.32	1.31	1.30	1.29	1.28
	.100	2.95	2.56	2.35	2.22	2.13	2.06	2.01	1.97	1.93	1.90	1.86	1.81	1.76	1.73	1.70	1.67	1.64	1.60	1.57
	.025	5.79	4.38	3.78	3.44	3.22	3.05	2.93	2.84	2.76	2.70	2.60	2.50	2.39	2.33	2.27	2.21	2.14	2.08	2.00
	.005	9.73	6.81	5.65	5.02	4.61	4.32	4.11	3.94	3.81	3.70	3.54	3.36	3.18	3.08	2.98	2.88	2.77	2.66	2.55
23	.250	1.39	1.47	1.47	1.45	1.43	1.42	1.41	1.40	1.39	1.38	1.37	1.35	1.34	1.33	1.32	1.31	1.30	1.28	1.27
	.100	2.94	2.55	2.34	2.21	2.11	2.05	1.99	1.95	1.92	1.89	1.84	1.80	1.74	1.72	1.69	1.66	1.62	1.59	1.55
	.025	5.75	4.35	3.75	3.41	3.18	3.02	2.90	2.81	2.73	2.67	2.57	2.47	2.36	2.30	2.24	2.18	2.11	2.04	1.97
	.005	9.63	6.73	5.58	4.95	4.54	4.26	4.05	3.88	3.75	3.64	3.47	3.30	3.12	3.02	2.92	2.82	2.71	2.60	2.48
24	.250	1.39	1.47	1.46	1.44	1.43	1.41	1.40	1.39	1.38	1.38	1.36	1.35	1.33	1.32	1.31	1.30	1.29	1.28	1.26
	.100	2.93	2.54	2.33	2.19	2.10	2.04	1.98	1.94	1.91	1.88	1.83	1.78	1.73	1.70	1.67	1.64	1.61	1.57	1.53
	.015	5.72	4.32	3.72	3.38	3.15	2.99	2.87	2.78	2.70	2.64	2.54	2.44	2.33	2.27	2.21	2.15	2.08	2.01	1.94
	.005	9.55	6.66	5.52	4.89	4.49	4.20	3.99	3.83	3.69	3.59	3.42	3.25	3.06	2.97	2.87	2.77	2.66	2.55	2.43

continued

TABLE 10.4 (Continued)

df	α	1	2	3	4	5	6	7	8	9	10	12	15	20	24	30	40	60	120	∞
25	.250	1.39	1.47	1.46	1.44	1.42	1.41	1.40	1.39	1.38	1.37	1.36	1.34	1.33	1.32	1.31	1.29	1.28	1.27	1.25
	.100	2.92	2.53	2.32	2.18	2.09	2.02	1.97	1.93	1.89	1.87	1.82	1.77	1.72	1.69	1.66	1.63	1.59	1.56	1.52
	.025	5.69	4.29	3.69	3.35	3.13	2.97	2.85	2.75	2.68	2.61	2.51	2.41	2.30	2.24	2.18	2.12	2.05	1.98	1.91
	.005	9.48	6.60	5.46	4.84	4.43	4.15	3.94	3.78	3.64	3.54	3.37	3.20	3.02	2.92	2.82	2.72	2.61	2.50	2.38
26	.250	1.38	1.46	1.45	1.44	1.42	1.41	1.39	1.38	1.37	1.37	1.35	1.34	1.32	1.31	1.30	1.29	1.28	1.26	1.25
	.100	2.91	2.52	2.31	2.17	2.08	2.01	1.96	1.92	1.88	1.86	1.81	1.76	1.71	1.68	1.65	1.61	1.58	1.54	1.50
	.025	5.66	4.27	3.67	3.33	3.10	2.94	2.82	2.73	2.65	2.59	2.49	2.39	2.28	2.22	2.16	2.09	2.03	1.95	1.83
	.005	9.41	6.54	5.41	4.79	4.38	4.10	3.89	3.73	3.60	3.49	3.33	3.15	2.97	2.87	2.77	2.67	2.56	2.45	2.33
27	.250	1.38	1.46	1.45	1.43	1.42	1.40	1.39	1.38	1.37	1.36	1.35	1.33	1.32	1.31	1.30	1.28	1.27	1.26	1.24
	.100	2.90	2.51	2.30	2.17	2.07	2.00	1.95	1.91	1.87	1.85	1.80	1.75	1.70	1.67	1.64	1.60	1.57	1.53	1.49
	.025	5.63	4.24	3.65	3.31	3.08	2.92	2.80	2.71	2.63	2.57	2.47	2.36	2.25	2.19	2.13	2.07	2.00	1.93	1.85
	.005	9.34	6.49	5.36	4.74	4.34	4.06	3.85	3.69	3.56	3.45	3.28	3.11	2.93	2.83	2.73	2.63	2.52	2.41	2.29
28	.250	1.38	1.46	1.45	1.43	1.41	1.40	1.39	1.38	1.37	1.36	1.34	1.33	1.31	1.30	1.29	1.27	1.27	1.25	1.24
	.100	2.89	2.50	2.29	2.16	2.06	2.00	1.94	1.90	1.87	1.84	1.79	1.74	1.69	1.66	1.63	1.59	1.56	1.52	1.48
	.025	5.61	4.22	3.63	3.29	3.06	2.90	2.78	2.69	2.61	2.55	2.45	2.34	2.23	2.17	2.11	2.05	1.98	1.91	1.83
	.005	9.28	6.44	5.32	4.70	4.30	4.02	3.81	3.65	3.52	3.41	3.25	3.07	2.89	2.79	2.69	2.59	2.48	2.37	2.25
29	.250	1.38	1.45	1.45	1.43	1.41	1.40	1.38	1.37	1.36	1.35	1.34	1.32	1.31	1.30	1.29	1.27	1.26	1.25	1.23
	.100	2.89	2.50	2.28	2.15	2.06	1.99	1.93	1.89	1.86	1.83	1.78	1.73	1.68	1.65	1.62	1.58	1.55	1.51	1.47
	.025	5.59	4.20	3.61	3.27	3.04	2.88	2.76	2.67	2.59	2.53	2.43	2.32	2.21	2.15	2.09	2.03	1.96	1.89	1.81
	.005	9.23	6.40	5.28	4.66	4.26	3.98	3.77	3.61	3.48	3.38	3.21	3.04	2.86	2.76	2.66	2.56	2.45	2.33	2.21
30	.250	1.38	1.45	1.44	1.42	1.41	1.39	1.38	1.37	1.36	1.35	1.34	1.32	1.30	1.29	1.28	1.27	1.26	1.24	1.23
	.100	2.88	2.49	2.28	2.14	2.05	1.98	1.93	1.88	1.85	1.82	1.77	1.72	1.67	1.64	1.61	1.57	1.54	1.50	1.46
	.025	5.57	4.18	3.59	3.25	3.03	2.87	2.75	2.65	2.57	2.51	2.41	2.31	2.20	2.14	2.07	2.01	1.94	1.87	1.79
	.005	9.18	6.35	5.24	4.62	4.23	3.95	3.74	3.58	3.45	3.34	3.18	3.01	2.82	2.73	2.63	2.52	2.42	2.30	2.18
40	.250	1.36	1.44	1.42	1.40	1.39	1.37	1.36	1.35	1.34	1.33	1.31	1.30	1.28	1.26	1.25	1.24	1.22	1.21	1.19
	.100	2.84	2.44	2.23	2.09	2.00	1.93	1.87	1.83	1.79	1.76	1.71	1.66	1.61	1.57	1.54	1.51	1.47	1.42	1.38
	.025	5.42	4.05	3.46	3.13	2.90	2.74	2.62	2.53	2.45	2.39	2.29	2.18	2.07	2.01	1.94	1.88	1.80	1.72	1.64
	.005	8.83	6.07	4.98	4.37	3.99	3.71	3.51	3.35	3.22	3.12	2.95	2.78	2.60	2.50	2.40	2.30	2.18	2.06	1.93
60	.250	1.35	1.42	1.41	1.38	1.37	1.35	1.33	1.32	1.31	1.30	1.29	1.27	1.25	1.24	1.22	1.21	1.19	1.17	1.15
	.100	2.79	2.39	2.18	2.04	1.95	1.87	1.82	1.77	1.74	1.71	1.66	1.60	1.54	1.51	1.48	1.44	1.40	1.35	1.29
	.025	5.29	3.93	3.34	3.01	2.79	2.63	2.51	2.41	2.33	2.27	2.17	2.06	1.94	1.88	1.82	1.74	1.67	1.58	1.48
	.005	8.49	5.80	4.73	4.14	3.76	3.49	3.29	3.13	3.01	2.90	2.74	2.57	2.39	2.29	2.19	2.08	1.96	1.83	1.69
120	.250	1.34	1.40	1.39	1.37	1.35	1.33	1.31	1.30	1.29	1.28	1.26	1.24	1.22	1.21	1.19	1.18	1.16	1.13	1.10
	.100	2.75	2.35	2.13	1.99	1.90	1.82	1.77	1.72	1.68	1.65	1.60	1.55	1.48	1.45	1.41	1.37	1.32	1.26	1.19
	.025	5.15	3.80	3.23	2.89	2.67	2.52	2.39	2.30	2.22	2.16	2.05	1.94	1.82	1.76	1.69	1.61	1.53	1.43	1.31
	.005	8.18	5.54	4.50	3.92	3.55	3.28	3.09	2.93	2.81	2.71	2.54	2.37	2.19	2.09	1.98	1.87	1.75	1.61	1.43
∞	.250	1.32	1.39	1.37	1.35	1.33	1.31	1.29	1.28	1.27	1.25	1.24	1.22	1.19	1.18	1.16	1.14	1.12	1.08	1.00
	.100	2.71	2.30	2.08	1.94	1.85	1.77	1.72	1.67	1.63	1.60	1.55	1.49	1.42	1.38	1.34	1.30	1.24	1.17	1.00
	.025	5.02	3.69	3.12	2.79	2.57	2.41	2.29	2.19	2.11	2.05	1.94	1.83	1.71	1.64	1.57	1.48	1.39	1.27	1.00
	.005	7.88	5.30	4.28	3.72	3.35	3.09	2.90	2.74	2.62	2.52	2.36	2.19	2.00	1.90	1.79	1.67	1.53	1.36	1.00

*Reprinted from "Tables of percentage points of the inverted beta (F) distribution," by Maxine Merrington and Catherine M. Thompson, Biometrika, 33, 73 (1943) by permission of the authors and the editor.

Source: Snedecor, G. W. and W. G. Cochran. 1967. *Statistical Methods, 6th ed.* Ames: The Iowa State University Press.

TABLE 10.5 Cumulative Normal Frequency Distribution (area under the standard normal curve from 0 to Z)

Z	0.00	0.01	0.02	0.03	0.04	0.05	0.06	0.07	0.08	0.09
0.0	0.0000	0.0040	0.0080	0.0120	0.0060	0.0199	0.0239	0.0279	0.0319	0.0359
0.1	.0398	.0438	.0478	.0517	.0557	.0596	.0636	.0675	.0714	.0753
0.2	.0793	.0832	.0871	.0910	.0948	.0987	.1026	.1064	.1103	.1141
0.3	.1179	.1217	.1255	.1293	.1531	.1368	.1406	.1443	.1480	.1517
0.4	.1554	.1591	.1628	.1664	.1700	.1736	.1772	.1808	.1844	.1879
0.5	.1915	.1950	.1985	.2019	.2054	.2088	.2123	.2157	.2190	.2224
0.6	.2257	.2291	.2324	.2357	.2389	.2422	.2454	.2486	.2517	.2549
0.7	.2580	.2611	.2642	.2673	.2704	.2734	.2764	.2794	.2823	.2852
0.8	.2881	.2910	.2939	.2967	.2995	.3023	.3051	.3078	.3106	.3133
0.9	.3159	.3186	.3212	.3238	.3264	.3289	.3315	.3340	.3365	.3389
1.0	.3413	.3438	.3461	.3485	.3508	.3531	.3554	.3577	.3599	.3621
1.1	.3643	.3665	.3685	.3708	.3729	.3749	.3770	.3790	.3810	.3830
1.2	.3849	.3869	.3883	.3907	.3925	.3944	.3962	.3980	.3997	.4015
1.3	.4032	.4049	.4066	.4082	.4099	.4115	.4131	.4147	.4162	.4177
1.4	.4192	.4207	.4222	.4236	.4251	.4265	.4279	.4292	.4306	.4319
1.5	.4332	.4345	.4357	.4370	.4382	.4394	.4406	.4418	.4429	.4441
1.6	.4452	.4463	.4474	.4434	.4495	.4505	.4515	.4525	.4535	.4545
1.7	.4554	.4564	.4573	.4532	.4591	.4599	.4608	.4616	.4625	.4633
1.8	.4641	.4649	.4656	.4654	.4671	.4678	.4686	.4693	.4699	.4706
1.9	.4713	.4719	.4726	.4732	.4738	.4744	.4750	.4756	.4761	.4767
2.0	.4772	.4778	.4783	.4738	.4793	.4798	.4803	.4808	.4812	.4817
2.1	.4821	.4826	.4830	.4834	.4838	.4842	.4846	.4850	.4854	.4857
2.2	.4861	.4864	.4868	.4871	.4875	.4878	.4881	.4884	.4887	.4890
2.3	.4893	.4896	.4898	.4901	.4904	.4906	.4909	.4911	.4913	.4916
2.4	.4918	.4920	.4922	.4925	.4927	.4929	.4931	.4932	.4934	.4936
2.5	.4938	.4940	.4941	.4943	.4945	.4946	.4948	.4949	.4951	.4952
2.6	.4953	.4955	.4956	.4957	.4959	.4960	.4961	.4962	.4963	.4964
2.7	.4965	.4966	.4967	.4968	.4969	.4970	.4971	.4972	.4973	.4974
2.8	.4974	.4975	.4976	.4977	.4977	.4978	.4979	.4979	.4980	.4981
2.9	.4981	.4982	.4982	.4983	.4984	.4984	.4985	.4985	.4986	.4986
3.0	.4987	.4987	.4987	.4988	.4988	.4989	.4989	.4989	.4990	.4990
3.1	.4990	.4991	.4991	.4991	.4992	.4992	.4992	.4992	.4993	.4993
3.2	.4993	.4993	.4994	.4994	.4994	.4994	.4994	.4995	.4995	.4995
3.3	.4995	.4995	.4995	.4996	.4996	.4996	.4996	.4996	.4996	.4997
3.4	.4997	.4997	.4997	.4997	.4997	.4997	.4997	.4997	.4997	.4998
3.6	.4998	.4998	.4999	.4999	.4999	.4999	.4999	.4999	.4999	.4999
3.9	.5000									

SOURCE: Snedecor, G. W., and W. G. Cochran. 1967. *Statistical Methods*, 6th ed. Ames, IA: The Iowa State University Press. Used with permission.

CASE CONTROL STUDIES

Steven T. Fleming

"Time crumbles things; everything grows old under the power of Time and is forgotten through the lapse of Time." Aristotle, Physics, *Bk. IV, 12*

One of the classic study designs used in epidemiological research is the retrospective or case control study. With this mode of investigation, one identifies a group of subjects with a particular outcome, such as a disease or condition (the cases), and compares them to a group without the disease or condition (the controls). The comparison is made by looking back in time—that is, retrospectively—at the risk(s) to which each group was exposed. Case control studies are sometimes referred to as retrospective observational studies. The warning of Aristotle above foreshadows the discussion of one of the major problems of case control studies: recall bias.

Most epidemiological studies compare one group to another to determine the effect of risk factors (i.e., exposures) or treatments (i.e., interventions) on the incidence or course of disease. The studies can be classified on the basis of (1) the date when the disease is identified, (2) the date of exposure or treatment recognition, and (3) the time frame used in conducting the analysis. Figure 11.1 illustrates this paradigm for the case control study.

The identification of cases (with a particular outcome) and controls (without the outcome) is done in the present. Researchers look to the past for exposure to a risk factor and classify each case and control into exposed or unexposed groups. The analysis is typically accomplished in the present.

Selection of Cases and Controls

In most case control studies, cases are patients who have developed a particular disease, condition, or disability. To be identified as such, most of these patients have had access to the healthcare system at some point. For example, they have been hospitalized or they have been seen by their primary care physician. It is important to be specific in terms of patient characteristics (age, diagnosis, even severity of illness) and the period during which patients present themselves for medical care. Cases may even be defined over an extended period.

FIGURE 11.1
Schematic
for Case
Control
Studies

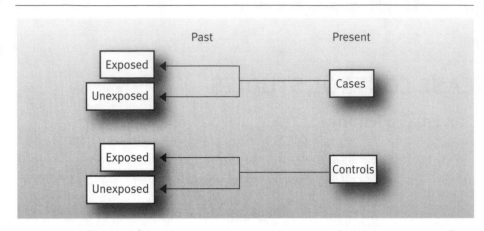

Control groups are necessary in most epidemiological studies to account for the underlying propensity of people to develop disease, even without a particular exposure, or recover from illness, even without a particular treatment. In a case control study, researchers determine the exposure status of the subjects in the case group (those who have developed disease) and compare it with the exposure status of the control group (those who have not developed disease). This measures the extent to which cases are more likely than controls to be exposed to risk factor(s).

The control group should be representative of the general population as far as exposure to the risk factor(s) is concerned and should have the same probability of selection into the sample as the cases have (Timmreck 1998). Control groups are typically matched to cases using a matching strategy. One strategy is to pair cases to controls along a number of relevant dimensions. This means the researcher matches one control (with specific characteristics, such as age and sex) with each case. Alternatively, the controls may be group or frequency matched. This strategy involves no one-to-one matching, but it requires that controls as a group be similar to the case group in terms of certain characteristics (e.g., the percentage of cases age 65 and older should be the same as that of the control group).

Typically, the desire to match cases to controls along a number of potentially relevant characteristics—the first strategy—must be balanced against the practicality of being able to locate controls who meet the necessary criteria for inclusion in the study. Thus, most studies employ the second strategy, and seek controls of the same age and gender, without the disease, and from the same general geographical area or with some history of treatment in the same facility. It should also be pointed out that the influence of a particular variable (e.g., income) can be measured later on, in the statistical analysis, and need not be included in the matching strategy (Lilienfeld and Stolley 1994).

Selection of a control group(s) is a critical component of the research. If the control group is not representative of the general population and/or is more likely to have characteristics associated with the disease under study, or if it is biased in any other way, the study is flawed. This means the results and interpretations may be misleading. For example, Grisso and colleagues (1991) studied risk factors for falls as a cause of hip fracture in women and recognized that the control group "may have a greater prevalence of risk factors for falls, such as neurologic illnesses, lower limb disability, use of psychoactive medications, and alcohol use, than the general population, thus the comparison of case patients with hospitalized controls is likely to underestimate the effect of these factors on the risk of hip fracture."

Exposure

Any characteristic or event that increases or decreases the probability of disease, disability, death, or other adverse outcome can be referred to as an *exposure* (Norell 1995).

Although an exposure can also be called a risk factor, note that exposures can either increase or decrease the risk of disease. Thus, some exposures are protective, whereas others are malicious. Exposures may be characterized in terms of magnitude and duration for the purpose of determining whether a dose-response relationship exists. A higher dose may be of higher magnitude, longer duration, or both. With a dose-response relationship, a higher dose of exposure results in a larger response (or effect), in terms of its impact on the outcome in question. Consider the following examples of exposures:

1. "We observed a positive association between adult height and breast cancer risk" (Swanson et al. 1996).
2. "[The] risk associated with obesity is, in most studies, limited to older postmenopausal women. In younger women....obesity appears to be inversely related to the risk of disease" (Swanson et al. 1996).
3. "Pregnancy has a dual effect on the risk of breast cancer: it transiently increases the risk after childbirth but reduces the risk in later years" (Lambe et al. 1994).
4. "Women with a family history of breast cancer, even if the nearest relative with breast cancer is a third-degree relative, are at increased risk of the disease" (Slattery and Kerber 1993).

Each of the above studies concerns an exposure that is associated with the risk of developing breast cancer. These studies illustrate the inherent complexity in defining exposure. Height is simply a characteristic that appears to be associated with the risk of breast cancer. The authors hypothesize that height may represent some other underlying risk factor, such as surface area or metabolic rate. Obesity is a risk factor that appears to be protective in younger women, but malicious in older women, with a possible underlying hormonal basis. With regard to pregnancy, the risk of breast cancer is initially higher immediately following the pregnancy, but lower thereafter. Thus, pregnancy changes from a malicious to a protective exposure with time. Finally, family history is an exposure related to one's pedigree, which may have underlying genetic and environmental components.

The diversity, definitions, and distinctions of exposure can be explored in the following studies. According to Perneger, Whelton, and Klag (1994), "Both heavy average intake...and medium-to-high cumulative intake...of acetaminophen [Tylenol] appeared to double the odds of ESRD [end stage renal disease]." The results of this study would indicate a dose-response relationship with the exposure (acetaminophen) and disease (ESRD) in terms of both magnitude ("average intake") and duration ("cumulative intake").

Grisso and colleagues (1994), who studied the risk of hip fracture in women, showed that "among black women, thinness, previous stroke, use of aids in walking, and alcohol consumption are associated with an increased risk of hip fracture." Here, the four exposures are a body characteristic, a medical history event, a therapeutic device, and a behavior.

Eskenazi, Fenster, and Sidney (1991) examined the risks of pre-eclampsia, which is a hypertensive disorder of pregnancy, and found that "being nulliparous [childless] and having a previous history of preeclampsia greatly increased a woman's risk for preeclampsia...working during pregnancy more than doubled the risk for preeclampsia....cigarette smoking tended to protect against preeclampsia...alcohol consumption was protective...having a history of spontaneous abortion may be protective and being black may be a risk." With this study the protective exposures are a condition (pregnancy), two behaviors (smoking and alcohol use), and a history of medical events (miscarriages).

The relationship between baldness in men and myocardial infarction (heart attack) was the topic of a study by Lesko, Rosenberg, and Shapiro (1993), who reported a dose-response relationship, since "the results support the hypothesis that MPB [male pattern baldness] is associated with an increased risk of MI [myocardial infarction] in men under the age of 55 years...the RR [relative risk] estimate for men with extreme vertex baldness compared with men with no baldness was approximately 3.0; for lesser degrees of hair loss, the risk was lower." Clearly, it is not baldness itself that predisposes one to these cardiovascular events, but rather some underlying physiological mechanism (e.g., level of testosterone) for which baldness is the observable measure.

These examples show the breadth of possible exposures and the difficulty of distinguishing exposures as derivative risks, in the sense that they represent a more cellular, biochemical, or physiological basis of disease than that found in the exposures themselves. It should also be clear that both exposure and risk operate within the context of time. A dose-response relationship may reflect either (or both) the magnitude or the duration of exposure. Further, the increase or decrease in the probability of disease brought about by an exposure may vary across time, as was the case with the effect of pregnancy on breast cancer.

FIGURE 11.2
Case
Control
Study
Design

		Cases	Control
Exposure	Yes	a	b
	No	c	d

Relative Risk in a Case Control Study

The purpose of most case control studies is to assess the degree of risk, in terms of disease, disability, or other adverse outcome, that is associated with a particular exposure to a risk factor. The data are typically presented in a two-by-two grid (Figure 11.2) with the presence or absence of a characteristic or risk factor (the exposure) as rows, and the presence (cases) or absence (controls) of disease as columns.

With most epidemiological studies, the interest is in measuring the number of times more likely one is to develop a disease after exposure to a particular risk factor. This concept is referred to as *relative risk*. With a case control study design, one can estimate the relative risk by the odds ratio (OR), which is defined as the cross-product of the entries in Figure 11.2, that is, a × d divided by b × c. Since a case-control study starts out with two groups—cases and controls—it makes the most sense to interpret the odds ratio as the increased (or decreased) odds that cases have been exposed to the risk factor as compared with controls. An algebraic equivalent, but perhaps less intuitive statement, would be that the odds ratio is the increased (or decreased) odds of disease of the exposed compared to the unexposed. In either case, the odds ratio is only an estimate of the relative risk (the incidence of disease in the exposed group divided by the incidence of disease in the unexposed group).

The degree to which the estimate of relative risk is valid depends on (1) whether cases and controls are truly representative of the population from which they are drawn and (2) whether the frequency of disease in the population is low (see Lilienfeld and Stolley 1994, on pages 316–317, for a derivation of the odds ratio as a good estimate of relative risk when the prevalence of disease in the population is low). Relative risk cannot be calculated directly from the data typically presented in case control studies, because to do so requires information on the incidence of disease in the exposed and unexposed groups, statistics that are not available in a case control study.

FIGURE 11.3
Family
History and
Breast
Cancer Risk

		Cases	Control
Exposure	Yes	123	51
	No	3,960	4,032

OR = 123 × 4,032/51 × 3,960 = 2.4.3

SOURCE: Slattery and Kerber (1993).

An odds ratio greater than 1.0 indicates that an individual who has the disease in question—that is, he or she falls into the "cases" column of the two-by-two grid—is more likely to have been exposed to the risk factor than someone without the disease; a value of 1.0 means that the likelihood of having the disease is unaffected by the risk factor; a value of less than one implies that the risk factor is actually protective—that someone with the disease is less likely to have the risk factor than someone without the disease (the "controls" in the 2 x 2 grid). For example, when Slattery and Kerber (1993) evaluated family history and breast cancer risk, they considered, among other things, the risk of having a mother who had suffered breast cancer. Figure 11.3 reports these results. In this example, the "exposure" is to have a mother who suffered breast cancer. According to the odds ratio, a woman with breast cancer has 2.4 times the odds of having a mother who also has (or had) breast cancer than a woman without breast cancer.

Figure 11.4 illustrates the risk of breast cancer reported by Daling and colleagues (1996) among nulliparous women associated with induced abortion. The exposure here is induced abortion, and a woman with breast cancer has 1.3 times the odds of having had an induced abortion than a woman without breast cancer. Figure 11.5, on the other hand, illustrates the protective effect of lactation on breast cancer risk as well as a dose-response relationship, from a study by Newcomb and colleagues (1994). In this study the hypothesis was that lactation duration may be associated with reduced risk of premenopausal breast cancer.

As the odds ratio decreases (from 1.0 toward 0), the protective effect increases. In other words, women with premenopausal breast cancer have only 0.71 times the odds to have lactated for a year or two than women without premenopausal cancer. The protective effect of lactation decreases (the odds ratio increases) as the dose of the exposure decreases.

FIGURE 11.4
Induced
Abortion
and Breast
Cancer Risk

		Cases	Control
Exposure	Yes	95	63
	No	208	181

OR = 95 × 181/63 × 208 = 1.3

SOURCE: Daling et al. (1996). Used with permission of Oxford University Press.

Confounding

Factors or variables other than the exposures in question may influence the probability of developing the disease under study. These confounding variables complicate and confuse the analysis. According to Timmreck (1998):

> Confounding variables can affect controls and may lead to biased or misguided association between disease and cause, the agents or risk factors. Any characteristic, trait, or other factor that can distort or slant the results of the study can be a confounding variable if not taken into account or considered.

Confounding variables must be associated with both the disease (outcome) and the exposure as indicated in Figure 11.6. Thompson (1994) makes four points with regard to confounding: (1) the size of the bias in the odds ratio depends on the level of confounder association with the exposure and the disease; (2) confounders may be causally related to the disease or associated with the exposure as proxies for unmeasured causes; (3) if an exposure has a causal effect on another variable, that variable is an intervening variable rather than a confounder; and (4) the aggregate effect of multiple confounders may be substantial even if the effect of each is small.

For example, consider the relationship between smoking (an exposure) and coronary heart disease (CHD). Confounders may include variables such as stress. Stress may be causally related to CHD, or it may be a proxy for some unmeasured variable such as personality. Moreover, stress may be related to the exposure, to the extent that smokers are more likely to smoke under stress. In any event, failure to measure stress could

FIGURE 11.5
Dose–
Response
Relationship
Between
Duration of
Lactation
and
Premenopausal
Breast
Cancer

		Cases	Control
Exposure ≤ 3 months	Yes	203	375
	No	602	1,009

OR = 0.91

		Cases	Control
Exposure 4–12 months	Yes	195	390
	No	602	1,009

OR = 0.84

		Cases	Control
Exposure 13–24 months	Yes	106	251
	No	602	1,009

OR = 0.71

SOURCE: Data from Newcomb et al. (1994).

distort or bias the results. If the exposed group (smokers) is more likely to be under stress than the unexposed group (nonsmokers), then an exaggerated incidence of CHD could be the result of both smoking and stress.

At least two ways have been developed to deal with confounding: multivariate analysis and stratification. The former is appropriate when many known risk factors can be measured and included in the analysis. The latter can be useful with a small number of risk factors.

Newcomb and colleagues (1994) studied the hypothesis that lactation may be a protective factor for breast cancer. These authors chose to use a multivariate logistic regression that includes a number of well-established risk factors for breast cancer, such as subjects' age at birth of first child and family history of breast cancer. Cases and controls may differ in exposure to these other risk factors (e.g., in the Newcomb study, 18 percent of cases had a family history of breast cancer compared with 11 percent of controls). If these confounding variables are not taken into account, the results may be biased or misleading. Suppose that older mothers are more likely to breast-feed their babies. The protective effect of lactation may be mitigated by delivery of the first child at a later age (a risk factor). The logistic regression calculates an adjusted odds ratio that compensates or controls for the influence of these other risk factors.

The other approach is to stratify the results by the confounding variable in question. Pershagen and colleagues (1994), for instance, were interested is residential radon exposure as a risk factor for lung cancer in Sweden. Strong evidence would suggest that smoking is a behemoth of a risk factor for lung cancer, the protests of the tobacco industry to the contrary notwithstanding. If radon is a risk factor for lung cancer (which it is), and smoking is associated with radon exposure (i.e., those who are exposed to radon are more likely to smoke), it would be difficult to disentangle the effects of smoking versus radon exposure in the analysis. One solution would be to stratify the analysis as in Figure 11.7. Although the authors used a multivariate logistic regression, the results are stratified by exposure to smoking.

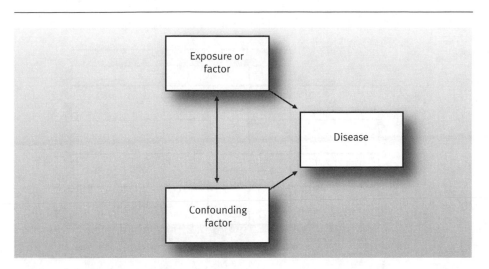

FIGURE 11.6
Confounding
Variables

Although there may be some increased risk of lung cancer with radon exposure, the risk of lung cancer for smokers who are exposed to radon grows exponentially. Since the results are stratified by smoking exposure, we are able to see the interaction (and potential confounding) of these two exposures.

Attributable Fraction

Earlier, the odds ratio (OR) was defined as an estimate of the relative risk of disease given exposure to a particular risk factor. To the extent that confounding may occur—especially if there are multiple risk factors, some of which may potentiate or mitigate each other—the odds ratio must be adjusted to compensate for this interaction. Also, one may be interested in determining the extent to which a particular risk factor is responsible for disease in the population. The proportion of disease attributed to a particular risk factor is called the *attributable fraction* (AF) and is estimated for case control studies here:

$$AF = p(OR - 1)/p(OR - 1) + 1 \times 100\%$$

where p is the proportion of the population with the risk factor and OR is the odds ratio. For example, in a study of the risk factors for lung cancer among young adults in Germany, Kreuzer and colleagues (1998) report odds ratios of 15.9 and 29.9 for males and females, respectively, who are 45 years old or less and current smokers. Assume that the prevalence of smoking in Germany is 36.8 percent for men and 21.5 percent for women (World Health Organization 1996). The attributable fraction would be:

FIGURE 11.7
Radon and
Risk of Lung
Cancer
Stratified by
Smoking
Exposure

		Level of radon in the home				
		1	2	3	4	5
Smoking exposure	Never smoked	1	1.1	1.0	1.5	1.2
	Ex-smoker	2.6	2.4	3.2	4.5	1.1
	Current smoker (< 10 cigarettes/day)	6.2	6.0	6.1	7.3	25.1
	Current smoker (≥ 10 cigarettes/day)	12.6	11.6	11.8	15.0	32.5

SOURCE: Data from Pershagen et al. (1994).

AF (males) = .368 (14.9)/.368 (14.9) + 1 × 100 = 84.6%
AF (females) = .215 (28.9)/.215 (28.9) + 1 × 100 = 86.1%

According to these results, men with lung cancer have 15.9 times the odds of being a current smoker compared to those without the disease, with smoking behavior being responsible for 84.6 percent of the disease. Females with lung cancer have 29.9 times the odds of being a current smoker compared to those without the disease, with smoking behavior being responsible for 86.1 percent of the disease.

The AF may be high, as in the case of smoking and lung cancer. Another study (Chaouki et al. 1998) reported an odds ratio of 61.6 for human papillovirus and cervical cancer in Morocco with an attributable fraction of 92 percent. These results would indicate that 92 percent of cervical cancer is attributed to the human papillovirus.

The risk factor may be only one of multiple causes of the disease, which would reduce the AF. The AF also may be low because of a low odds ratio, or a low prevalence of the risk factor in the population, or both. In the Daling study discussed earlier, the risk of breast cancer among childless women who had an induced abortion was 1.3. If we assume that about 30 percent of women in this age group report an induced abortion, the attributable fraction would be [0.3(0.3)/(0.3)(0.3) + 1] × 100 = 8.3%.

Attributable risk is also a measure of the degree to which eliminating a particular risk factor would decrease the incidence of disease. Since it is calculated as a rate difference (incidence in the exposed group minus incidence in the unexposed group), it is more appropriate to discuss this in the cohort study (Chapter 12), where incidence rates can be calculated directly.

Sources of Bias

A study design may be subject to one or more sources of bias, which means the results either underestimate or exaggerate the true effect of the risk factor.

Selection bias means the study participants—both cases and controls—are not chosen randomly. This source of bias is especially pronounced in hospital studies where cases (e.g., patients with a hip fracture or hip replacement) are typically compared to a control group of hospitalized patients without that condition. But it can also occur in other settings (e.g., physician offices) where the control group is derived from patients who are seen in that same setting. It can be demonstrated (Lilienfeld and Stolley 1994) that this source of bias, also referred to as *Berksonian bias*, may either underestimate or overestimate the relationship between a risk factor and disease (Kraus 1954) if either (1) the rates of admission to the hospital (or visits to a physician) are different for cases and controls or (2) people are hospitalized (or see a physician) simply because they have a particular risk factor. The former is probably true most of the time; the latter is difficult to prove. Case Study 11.1 presents a classic case of selection bias involving the alleged link between coffee drinking and pancreatic cancer.

Case Study 11.1. Coffee and Pancreatic Cancer

MacMahon and colleagues (1981) caused a stir when they published a report in the prestigious *New England Journal of Medicine* in which they linked coffee drinking to cancer of the pancreas. The study has been criticized by many, including Feinstein and colleagues. (1981). MacMahon conducted a hospital-based case control study in 11 large hospitals in Boston and Rhode Island. The study included 369 patients with histologically confirmed cancer of the pancreas and 644 control patients. Controls comprised two groups of patients: (1) patients with other cancers and (2) patients with other conditions, with an overrepresentation of patients with gastroenterologic conditions such as colitis, enteritis, diverticulitis, and gastritis. Figure 11.8 summarizes the results for men and women for each of the three levels of coffee drinking and the unexposed group.

QUESTIONS

1. What is the overall crude odds ratio for the risk of pancreatic cancer from using coffee for men and women?
2. Why can't we calculate a relative risk directly?
3. What is the odds ratio for each level of coffee consumption?
4. Is there a dose-response relationship for either men or women?

FIGURE 11.8. COFFEE AND PANCREATIC CANCER, BY GENDER AND DOSE

Men	Pancreatic cancer		Women	Pancreatic cancer	
	Yes	No		Yes	No
Exposure coffee drinking — > 4 cups	60	82	Exposure coffee drinking — > 4 cups	28	48
3–4 cups	53	74	3–4 cups	53	80
1–2 cups	94	119	1–2 cups	59	152
None	9	32	None	11	56

SOURCE: MacMahon et al. (1981).

5. Nearly 40 percent of the controls had a gastroenterologic diagnosis such as gastritis or colitis. One might suspect that many of these controls would have reduced or eliminated coffee consumption to reduce the symptoms of their disease. What effect would this have on the study results?

6. This study is based on 369 (64 percent) of a total of 578 patients who were identified as potential cases with pancreatic cancer. Most of these "lost" cases were not interviewed, but 98 (47 percent) were either too sick to be interviewed or dead. Suppose that the group of lost cases had a higher incidence of smoking than either the 369 remaining cases or the controls and that smoking increases the risk of pancreatic cancer. What kind of bias exists here, and what is the effect on the odds ratio?

ANSWERS

1. Figure 11.8 can be collapsed into Figure 11.9 by adding together counts of the three exposure groups. Since each of the exposure levels is compared to the unexposed group in each table, the unexposed counts remain the same. Based on this table the crude odds ratio for men would be $(207 \times 32)/(275 \times 9) = 2.68$. For women the crude odds ratio would be $(140 \times 56)/(280 \times 11) = 2.55$.

2. We can't calculate the relative risk directly because the "relative risk" is the ratio of the incidence of disease in the exposed group divided by the incidence of disease in the unexposed group. With a case control study, we do

FIGURE 11.9. COFFEE AND PANCREATIC CANCER, BY GENDER

		Men		Women	
		Cases	Control	Cases	Control
Coffee	Yes	207	275	140	280
	No	9	32	32	11

SOURCE: MacMahon et al. (1981).

not start out with a group of exposed and unexposed subjects, so there is no way to directly calculate relative risk.

3. Based on Figure 11.8, the crude odds ratio for each level of use is calculated as follows

Men
1–2 cups $(94 \times 32)/(119 \times 9) = 2.8$
3–4 cups $(53 \times 32)/(74 \times 9) = 2.5$
>5 cups $(60 \times 32)/(82 \times 9) = 2.6$

Women
1–2 cups $(59 \times 56)/(152 \times 11) = 2.0$
3–4 cups $(53 \times 56)/(80 \times 11) = 3.4$
>5 cups $(28 \times 56)/(48 \times 11) = 3.0$

4. For men there is clearly no dose-response relationship. Among women, one could argue that there is a dose-response relationship for low (1–2 cups) compared to higher doses of coffee drinking.
5. If the number of exposed controls was artificially lower than it should be because subjects had reduced/eliminated coffee consumption to treat symptoms, then the odds ratio would be exaggerated. Feinstein and colleagues (1981) demonstrate how very modest changes in this misclassification of exposure would result in an odds ratio of 1.09.
6. The lost cases result in a form of selection bias, since the remaining cases are unlike the eligible population of pancreatic cancer patients, e.g., they have a lower prevalence of smoking. For smoking to be a confounding variable, it must

be associated with coffee drinking (e.g., smokers drink more coffee than non-smokers), and the outcome (e.g., smokers have a higher risk of pancreatic cancer). If smoking were a confounding variable, and the remaining cases had a lower prevalence of smoking than the controls, then the cases would also have a lower prevalence of coffee drinking, and the crude odds ratio would be lower than it should be. The authors of this paper actually stratified by smoking behavior and showed that never smokers, ex-smokers, and current smokers all had an increased risk of pancreatic cancer that was related to coffee drinking.

Another important source of bias is referred to as *misclassification bias*. As shown in Figure 11.1, past exposure must be taken into account in both the cases and controls. Subjects must be classified as either cases or controls, all of whom either were exposed or not exposed to the particular risk factor. If a subject is misclassified as a case (when he or she should have been a control) or a control (when he or she should have been a case), the true effect of the risk factor may be underestimated or exaggerated. Likewise, if either a case or a control has been erroneously classified as having been exposed to a risk factor (when he or she was not) or unexposed (when he or she was), the true effect may be underestimated or exaggerated. Thus, subjects may be misclassified on the basis of disease, exposure, or both. In short, with the typical 2 × 2 table (Figure 11.10) used to summarize most kinds of observational studies, such as the case control study, misclassification bias occurs when subjects are incorrectly categorized into any of the four cells of the table. See Norell (1995) for an excellent expostulation of these concepts.

Sensitivity and specificity were defined in Chapter 3 as characteristics of screening or diagnostic tests. *Sensitivity* is the probability that someone with disease will test positive (tests positive/all those with disease). *Specificity* is the probability that someone without the disease will test negative (tests negative/all those without the disease). We can also measure the sensitivity

FIGURE 11.10
Typical 2 x 2
Table

		Disease	
		Yes	No
Exposure	Yes	a	b
	No	c	d

and specificity of tests for exposure. Consider such measures of exposure as laboratory tests, questionnaires, or interviews. The sensitivity of such instruments would be the probability that someone who actually is exposed tests positive (tests positive for exposure/truly exposed). The specificity is the probability that someone who actually is not exposed tests negative (tests negative/truly not exposed).

Suppose that a questionnaire that assesses smoking status has a sensitivity of 90 percent and a specificity of 80 percent. This means that 90 percent of those who smoke are classified as smokers on the basis of this questionnaire, and 80 percent of those who do not smoke are correctly classified as nonsmokers.

Misclassification bias may be differential or nondifferential, depending on the sensitivity and specificity of the tests used to measure either disease or exposure. For nondifferential bias, the test has the same sensitivity and specificity for the two groups under study. For example, if a test measuring exposure status (e.g., questionnaire) has the same sensitivity and specificity for both cases and controls, the bias may be nondifferential. If a diagnostic test (or "diagnostic workup") measuring disease status has the same sensitivity and specificity for those with and without an exposure, then the bias may be nondifferential.

With differential bias, the sensitivity and/or specificity of the test may be different for the two groups under study. That is, the measure of exposure may have a different sensitivity and/or specificity for cases and controls, or the diagnostic test may have a different sensitivity and/or specificity for the exposed and unexposed groups. For example, if both cases and controls tend to underreport exposure history (e.g., each group understates the number of sexual contacts they've had to the same degree), the bias is nondifferential. If the sensitivity and/or specificity of the measure is different (e.g., cases more accurately report exposure [higher sensitivity] than controls [lower sensitivity]), then the bias is differential. The four types of misclassification bias can be illustrated and described as follows:

1. nondifferential misclassification bias of disease;
2. differential misclassification bias of disease;
3. nondifferential misclassification bias of exposure; and
4. differential misclassification bias of exposure.

One issue that can affect the nondifferential misclassification bias of disease (or condition) is the potential gap between the theoretical and empirical definitions of a disease, which may relate to issues of either definition or measurement. The criteria used to diagnose the disease may be either too narrow or too wide, or the definition of disease may be too narrow or too wide.

Consider the definition of AIDS, for example, which has widened over the years to include some of the common symptoms of immunodeficiency manifested in women (e.g., invasive cervical cancer). Suppose you are engaging in a case control study to determine if promiscuity is a risk factor for AIDS in women. If the definition of AIDS is too narrow (i.e., does not include invasive cervical cancer), then both exposure groups (sexually overactive and never active) are more likely to be classified as controls. The bias is nondifferential if the sensitivity and specificity of the tests used to diagnose disease (Chapter 3) are the same for both the exposed and unexposed groups. In the case of AIDS, both exposed and unexposed subjects would tend to be classified as controls rather than cases. This type of bias typically results in underestimating the effect by shifting the relative risk (or odds ratio) toward 1.0.

With differential misclassification bias of disease (condition), the tendency to classify subjects as either cases or controls depends on the exposure status with a different sensitivity and/or specificity. For example, people who are exposed may be more likely be recognized as having the disease, simply because the medical staff who differentiate between cases and controls had prior knowledge of the exposure. Without blinding, the staff would tend to classify the exposed subject with symptoms as a case, and the unexposed subject as a control. The staff may even engage in more thorough diagnostic inquiry for exposed subjects, presupposing that they are cases.

Abenhaim and colleagues (1996) studied the risk of primary pulmonary hypertension associated with appetite-suppressant drugs (e.g., Fen-Phen). Had they not blinded the panel of reviewers to the patients' exposure to anorexic drugs, the reviewers might have had a tendency to misclassify patients as either cases or controls, based on presuppositions. With this type of bias the effect is either exaggerated or underestimated, and thus it becomes difficult to estimate the direction of the true odds ratio.

Nondifferential misclassification bias of exposure occurs when cases and controls tend to misrepresent (i.e., forget, omit, do not want to reveal) their exposure status to the same degree. Cases and controls may both overestimate or underestimate their exposure as a result of forgetfulness, embarrassment, or

Low Roman Catholic		
	Cases	Controls
Exposure — Yes	23	22
Exposure — No	292	326

High Roman Catholic		
	Cases	Controls
Exposure — Yes	12	1
Exposure — No	213	229

SOURCE: Rookus and Van Leeuwen (1996). Used with permission.

social expectations. This type of bias results in underestimating the effect by shifting the relative risk (or odds ratio) toward 1.0. For example, in a hypothetical study that attempts to link vitamin intake during early childhood with colon cancer, both cases and controls may underestimate the exposure (vitamins) due to recall bias (they forgot).

Differential misclassification bias of exposure occurs if the tendency of cases to misrepresent (i.e., forget, omit, not want to reveal) their exposure status differs from that of controls. In other words, the measure of exposure has a different sensitivity and/or specificity for cases and controls. For example, earlier we reported that women with breast cancer have 1.3 times the odds of having had an induced abortion compared to those without the disease (Daling et al. 1996). Suppose that both cases and controls tended to misrepresent this type of exposure for different reasons. Rookus and Van Leeuwen (1996) examined this question using data from four regions in the Netherlands, two in which Roman Catholics composed about 63 percent of the population, and two in which the Roman Catholic population composed only 28 percent of the residents. Presumably, Roman Catholics would be less willing to report an induced abortion (lower sensitivity) because church teaching outlaws the act. Figure 11.11 reports these results.

Notice that the odds ratio in the Roman Catholic areas is probably exaggerated because the authors "found evidence that the...increased risk for breast cancer after induced abortion was largely attributable to underreporting of abortion by healthy control subjects." They conclude that cases may be more likely to report an exposure despite social norms and criticism—perhaps because of their desire to understand the perils of the disease—whereas controls may misrepresent exposures that are not consistent with social norms of behavior. With this type of bias the effect is either exaggerated or underestimated, making it difficult to estimate the direction of the true odds ratio. Case Study 11.2 is an example of misclassification bias in a study involving smoking and low birth weight newborns.

Case Study 11.2. Smoking and Low Birth Weight Newborns

Smoking has been shown to be a risk factor for low birth weight (LBW) newborns with an odds ratio of about 2.0 (see Table 11.1). Suppose that you want to engage in a nested case control study with 450 cases of mothers with LBW newborns and 500 controls (mothers with normal weight infants). Since your study is nested within an ongoing cohort study, you have access to both urine and serum samples from these women.

QUESTIONS

1. Suppose that the "true" exposure status is 150 smokers among the cases and 100 smokers among the controls. What is the true crude odds ratio?
2. Both thiocyanate and cotinine are biological markers for smoking. Even biological markers are not perfect measures of exposure. Suppose you measure smoking status with serum thiocyanate, and assume a sensitivity of 86 percent and a specificity of 79 percent. If these characteristics of the test apply to women with LBW and normal birth weight infants, will there be a bias, what kind, and how does it affect the odds ratio?
3. If one knows the sensitivity and specificity of the test for exposure, is there a way to predict what the "observed" odds ratio would be under these circumstances of an imperfect test?
4. What would be the observed odds ratio using the serum thiocyanate measure for smoking status with a sensitivity of 86 percent and specificity of 79 percent?
5. You review the study by Russell, Crawford, and Woodby (2004) and notice the variability in sensitivity and specificity among the eight different biological markers for smoking. You are curious how differences in sensitivity and specificity, particularly those that affect cases and controls differently, would affect the observed odds ratio. How might you do a sensitivity analysis to predict such changes in the odds ratio?
6. So far we have been considering how the observed odds ratio may be different from the true odds ratio under conditions of an imperfect test to measure exposure. How might we do the opposite—adjust the observed odds ratio to the true odds ratio, taking into consideration the characteristics of the test of exposure?
7. Use the 2 × 2 table derived from question 4 to convert the observed odds ratio back to the true odds ratio.

ANSWERS

1. The true crude odds ratio is $(150 \times 400)/(100 \times 300) = 2.0$.
2. This imperfect measure of exposure would create a nondifferential misclassification bias of exposure. Because the specificity is higher than the sensitivity, more nonsmokers would be classified as smokers than the other way around. This would cause the observed odds ratio to be less than the true odds ratio, which we assume to be about 2.0.

TABLE 11.1 SMOKING STATUS AND NEWBORN WEIGHT

Smoking	LBW	Normal
Yes	150	100
No	300	400
Total	450	500

FIGURE 11.12. SMOKER CASE STUDY 2X2

		Truly exposed	Truly unexposed
Test results	Positive	120	60
	Negative	30	240

---

3. Consider the typical 2 × 2 table for a case control study (Figure 11.2) where a is the number of exposed cases, b is the number of exposed controls, c is the number of nonexposed cases, and d is the number of nonexposed controls. Suppose these numbers represent the true values for each of these cells. We can adjust the values in cells a and b if we know the sensitivity and specificity of the test used to measure exposure for cases and controls, respectively. Suppose the measure has a sensitivity and specificity of 80 percent for both cases and controls. In our example here (see figure 11.12), we should be observing 150 cases who smoke. Since the sensitivity of the measure is 80 percent, however, we will only observe $0.80 \times 150 = 120$ of these cases. Since the specificity is 80 percent, we will also pick up ($1 - 0.8 = 0.20$ or 20%) of those who are truly not exposed (300), but tested positive. Therefore, in this situation the observed number of exposed cases would be $0.80 \times 150 + (1 - 0.8) \times 300 = 120 + 60 = 180$. If we have 180 cases who smoke, then we will have $450 - 180 = 270$ cases who don't smoke. Since the sensitivity and

---

TABLE 11.2. SENSITIVITY ANALYSIS FOR SMOKING AND NEWBORN WEIGHT

Controls Sensitivity (%), Specificity (%)	Cases Sensitivity (%), Specificity (%)				
	100, 100	75, 75	50, 50	75, 25	25, 75
100, 100	2.00	2.86	4.00	12.00	1.33
75, 75	0.93	1.33	1.86	5.57	0.62
50, 50	0.50	0.71	1.00	3.00	0.33
75, 25	0.17	0.24	0.33	1.00	0.11
25, 75	1.50	2.14	3.00	9.00	1.00

specificity of the measure also apply to controls, the same procedure results in $0.80 \times 100 + (1 - 0.8) \times 400 = 80 + 80 = 160$ smoker controls, and $500 - 160 = 340$ nonsmoker controls. The observed odds ratio of $(180 \times 340)/(160 \times 270) = 1.42$ is less than the true odds ratio of 2.0, indicating the typical effects of a nondifferential misclassification bias of exposure. See Elwood (1998) for more information on this process.

4. There would be $0.86 \times 150 + (1 - 0.79) \times 300 = 192$ smoking cases, and $450 - 192 = 258$ nonsmoking cases, and $0.86 \times 100 + (1 - 0.79) \times 400 = 170$ smoking controls, and $500 - 170 = 330$ nonsmoking controls, for an odds ratio of $(192 \times 330)/(170 \times 258) = 1.44$.

5. Table 11.2 summarizes a sensitivity analysis that uses the procedure described above with sensitivities and specificities that are either nondifferential or differential. The nondifferential bias results from sensitivities and specificities being the same for cases and controls and results in odds ratios that move toward 1.0. If the sensitivity and specificity of an exposure measure are different for cases and controls, the odds ratio is unpredictable. In some cases it is exaggerated (odds ratio of 12.0 if the measure works perfectly for controls but less than perfectly for cases) and in some cases it becomes protective (odds ratio of 0.50 if the measure works perfectly for cases but with a sensitivity and specificity of 50 percent for controls).

6. We have used the following equation from earlier questions where e_{obs} is the number of observed exposed cases (or controls), e_{true} is the number of truly exposed cases (or controls), and u_{true} is the number of truly unexposed cases (or controls).

$$e_{obs} = e_{true} \text{ (sensitivity)} + u_{true} \text{ (1 - specificity)}$$

Since we know that the total number of either cases or controls (N) is the sum of the truly exposed (e_{true}) plus the truly unexposed (u_{true}), we can use these two equations, rearrange terms, and solve for e_{true} in order to manipulate an observed 2 × 2 table that has been derived from a study that uses a measure of exposure that is imperfect (sensitivity and/or specificity is less than 100 percent). The following formula is the result, where N is the total number of either cases or controls.

$$e_{true} = [e_{obs} - (1 - \text{specificity}) \times N]/[\text{sensitivity} + \text{specificity} - 1]$$

7. With question 4 we had 192 smoking cases, 258 nonsmoking cases, 170 smoking controls, and 330 nonsmoking controls, with N = 450 cases and N = 500 controls. The number of truly exposed cases can be derived from the formula above, $e_{true} = [192 - (1 - 0.79) \times 450]/[0.86 + 0.79 - 1] = 150$ truly exposed cases, and $450 - 150 = 300$ truly unexposed cases. For the controls, we have, $e_{true} = [170 - (1 - 0.79) \times 500]/[0.86 + 0.79 - 1] = 100$ truly exposed controls, and $500 - 100 = 400$ truly unexposed controls. These are exactly the same numbers of exposed/unexposed cases and controls reported in Table 11.1 (as expected).

Recall bias is a common type of misclassification bias of exposure. This bias is associated with the method by which subjects are asked to report on past exposures, and the period of time between the actual exposure and the information-gathering process. Subjects are often asked to "remember" their history of exposure to risk factors. If subjects misrepresent their exposure history, either intentionally (because of fears, embarrassment, or social expectations) or unintentionally (because of forgetfulness), recall bias can occur.

The issue with each of the four biases is whether cases/controls or exposures are misclassified in the same way or to the same degree. Ultimately this depends on whether the tests, clinical exams, or other measures used to determine either disease or exposure status are (a) accurate in their ability to measure disease or exposure (sensitivity and specificity) and (b) applied in the same way to the two groups being evaluated (exposed and unexposed subjects, in the case of disease misclassification, and cases and controls in the case of exposure misclassification). Case Study 11.3 illustrates both selection and recall bias in a study involving the diet pills Fen-Phen.

Case Study 11.3. Fen-Phen and Primary Pulmonary Hypertension

The popular diet pills Fen-Phen were removed from the market after millions of prescriptions were written, based on several studies that indicated serious complications. One study examined whether appetite suppressants (mostly related to fenfluramine, i.e., Fen) are a risk factor in the development of primary pulmonary hypertension (PPH), a rare but often fatal disease (Abenhaim et al. 1996). The study used a case control design conducted in four European countries. The 95 cases were patients diagnosed with primary pulmonary hypertension between September 1992 and September 1994. Four control patients were randomly selected for each case with PPH, based on lists of patients seen by the same physician as the case, and of these, 355 actually participated in the study. Interviewers of each subject were blinded to the study objectives and asked questions relating to health status and various other exposures.

QUESTIONS

1. In the analysis, the authors controlled for systemic hypertension and body mass index ≥ 30. What would have to be true for these variables to be confounding variables, and how could this affect the analysis?
2. Explain some of the problems with this study design, particularly the issues of selection and misclassification bias.

3. Some have suggested that because there "was considerable publicity about the possible association between appetite-suppressant drugs with primary pulmonary hypertension, this publicity is likely to have increased the referral of patients treated with such drugs to study hospitals" (Manson and Faich 1996; Brenot et al. 1993; Atanassoff et al. 1992). What kind of bias would be introduced into the study if this were true?

4. Suppose women with PPH were more likely to accurately recall having taken the appetite suppressants used in this study than women without PPH who took these drugs. What would be the name and effect of this kind of bias?

ANSWERS

1. For each variable to be a confounding variable it would have to be a risk factor for PPH, as well as be associated with Fen-Phen use. If users of Fen-Phen tended to be more obese or hypertensive, and if either of these conditions were associated with an increased risk of PPH, the risk of developing PPH due to Fen-Phen use would be higher than it should be. Their analysis did not show either variable to be significant.

2. In a case control study, selection bias occurs if the cases and controls are not representative of the same population, or the population to which generalizations are made. One could argue that since both cases and controls were selected based on having seen the same physician in the study hospitals, selection bias is minimized. However, selection bias may occur if cases and controls seen by these physicians are not representative of those with and without disease in the community. The authors of the study also mentioned that selection bias could occur if patients with PPH who used anorexic drugs were more likely to have their disease recognized.

3. This would be a form of selection bias because the prevalence of the exposure in both cases and controls would be higher than (and not representative of) the populations from which they are drawn.

4. Such differential recall would represent a differential misclassification bias of exposure, because the measure used to assess exposure status (face-to-face interview) had a higher sensitivity for those with PPH than those without. This would tend to exaggerate the observed odds ratio.

Cross-Sectional Studies

Cross-sectional studies, or *prevalence surveys*, associate the presence or absence of disease in a population with potential risk factors such as age or gender (Lilienfeld and Stolley 1994). Such studies could be conducted based on data gathered from national surveys, such as the United States National Health Interview Survey (NHIS), and other surveys conducted by the National Center for Health Statistics. The findings of these surveys are routinely reported in the popular "rainbow series" booklets.

FIGURE 11.13
Cross–
Sectional
Study of
Ulcers and
Divorce

		Divorce	
	Ulcers	Yes	No
Exposure	Yes	100	50
	No	400	450

The main difference between cross-sectional studies and case control studies is that case control studies look back in time to determine exposure history. Presumably, exposure precedes the onset of disease, as assumed in the study design. With the cross-sectional study, typically based on survey information, one is attempting to estimate the prevalence of disease and to associate disease patterns with demographic, health behavior, and other information.

For example, the NHIS collects data on various acute and chronic conditions, such as ulcers, and on demographic data, including marital status. While it may be possible to associate ulcers with stressful events such as divorce and losing a spouse, it is impossible with cross-sectional studies to establish causality. Stomach problems may have preceded or followed the stressful event. The case control study is more robust than the cross-sectional study to the extent that causality can be demonstrated.

Suppose that you conduct a cross-sectional study using national survey data, and report the results in Figure 11.13.

It would be inappropriate to calculate the odds ratio $(100 \times 450)/(50 \times 400) = 2.25$, because one cannot infer causality from a cross-sectional study. That is, it is unclear whether ulcers were a causal factor in precipitating a divorce, or a divorce led to the development of ulcers. It would be appropriate to make two sets of comparisons, and test for statistically significant differences within each set. We could compare the proportion of divorced subjects who have ulcers to the proportion of non-divorced subjects who have ulcers $(100/500 = 0.2$ compared to $50/500 = 0.1)$, and compare the proportion of subjects with ulcers who are divorced to the proportion of subjects without ulcers who are divorced $(100/150 = 0.67$ compared to $400/850 = 0.47)$. In both cases, we could test for statistical significance using the test of proportions described in Chapter 10.

Case Control Advantages and Disadvantages

The case control study is an inexpensive, relatively efficient approach to measuring the effect of exposures, and it is particularly suited for rare diseases with long latency periods or exposures over a long period. For example, in a study of the effects of environmental tobacco smoke (passive smoking) on lung cancer in nonsmoking women (Fontham et al. 1994), the authors describe the process:

> In-person interviews followed by an extensive structured questionnaire were designed to obtain information on household, occupational, and other exposures to ETS [environmental tobacco smoke] during each study subject's lifetime, as well as other exposures associated with lung cancer. Exposure to ETS was examined by source during childhood...and during adult life.

> Lung cancer is a relatively rare disease (incidence of 56 per 100,000 population in 1994) with a long latency period. Exposure to environmental tobacco smoking was measured over the entire lifetime of the subjects. A cohort study would have to be much larger (because of the low incidence of disease) and more expensive, and it would take years to accomplish given the long-term latency of the disease.

Case control studies are not without disadvantages, however. The configuration of the control group, a critical element in this design, may become the Achilles' heel of study validity if it is not structured correctly. Moreover, a sufficient number of controls willing to participate in the study may be difficult to find. Furthermore, whether the exposure preceded the disease may be difficult to ascertain in many studies; that is, the extent to which causality can be inferred from the results may be limited. The classic example of the latter is whether inactivity leads to heart disease or whether heart disease results in an inactive lifestyle. In another example the authors state:

> Establishing the causality of the association between acetaminophen [Tylenol] use and ESRD [end-stage renal disease] is critical. The association was dose-dependent, specific...consistent with several previous reports, and biologically plausible.... Thus several criteria for causality were fulfilled. Nevertheless, the temporal precedence of the presumed cause still needs to be demonstrated. (Perneger, Whelton, and Klag 1994)

The case control study may be subject to a number of biases discussed earlier: selection, recall, and misclassification biases, for example. Many researchers recognize these as potential flaws and try to ascertain whether these biases are real and the degree to which these biases could have affected the results.

We also examined potential sources of misclassification of the exposure to anorexic agents. Patients with primary pulmonary hypertension might be more likely to remember using anorexic agents than controls (recall bias) (Abenhaim et al. 1996).

It could be that those women with breast cancer whom we were unable to interview because of serious illness or death may have been more likely to have had an induced abortion than the women we did interview (Daling et al. 1996).

It is possible that a woman diagnosed with a life-threatening disease such as breast cancer might report a history of induced abortion more completely than a healthy control woman contacted at random (Daling et al. 1996).

Other data suggest that lung cancer cases who are never smokers may be less inclined to misreport smoking status than others in the general population. (Fontham et al. 1994)

The case control study does not directly report the incidence of disease among those exposed and not exposed to a presumed risk factor, as the cohort study does. Thus, the odds ratio is only an estimate of relative risk, the validity of which depends on the incidence of disease in the population.

The validity of inferences drawn from case control studies depends on the purity of the study design. Flawed studies can be somewhat biased at best and seriously misleading at worst. Armenian and Shapiro (1998) have suggested asking eight questions to assess the integrity of any particular case control study with respect to the following issues:

1. clarity of problem definition;
2. consistency between the definition of cases and the problem;
3. selection of cases and controls from the same base population;
4. validity of the measurement of exposure;
5. case/control selection independent of exposure assessment;
6. alternative explanations, such as confounding;
7. factor interactions; and
8. value of the study for health services decision making.

Summary

Although the case control study is not the gold standard approach to determining causality in epidemiological research (that distinction belongs to the randomized clinical trial), it is an efficient, inexpensive approach to determining the extent of relationships between risk factors and outcomes. With this study design, a group of subjects with a particular outcome is compared—on the basis of exposure (in the past) to specific risk factors—to a group of subjects selected because of the absence of the outcome. The odds ratio, which is an estimate of relative risk, measures the number of times more likely a case is exposed to a risk factor compared to a control. Although these studies are inexpensive and particularly appropriate for rare outcomes with long latency periods and lengthy exposures, they may be flawed by various types of bias such as misclassification bias, which occur when subjects are incorrectly classified in terms of either outcome or exposure. Despite these shortcomings, the case control study remains a fundamental element of epidemiological research.

References

Abenhaim, L., Y. Moride, F. Brenot, S. Rich, J. Benichou, X. Kurz, T. Higenbottam, C. Oakley, E. Wouters, M. Aubier, G. Simonneau, and B. Begaud. 1996. "Appetite Suppressant Drugs and the Risk of Primary Pulmonary Hypertension. International Primary Pulmonary Hypertension Study Group." *New England Journal of Medicine* 335 (9): 609–16.

Armenian, H. K., and S. Shapiro. 1998. *Epidemiology and Health Services.* New York: Oxford University Press.

Atanassoff, P. G., B. M. Weiss, E. R. Schmid, and M. Tornic. 1992. "Pulmonary Hypertension and Dexfenfluramine." [Letter.] *Lancet* 339 (8790): 436.

Brenot, F., P. Herve, P. Petitpretz, F. Parent, P. Duroux, and G. Simonneau. 1993. "Primary Pulmonary Hypertension and Fenfluramine Use." *British Heart Journal* 70 (6): 537–41.

Chaouki, N., F. X. Bosch, N. Munoz, C. J. Meijer, B. El-Gueddari, A. El-Ghazi, J. Deacon, X. Castellsague, and J. M. Wallboomers. 1998. "The Viral Origin of Cervical Cancer in Rabat, Morocco." *International Journal of Cancer* 75 (4): 546–54.

Daling, J. R., L. A. Brinton, L. F. Voigt, N. S. Weiss, R. J. Coates, K. E. Malone, J. B. Schoenberg, and M. Gammon. 1996. "Risk of Breast Cancer Among White Women Following Induced Abortion." *American Journal of Epidemiology* 144 (4): 373–80.

Elwood, M. 1998. *Critical Appraisal of Epidemiological Studies and Clinical Trials*, 2nd ed. New York: Oxford University Press.

Eskenazi, B., L. Fenster, and S. Sidney. 1991. "A Multivariate Analysis of Risk Factors for Preeclampsia." *Journal of the American Medical Association* 266 (2): 237–41.

Feinstein, A. R., R. I. Horwitz, W. O. Spitzer, and R. N. Battista. 1981. "Coffee and Pancreatic Cancer: The Problems of Etiologic Science and Epidemiologic Case-Control Research." *Journal of the American Medical Association* 246 (9): 957–61.

Fontham, E. T., P. Correa, P. Reynolds, A. Wu-Williams, P. A. Buffler, R. S. Greenberg, V. W. Chen, T. Alterman, P. Boyd, D. F. Austin, and J. Liff. 1994. "Environmental Tobacco Smoke and Lung Cancer in Nonsmoking Women: A Multicenter Study." *Journal of the American Medical Association* 271 (22): 1752–59.

Grisso, J. A., J. L. Kelsey, B. L. Strom, G. Y. Chiu, G. Maislin, L. A. O'Brien, S. Hoffman, and F. Kaplan. 1991. "Risk Factors for Falls as a Cause of Hip Fracture in Women. Northeast Hip Fracture Study Group." *New England Journal of Medicine* 324 (19): 1326–31.

Grisso, J. A., J. L. Kelsey, B. L. Strom, L. A. O'Brien, G. Maislin, K. LaPann, L. Samelson, and S. Hoffman. 1994. "Risk Factors for Hip Fracture in Black Women. The Northeast Hip Fracture Study Group." *New England Journal of Medicine* 330 (22): 1555–59.

Kraus, A. S. 1954. "The Use of Hospital Data in Studying the Association Between a Characteristic and a Disease." *Public Health Report* 69 (December): 1211–14.

Kreuzer, M., L. Kreienbrock, M. Gerken, J. Heinrich, I. Bruske-Hohlfeld, K. Muller, and E. Wichmann. 1998. "Risk Factors for Lung Cancer in Young Adults." *American Journal of Epidemiology* 147 (11): 1028–37.

Lambe, M., C. Hsieh, D. Trichopoulos, A. Ekbom, M. Pavia, and H. O. Adami. 1994. "Transient Increase in the Risk of Breast Cancer After Giving Birth." *New England Journal of Medicine* 331 (1): 5–9.

Lesko, S. M., L. Rosenberg, and S. Shapiro. 1993. "A Case Control Study of Baldness in Relation to Myocardial Infarction in Men." *Journal of the American Medical Association* 269 (8): 998–1003; published erratum appears in *Journal of the American Medical Association* 269 (19): 2508.

Lilienfeld, D. E., and P. D. Stolley. 1994. *Foundations of Epidemiology*, 3rd ed. New York: Oxford University Press.

MacMahon, B., S. Yen, D. Trichopoulos, K. Warren, and G. Nardi. 1981. "Coffee and Cancer of the Pancreas." *New England Journal of Medicine* 304 (11): 630–33.

Manson, J. E., and G. A. Faich. 1996. "Pharmacotherapy for Obesity: Do the Benefits Outweigh the Risks?" *New England Journal of Medicine* 335 (9): 659–60.

Newcomb, P. A., B. E. Storer, M. P. Longnecker, R. Mittendorf, E. R. Greenberg, R. W. Clapp, K. P. Burke, W. C. Willett, and B. MacMahon. 1994. "Lactation and a Reduced Risk of Premenopausal Breast Cancer." *New England Journal of Medicine* 330 (2): 81–87.

Norell, S. E. 1995. *Workbook of Epidemiology*. New York: Oxford University Press.

Perneger, T. V., P. K. Whelton, and M. J. Klag. 1994. "Risk of Kidney Failure Associated with the Use of Acetaminophen, Aspirin, and Nonsteroidal Anti-Inflammatory Drugs." *New England Journal of Medicine* 331 (25): 1675–79.

Pershagen, G., G. Akerblom, O. Axelson, B. Clavensjo, L. Damber, G. Desai, A. Enflo, F. Lagarde, H. Mellander, M. Svartengren, and G. A. Swedjemark. 1994. "Residential Radon Exposure and Lung Cancer in Sweden." *New England Journal of Medicine* 330 (3): 159–64.

Rookus, M. A., and F. E. Van Leeuwen. 1996. "Induced Abortion and Risk for Breast Cancer: Reporting Recall Bias in a Dutch Base-Control Study." *Journal of the National Cancer Institute* 88 (23): 1759–64.

Russell, T. V., M. A. Crawford, and L. L. Woodby. 2004. "Measurements for Active Cigarette Smoke Exposure in Prevalence and Cessation Studies: Why Simply Asking Pregnant Women Isn't Enough." *Nicotine and Tobacco Research* 6 (Suppl. 2): S141–S151.

Slattery, M. L., and R. A. Kerber. 1993. "A Comprehensive Evaluation of Family History and Breast Cancer Risk. The Utah Population Database." *Journal of the American Medical Association* 270 (13): 1563–68.

Swanson, C. A., R. J. Coates, J. B. Schoenberg, K. E. Malone, M. D. Gammon, J. L. Stanford, I. J. Shorr, N. A. Potischman, and L. A. Brinton. 1996. "Body Size and Breast Cancer Risk Among Women Under Age 45 Years." *American Journal of Epidemiology* 143 (7): 698–706.

Thompson, W. D. 1994. "Statistical Analysis of Case-Control Studies." *Epidemiologic Reviews* 16 (1): 33–50.

Timmreck, T. C. 1998. *An Introduction to Epidemiology*, 2nd ed. Sudbury, MA: Jones and Bartlett.

World Health Organization. 1996. "Substance Abuse Alert." [Online information; not retrievable at time of publication.] http://www.who.ch/psa/toh/Alert/apr96/gifs/table3.gif.

12

COHORT STUDIES

John Lewis and Steven T. Fleming

> *"The beginning is the most important part of the work."* Plato, *The Republic*, Bk. 1, 377

Chapter 11 details the retrospective case control study. A different approach to epidemiologic research is the cohort study, which is usually conducted prospectively. A *cohort* is defined formally by *The American Heritage Dictionary* (1985, 289) as 1. One of the ten divisions of a Roman legion, consisting of 300 to 600 men. 2. A group or band united in a struggle. Epidemiologists use this word to identify a group of people who are identified at the beginning of a study and followed prospectively for a period to observe what happens to them. Variations on this theme are cohorts that acquire new members over time and cohorts that are identified retrospectively (Mantel 1973).

Cohort studies may be contrasted graphically to case-control studies by comparing Figures 12.1 and 12.2 to Figure 11.1 in Chapter 11. The cohort is observed to have exposed members and unexposed members. These groups may be referred to as the *exposed cohort* and the *unexposed cohort*.

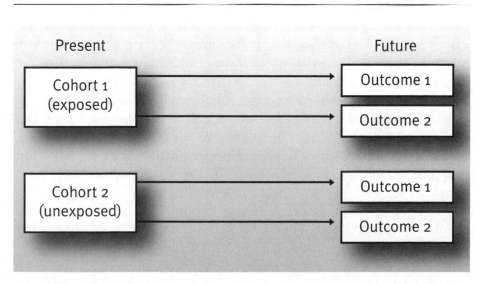

FIGURE 12.1
Schematic for Prospective Cohort Studies

FIGURE 12.2
Schematic for
Retrospective
Cohort
Studies

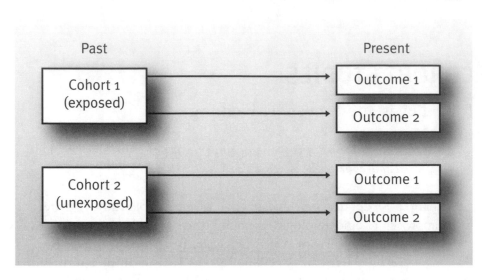

A classic example is the Framingham Study (Haider et al. 1999; Truett, Cornfield, and Kannel 1967). Framingham is a town to the west of Boston, at the starting point of the Boston Marathon. In the late 1940s, a large sample of the adult population of Framingham was recruited into the study. They received complete medical examinations that identified factors such as blood pressure, smoking, cholesterol, and other characteristics thought to be relevant to risk of cardiovascular disease. Over many years (the study is still going on) members of the cohort have been regularly examined. Comprehensive records of medical events and deaths have been meticulously collected. This large cohort study provided the definitive early findings on the relationship of cardiovascular risk factors to cardiovascular outcomes, including mortality and incidence of atherosclerotic disease, myocardial infarction, and stroke, among others. The Framingham Study has been able to change with time, adding new members of the cohort and producing answers to important new questions.

The less common retrospective cohort study is displayed graphically in Figure 12.2. Variations can be extended even further by designing a cohort study that looks from the present to both the past and the future. The arrows point from past to present because the study begins by identifying one or more cohort(s) in the past and then examines data in the present to see what has happened to members of the cohort(s).

A good example of a retrospective cohort study is a study of cancer in rubber workers (Delzell et al. 1981). This study was conducted entirely in the present. Past employment records were obtained from a rubber tire factory. These records provided worker identification information data on jobs/tasks that were relevant to exposure within the factory, and details on length of exposure and employment. These records were then linked to a statewide cancer registry and to death certificate records to measure specific outcomes, particularly cancer incidence and mortality. This study focused on cancer outcomes. The same cohort data could also have been used to examine other outcomes such as heart or lung disease. Some sort of reliable disease registry would have been required for that purpose. Of course, as in the Framingham Study, the individual workers could have been tracked down and their outcomes examined over time, but this approach would have been far more expensive in terms of time and resources.

To compare and contrast retrospective cohort studies with case control studies, consider how the relationship of rubber work to cancer could have been examined in a case control study (Table 12.1). The same cancer registry could have been used to select persons with incident cancer or death due to cancer. These could have been matched to controls (e.g., persons of the same age, gender, residence) who did not have cancer. The investigators could then obtain and examine data on which cases and controls had past exposure as employees in rubber factories.

The retrospective cohort study of rubber workers used available exposure data to subdivide the cohort based on duration of work in the rubber factory, job descriptions in making rubber tires, and the like. Other desirable data such as tobacco smoking history were not available. Approached as a case control study, such research could easily look at a variety of other past exposures as well (e.g., smoking, asbestos work, diet, alcohol consumption, genetic history, etc.), so long as those data were available.

Each study method has advantages and disadvantages. If the intention is to focus on a particular population or on people with particular exposures, the retrospective cohort design is preferable (the rubber workers study was

	Tasks	
Order of Tasks	Retrospective Cohort Study	Case Control Study
First	Identify past rubber workers	Identify cancer cases
Second	Determine past exposure history; identify controls (persons without cancer)	Identify cancer cases
Third	Determine cancer incidence	Determine past exposure history (rubber work, etc.)
Fourth	Analyze relationship of exposures to outcomes	Analyze relationship of exposures to outcomes

TABLE 12.1
Comparison of Retrospective Cohort Study and Case Control Study of Cancer in Rubber Workers

supported by the rubber industry and rubber workers union, and could have been expanded to look at outcomes for rubber workers other than cancer). If, on the other hand, the focus is on a particular disease, then case control design has advantages. For example, a case control cancer study could examine exposures of much wider scope than just the rubber industry.

Even when a cohort design might be a desirable choice, putting together the needed resources may be difficult and expensive. Prospective cohort studies usually require long-term commitment and are relatively expensive. In a retrospective cohort study, on the other hand, it may be difficult or impossible to obtain sufficiently comprehensive information from the past. Such studies need to be carefully designed and constructed based on the availability of complete retrospective cohort data (defining the cohort and its exposures), and the availability of appropriate outcomes data to which the cohort data can be linked. An important strength of the cohort design is the ability to directly measure relative and attributable risk.

Availability of good outcomes data (such as a cancer registry) can make case control design a good choice. This is especially true if an outcome being measured is not common (e.g., an uncommon cancer). In such situations, the case control design is highly efficient, since studying a relatively small number of cases and controls with appropriate exposure information can lead to important results not easily detected in cohort studies.

A difficulty inherent in case control studies is that controls must be chosen very carefully. An unexpected link may exist between the controls and the exposure being studied, which can bias the results and compromise the value of the study. An example is an unsuccessful study of the relationship of carbon dioxide exposure to myocardial infarction (heart attack) in the workplace (Lewis 1975). Cases—workers who had onset of myocardial infarction (from worker's compensation data)—were matched with controls—workers who had workman's compensation claims for skin conditions. It was assumed incorrectly that there was no link between the skin conditions and carbon monoxide in the workplace, the exposure being studied. The data showed that workers with skin conditions were more likely to be exposed to carbon monoxide than workers with myocardial infarction. The unexpected association that upset this study was that skin conditions in the workplace were frequently caused by oils and other environmental exposures in "dirty" industries, whereas myocardial infarctions were common among all workers, most of whom work in "clean" environments. The poor choice of controls made a sensitive analysis of a relationship between carbon monoxide and myocardial infarction impossible. A better choice of controls might have been workers randomly selected from all workplaces. Fortunately, this study was done quickly and at low cost, which are advantages of case control studies.

Just as the ability to directly measure relative and attributable risk is a strength of cohort studies, the need to estimate the same rates is a weakness of case control studies. There have been many examples in which a case control study has been a cost-effective way to gain preliminary support of a hypothesis, leading to a cohort study and/or intervention study performed at greater expense to provide more definitive evidence.

Selection of Cohorts

Cohort studies begin with the selection of a group or population that will be traced to particular outcomes at later times. Details are gathered about different exposures and/or risk categories of the cohort. When data on outcomes have been collected, the original cohort is usually divided in the analysis into different cohorts based on exposure or risk category. Examples of cohort selection are as follows:

1. "A private census of the population of Beaver Dam, Wisconsin, was performed from September 15, 1987 to May 4, 1998 to identify all residents in the city or township of Beaver Dam who were aged 43–84 years. Of the 5,927 eligible individuals, 4,926 participated in the baseline examination..." (Klein, Klein, and Moss 1998, 103).
2. "All boys with a Canadian Institute for Health Information entry code of NB (newborn) born to residents of Ontario in fiscal year 1993 were included. Two cohorts of male infants were identified—circumcised... and uncircumcised..." (To et al. 1998, 1814).
3. "In June 1976, questionnaires were sent to all married, female, registered nurses born between 1921 and 1946 and living in eleven U.S. states... Of the 172,413 who were sent this questionnaire, 120,557 completed information about whether they had used permanent hair dyes or smoked cigarettes..." (Hennekens et al. 1979, 1390).
4. "In 1975, at baseline, 7,925 healthy men and 7,977 healthy women of the Finnish Twin Cohort aged 25 to 64 years...responded to a questionnaire on physical activity habits and known predictors of mortality" (Kujala et al. 1998, 440).

As can be seen in these examples, characteristics of the cohort must be carefully defined. Usually the population from which the cohort is determined is larger than the cohort. In the Beaver Dam study, for example (Klein, Klein, and Moss 1998), the eligible population of 5,927 reduced to a cohort of 4,926. Nine hundred ninety-eight individuals were not included because some died prior to the baseline examination, some declined participation, and there were other exclusions carefully detailed in the text.

The eligible population in the hair dyes and cancer study (Hennekens et al. 1979) was the same as that in another study of coffee consumption and coronary heart disease (Willett et al. 1996). The cohort selection and size of the two studies are slightly different due to differences in completeness of data for the different exposure/risk categories.

Exposure

Exposure measures in case control studies and the relationship of "exposure" and "risk factor" are discussed in Chapter 11. We defined *exposure* as something that increased or decreased the probability of disease. Cohort studies frequently include fine detail in the definition and evaluation of exposures. Exposures may be external agents (infectious and otherwise), behaviors (both protective and malevolent), and other risk factors such as genetic predisposition.

It is also important to conceptualize the *active agent*, which is hypothesized to be the cause of disease, and the best construct of *dose*, which captures intensity, frequency, and duration (White, Hunt, and Casso 1998). Moreover, one should distinguish between past and present exposures, and deal with exposures that change over the course of the cohort study. If the literature suggests an "etiologically relevant time window" during which time exposure is most relevant, then it would be important to measure exposures only during this period; otherwise, exposure measurement error would occur (White, Hunt, and Casso 1998).

The etiology of cancer, for instance, is rather complicated and may include an initial exposure stage followed by a promotion stage during which the cancer progresses. In this case, there may be a particular window of time in which the initial exposure is causally related to disease. Consider the relationship between sun exposure and skin cancer, for instance. The active agent has been recast recently to include both ultra-violet (UV) A and UV B radiation. The dose could be conceptualized to include intensity (early morning, mid-day, or afternoon sun exposure), frequency (daily, weekends, or once a year), and duration (summer months versus year-round). We could assess current and past sun exposures, and determine if there is an etiologically relevant time window during which time sun exposure is causally related to skin cancer—early childhood, for instance.

To elaborate further the complexities of exposure definition and assessment, consider the following examples of exposure in cohort studies:

1. Hu and colleagues (1999) carefully measured levels of egg consumption and other factors such as presence of diabetes and other known risk factors for cardiovascular disease. They assessed the relationship of egg consumption to cardiovascular disease outcomes.
2. In the Framingham Study, chronic cough was found to be associated with risk of myocardial infarction (Haider et al. 1999).

3. Following the bombing of Hiroshima and Nagasaki, Japan, epidemiologists used careful measurements of radiation exposure to evaluate the relationship to long-term survival and cancer incidence (Schull 1995).
4. Studies of prostate cancer in cohorts of men have examined various characteristics of the men and lab tests performed prior to cancer incidence, in an effort to determine predictive factors for cancer outcomes (Gann, Hennekens, and Stampfer 1995; Johansson et al. 1997; Rodríguez et al. 1997).

Before the study by Hu and colleagues (1999) of the association of egg consumption (exposure) to cardiovascular disease incidence (outcome), there was a popular assumption that cholesterol in eggs increased the risk of cardiovascular disease (CD). Other cohort studies had demonstrated a strong association of elevated serum cholesterol with cardiovascular outcomes. The findings of Hu and colleagues were a surprise, as there was no association demonstrated in most persons between egg consumption and CD incidence. An exception was an association observed between egg consumption and CD incidence in persons with diabetes. This is a good example of how cohort studies can provide fresh insight.

Hu and colleagues (1999) also demonstrated how complex exposure information can be gathered and analyzed in cohort studies to produce precise results relating a specific exposure (eating eggs) to the outcome being studied (incidence of CD). This report was based on two prospective cohort studies, the Health Professionals Follow-up Study of men (1986–1994) and the Nurses Health Study of women (1980–1994) (Colditz, Manson, and Hankinson 1997). Comparable exposure data had been collected. These included details on more than 30 exposure types or risk factors known or suspected to be associated with CD incidence. Participants were asked how many eggs they had eaten in the past year, using nine options from never to six or more per day. In the analysis, they were divided into five levels of egg exposure. Questionnaires were completed by participants at the beginning and at regular intervals throughout the studies. If exposure for an individual was different in different questionnaires, the exposure levels were averaged on the the basis of length of time for each exposure.

Participants with diabetes were analyzed separately from others. The diabetic participants had a significantly elevated incidence of CD in the highest egg consumption category compared to the lowest, and there was a significant trend as well.

Other participants had no significant association between egg exposure and disease incidence. The analysis adjusted for more than ten variables known to affect or be associated with disease risk, including smoking history, hypertension, age, body mass index, menopausal status, and physical activity. As with egg exposure, many of the other exposures were measured using multiple possible levels. The ability to design a study with this extent of exhaustive exposure data is a major advantage of prospective cohort studies. Retrospective cohort studies and case control studies usually do not include exposure data in this detail, as those studies are typically designed after the exposures occurred.

The report by Haider and colleagues (1999) detailed a positive association between chronic cough and incidence rate of myocardial infarction. (The word *association* is appropriate to most epidemiologic studies. Conclusions about cause and effect, on the other hand, are rarely justified by the data and should be speculated upon only in the discussion section.)

Two possible ways that chronic cough can be considered an exposure in this study are:

1. the cough relates directly to heart disease, perhaps an early symptom of heart failure; and
2. the cough is an intervening variable. It is a pulmonary symptom of tobacco smoking, which is an important risk factor for myocardial infarction. If tobacco smoking history were not adequately measured in the study, then tobacco smoking would be a confounding factor (confounding is discussed in detail in Chapter 11).

A simpler example of confounding would be an association between yellow fingers and lung cancer. Cigarette smoking is the confounding factor, as it is closely associated with both yellow fingers and lung cancer.

Schull (1995) reported extensive studies of radiation exposure in the bombing of Hiroshima and of the outcomes of exposed residents over a long period. The persons in this cohort were the survivors of the nuclear explosion. The various radiation exposures and other factors such as the effects of fire were studied carefully. Much of this exposure information was not measured directly, but was estimated after the fact through modeling of the event using detailed knowledge of the radiation produced by an atomic bomb. Much of this knowledge was based on measurements made of other bombs long after the bombing of Hiroshima. Comparably detailed information was gathered on the lives, disease incidence, and deaths of the survivors, some of whom are still alive today. Cancer incidence was the outcome of greatest interest. In addition to information and estimates of radiation exposure of individual survivors, it was possible to analyze risk factors such as age, gender, and genetic differences. This prospective cohort study was, in fact, the combination of many studies in a variety of fields, including physics, clinical medicine, and epidemiology. The scope of this work was so great and took so long that an appropriate overview required a book published 40 years after the exposure occurred and the diverse studies began.

The prostate cancer cohort studies cited above (Gann, Hennekens, and Stampfer 1995; Johansson et al. 1997; Rodríguez et al. 1997) explored the important unknown areas of the usefulness of a screening test in predicting cancer outcomes, the role of family history as a risk factor, and other observations of exposure that cast new light on the management of this disease.

Gann, Hennekens, and Stampfer conducted a retrospective cohort study based on an ongoing randomized double-blind intervention study of aspirin and beta carotene (Steering Committee of the Physicians' Health Study Research Group 1989). Participants had provided a blood sample in 1982 that was frozen and saved. These samples had a prostate-specific antigen (PSA) test performed retrospectively, and occurrence of prostate cancer in the participants was examined retrospectively for a ten-year period beginning in 1982.

A nested case control design was used in the analysis. With this type of design one compares the exposure(s) of subjects who develop the disease (cases) to a sample of subjects who do not (controls). The case control study is nested into the cohort study in the sense that one can conduct a retrospective analysis once a sufficient number of cases of disease emerge out of the cohort study. The exposures of interest were the PSA levels and the duration of observation, ending in the diagnosis of prostate cancer. An elevated PSA could be considered a risk factor for prostate cancer or an indicator of pre-clinical cancer. Exposures were measured as a specific PSA level at the beginning of the cohort study and the length of exposure (duration of observation). The study concluded that "A single PSA measurement had a relatively high sensitivity and specificity for detection of prostate cancers that arose within 4 years" (Gann, Hennekens, and Stampfer 1995, 289).

Johansson and colleagues (1997) followed a group of men in a Swedish county diagnosed with prostate cancer between 1977 and 1984. Measurement of outcomes (deaths) was complete through 1994. Exposures were the presence at enrollment (diagnosis) of cancer of different stages, and the presence of either treatment or no treatment. The findings of greatest interest were that "Patients with localized prostate cancer have a favorable outlook following watchful waiting" (Johansson et al. 1997, 467) and that treatment of localized cancer with surgery, radiation, or hormonal therapy had no advantage over watchful waiting. As expected, cancers that were more advanced at diagnosis had worse outcomes.

There have been many cohort studies of the association of tobacco exposure with cancer incidence and other outcomes (Cornuz et al. 1999; Klein, Klein, and Moss 1998). Such studies emphasize the importance of defining exposure in great detail. This includes route of exposure and variation of tobacco products (smoking, chewing, cigarettes, cigars, mainstream smoke, sidestream smoke, "smokeless tobacco"), the variation of active substances that are not uniform (nicotine, tars, carbon monoxide, etc.), and dose (duration and amount of exposure).

The term *pack-years of exposure to cigarettes* has frequently been used as a dose indicator (years of exposure multiplied by packs smoked per day). This provides a cumulative dose, but it has also been shown that years of exposure and daily dose at any point in time may have independent effects on outcomes. The situation is further complicated by current thinking about carcinogens, in which some exposures may be necessary to initiate a long interval of cancer development, while other exposures may function independently as facilitators, so that their effects may appear quickly. As in the study of eggs by Hu and colleagues (1999), cohort studies, and particularly prospective cohort studies, provide the best methods to include exposure measurement in great detail.

Relative Risk in a Cohort Study

The cohort study design is illustrated in Figure 12.3, where the incidence of disease in the exposed cohort is $a/(a + b)$, and the incidence of disease in the unexposed cohort is $c/(c + d)$. Unlike the case control study (which uses the odds ratio as an estimate of relative risk), the incidence of disease in the exposed and unexposed groups can be calculated directly because there are

FIGURE 12.3
Cohort Study
Design

		Disease		
		Yes	No	
Cohort	Exposed	a	b	a + b
	Unexposed	c	d	c + d

FIGURE 12.4
Smoking and
Coronary
Heart Disease

		CHD		
		Yes	No	
Smokers	Yes	40	960	1,000
	No	50	1,950	2,000

Incidence (smokers): 40/1,000 = .04
Incidence (nonsmokers): 50/2,000 = .025
Relative risk: .04/.025 = 1.6

defined cohorts from the onset of the study. Thus, the relative risk is simply the ratio of the exposed and unexposed incidence: $(a/[a + b]) / (c/[c + d])$.

For example, suppose a prospective cohort study were designed to test the association of smoking to coronary heart disease (CHD). Of the 1,000 men who smoked, 40 developed coronary heart disease. Of the 2,000 nonsmoking (or unexposed) members, 50 developed CHD. Figure 12.4 summarizes the results including those with the relative risk of 1.6, indicating that smokers are 1.6 times as likely to develop CHD as nonsmokers.

Case Study 12.1 is a large cohort study that examines the relationship between dietary factors and cardiovascular disease.

Case Study 12.1. Scottish Heart Study

The Scottish Heart Health Study is a large cohort study that evaluated the relationship between dietary factors, cardiovascular disease incidence (or death), and mortality (Todd et al. 1999). In that study the relationship of dietary fiber to outcomes in men was displayed (Table 12.2). Todd and colleagues concluded that dietary "fiber will impact on both CHD risk and the general health of the population."

TABLE 12.2. RELATIONSHIP OF DIETARY FIBER TO CHD OUTCOMES

	Number	Fiber (g/4.18 MJ)
No event	5,076	8.8 (8.7, 8.9)[*]
CHD[**] case	454	8.4 (8.1, 8.6) $p = 0.002$[***]
No-CHD death	224	7.7 (7.3, 8.0) $p < 0.001$

NOTES: * numbers in parenthesis, 95% confidence interval; ** CHD, coronary heart disease; *** p values are presented for comparisons of mean values with that of the no-event group.

SOURCE: Todd et al. (1999). Used with permission of Oxford University Press.

QUESTIONS

1. Does dietary fiber appear to be more protective against CHD risk or against non-CHD death?
2. The authors do not detail the causes of "non-CHD death." Speculate about what those causes could be and what they might have to do with dietary fiber.
3. If the 95 percent confidence interval for "CHD case" was (8.1, 9.0) instead of (8.1, 8.6), how would it affect the conclusions?

ANSWERS

1. Those who had CHD had a lower fiber intake than those who had no event (compare 8.4 to 8.8), meaning the fiber intake level is protective against the risk of CHD. Those who died from a cause other than CHD had a lower fiber intake than those with no event (compare 7.7 to 8.8). It would appear that fiber level is also protective against non-CHD death.
2. Non-CHD deaths could be caused by cancer or cerebrovascular disease. Fiber level may be protective for mortality from these causes.
3. The confidence interval would span the fiber intake for no event, meaning that the fiber intake level of CHD cases was not statistically significantly different from the fiber intake level of those without an event.

Attributable Fraction

As described in the previous chapter, *attributable fraction* (AF) is the proportion of disease that is attributed to a particular risk factor. In case-control studies the odds ratio is used to estimate the attributable fraction because risk (the rate of an outcome) is not measured directly in a known population. In a cohort study the risk in a known population (the cohort) is measured directly. Furthermore, the cohort may be an entire population or a random sample of a larger population. For a cohort study the attributable fraction formula is the same as for the case control study except that relative risk (RR) is used instead of the odds ratio. In this case p is the proportion of the population with the risk factor and RR is the relative risk.

$$AF = \frac{p\,(RR-1) \times 100\%}{p\,(RR-1) + 1}$$

The attributable fraction for the CHD and smoking example above can be calculated as follows if one assumes that 25 percent of the population smokes:

$$\frac{0.25\,(1.6-1) \times 100}{0.25\,(1.6-1) + 1} = 13\%$$

The attributable fraction points out one of the strengths of a cohort study. If the cohorts are representative of the general population, then the incidence of disease in the exposed and unexposed groups is also representative. The CHD and smoking study would enable us to conclude that 13 percent of all heart disease is attributable to smoking. This is a critical conclusion in planning how best to expend resources to prevent heart disease.

Another value of attributable fraction concerns exposures that are highly associated with bad outcomes (high relative risk) but are themselves uncommon or rare. For example, vinyl chloride exposure as a risk factor for cancer has a high relative risk. In fact, its relative risk is even greater than that of tobacco smoking. But very few people in the general population are exposed to vinyl chloride. So the attributable fraction of cancer risk associated with vinyl chloride is very low. Eliminating vinyl chloride exposure would likely have a very small impact on cancer outcomes in the general population. Eliminating tobacco exposure, by contrast, would likely have a very large impact.

The attributable risk is a measure of the potential savings that would occur if the risk factor were eliminated in a population, and is calculated as the difference between the incidence of disease in the exposed group minus the incidence of disease in the unexposed group. Referring to Figure 12.3, the attributable risk would be calculated as follows:

$$\text{Attributable risk} = a/(a + b) - c/(c + d)$$

In the case of the preceding smoking and CHD example, this would be 0.04 – 0.025 or 0.015. This means that more than a third—15 out of 40—of CHD cases among smokers are caused by smoking. If no one in that population smoked, CHD cases would be 25 per thousand. In this population, where 25 percent smoke, it is 29 cases per thousand. Thus, smoking causes four extra CHD cases per thousand, or 13.8 percent of the total (note that this is essentially the attributable fraction, as calculated above).

Case Study 12.2 presents the results of an "unknown cohort study" with a high mortality rate.

Case Study 12.2. The "Unknown Cohort Study"

The following table (Table 12.3) displays data from an unknown cohort study with a high mortality rate. All of the subjects experienced life-threatening exposures, although risk varied by class, employment, age, and gender.

TABLE 12.3. DATA FOR AN UNKNOWN COHORT STUDY WITH A HIGH MORTALITY RATE

	Male			Female			Total		
	No. in Group	No. Died	Mortality	No. in Group	No. Died	Mortality	No. in Group	No. Died	Mortality
Upper class									
Adult	175	118	67%	144	4	3%	319	122	38%
Child	5	0	0%	1	0	0%	6	0	0%
Middle class									
Adult	168	154	92%	93	13	14%	261	167	64%
Child	11	0	0%	13	0	0%	24	0	0%
Lower class									
Adult	462	387	84%	165	89	54%	627	476	76%
Child	48	35	73%	31	17	55%	79	52	66%

(Continued)

(Continued from previous page)

	Male			Female			Total		
	No. in Group	No. Died	Mortality	No. in Group	No. Died	Mortality	No. in Group	No. Died	Mortality
Employees									
Class									
Adult	862	670	78%	23	3	13%	885	673	76%
Child	0	0		0	0		0	0	

SOURCE: Great Britain, Parliament (1999).

QUESTIONS

1. What was the size of the cohort, the number with a bad outcome, and the mortality rate?
2. Was it more protective to be upper class or to be female?
3. What is the relative risk of adult men compared to adult women? Compared to upper-class adult females, what was the relative risk for lower-class adult males?
4. Though it is unnamed in Table 12.3, you are probably familiar with this event. Draw conclusions about its characteristics. Can you guess what actually happened?

ANSWERS

1. There were 2,201 in the cohort: 325 (upper class) + 285 (middle class) + 706 (lower class) + 885 (employees). There were 1,490 deaths in this cohort: 122 (upper class) + 167 (middle class) + 528 (lower class) + 673 (employees). The overall mortality rate would be (1,490/2,201) × 100 = 68 per 100, or 68%.
2. The upper-class mortality rate was 38 percent. The female mortality rate (adults and children), 126 deaths out of 470 females, was (126/470) × 100 = 26.8%. Females had a lower mortality rate, so it was more protective to be a female than an upper-class member.
3. The mortality rates of adult men and women were 79.7 percent and 25.6 percent, respectively. The relative risk of being an adult male compared to an adult female was 79.7/25.6 = 3.1. Adult males were 3.1 times as likely to die as adult females. The mortality rate for upper-class adult females was 3 percent and for lower-class adult males was 84 percent. The relative risk of dying 84%/3% = 28. Thus, lower-class adult males were 28 times as likely to die as upper-class adult females. The attributable risk of 84% − 3% = 81%. Therefore, a mortality rate of 81 percent can be attributed to being a lower-class adult male rather than an upper-class adult female.
4. These results summarize the Titanic disaster. Preference was given to women and children over men, although lower-class passengers (men and women) had high mortality rates.

Measuring Incidence

The simplest way of calculating an incidence rate is to divide the number of subjects who develop a disease by the number of subjects in the cohort. Thus, 40 smokers out of a cohort of 1,000 developed CHD in the preceding example, for an incidence rate of 40 per 1,000 or 0.04. A related but somewhat more complicated method of calculating incidence is with incidence density. Most prospective cohort studies span multiple years, during which time the cohorts change in size as subjects enter or drop out of the study. Subjects may become disengaged from the research due to death, disinterest, side effects, or many other reasons that are collectively referred to as *loss to follow-up*. One solution to this problem is to calculate incidence in terms of density, such as person-years or person-months of exposure.

Consider the following hypothetical case as illustrated in figures 12.5 and 12.6: a five-year study with five subjects in each group. Notice that of the five exposed subjects (Figure 12.5), three develop the condition, say coronary heart disease. Subject 1 finishes the study; subject 2 dies (D) after two years; subject 3 gets the disease after two years (X); subject 4 gets CHD and dies in year 3 (XD); subject 5 gets CHD in year 1 and dies in year 4. Of the unexposed subjects (Figure 12.6), subject 1 finishes the study, while subject 2 is lost to follow-up in year 4. Subjects 3 and 5 get CHD in year 4 but only one dies at the end of the study. Subject 4 gets CHD and dies in year 3.

The cumulative incidence over five years would be 3/5 = 60% for each group. Incidence density, on the other hand, takes into consideration both loss to follow-up and disease onset. In other words, the "at-risk" period would end if the subject drops out of the study, develops the disease, or dies. Thus, there are 13 person-years of exposure for the exposed group

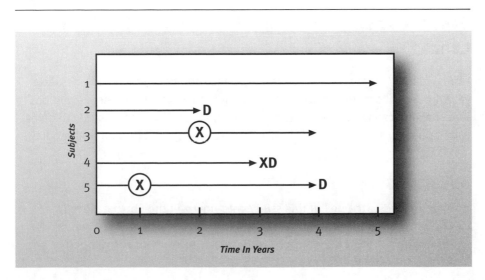

FIGURE 12.5
Cumulative Incidence vs. Incidence Density— Exposed

FIGURE 12.6
Cumulative
Incidence vs.
Incidence
Density—
Unexposed

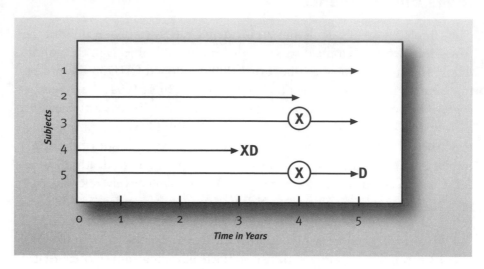

and 20 person-years of exposure for the unexposed group. The incidence density for the exposed group would be 3/13, or 3 cases of CHD for every 13 person-years of exposure. For the unexposed group, the incidence density would be 3/20, or 3 cases of CHD for every 20 person-years of exposore. Relative risk with cumulative incidence would be $\frac{3}{5} \div \frac{3}{5} = 1.0$, indicating no increased risk of CHD with exposure. With incidence density, the relative risk would be $\frac{3}{13} \div \frac{3}{20} = 1.54$, indicating that one is 1.54 times as likely to develop CHD with an exposure.

Case Study 12.3 challenges you to design a study that links smoking to heart disease and lung cancer.

Case Study 12.3. Smoking, Heart Disease, and Lung Cancer

You have been motivated by the recent tobacco company settlements to design yet another cohort study that will test the hypothesis that both active and passive smoking cause heart disease and lung cancer. You want this study to be as valid as possible, and to be practically flawless in terms of bias and confounding.

QUESTIONS

1. What are the outcomes of this study, and how will they be measured?
2. How will you minimize misclassification bias of disease (see Chapter 11)?
3. What would be the advantages and disadvantages of retrospective and prospective study designs?

4. You would like to confirm a dose-response relationship. How will you conceptualize the "active agent" and measure dose in terms of intensity, frequency, and duration?
5. Does the concept of dose differ for active versus passive smoking?
6. What are the confounding variables that you need to measure?
7. What are the sources of misclassification bias of exposure?
8. How will you minimize selection bias?
9. How will you deal with dropouts?

Assume that you design a prospective cohort study to test the effect of active smoking only on lung cancer. You have assembled two groups of middle-aged adults—2,000 smokers and 2,000 nonsmokers. You follow them for ten years, and then divide your exposed subjects into three categories. You measure lung cancer by positive biopsy. The cumulative ten-year incidence of CHD for the various cohorts is given below (Table 12.4). Exposure is defined as average packs per day over the period of observation, while person-years of exposure is accumulated during the ten-year observation period.

TABLE 12.4. ACTIVE SMOKING AND LUNG CANCER

Exposure	No. Subjects	Incidence	Person-Years
Nonsmoker	2,000	50	18,000
<1 pack/day	1,000	70	7,000
1–2 packs/day	500	80	6,000
>2 packs/day	500	100	3,000

10. What is the relative risk of CHD for various levels of smoking using cumulative incidence and incidence density?
11. How might we use pack-years of exposure as an alternative to this approach?
12. Is there a dose-response relationship?
13. What is the attributable fraction if approximately 30 percent of the population smokes?

ANSWERS

1. The two outcomes in the study would be heart disease and lung cancer. Histologically confirmed lung cancer could be measured by biopsy. Heart disease is a bit more problematic. There are a number of tests for heart disease with different levels of specificity and sensitivity, for example, treadmill test and angiogram.

2. Misclassification bias of disease would be minimized by employing a diagnostic test with both high sensitivity and high specificity, for example, a coronary angiogram.

3. The prospective cohort design has the advantage of being able to ensure that exposure preceded outcome. Subjects could be tested at the onset of the study to ensure that they were disease free. The design also has the advantage of being able to follow subjects over time to collect measures of outcome and determine if there are any changes to exposure status, such as whether subjects changed their level of smoking. The disadvantages would include expense and long follow-up. The retrospective design has the advantage of much lower expense and time of completion, with the disadvantage of not knowing for sure that smoking preceded the onset of disease, and not being able to collect measures of outcome over time.

4. It is difficult to specifically measure the active agent with smoking since tobacco smoke contains hundreds of carcinogens. Dose is typically measured in pack-years of exposure for active smoking. You could measure both past exposure (pack-years) as well as current exposure (packs/day) and stratify your analyses by some categorization of these two variables.

5. The concept of dose would be different for active and passive smoking. Dose for active smoking has been described in the previous question. For passive smoking, one could measure dose in months/years of exposure in a passive smoking environment.

6. Confounding variables would include any variable that is associated with both smoking and either heart disease or lung cancer. Such variables could include measures of stress, obesity, and alcohol use.

7. Sources of misclassification bias of exposure would include factors that make classification of smoking status inaccurate. For example, if subjects are reluctant to admit smoking status because it is socially undesirable, they may be incorrectly classified as nonsmokers.

8. Selection bias could be minimized by selecting exposed and unexposed subjects from the same source population, for example, residents of Kentucky, by maintaining good follow-up of subjects, and by minimizing dropouts.

9. Dropouts are difficult to deal with in any study. One approach is to collect descriptive information on those who drop out of the study, and compare such information to those who remain in the study, particular for exposure variables and confounders. By comparing dropouts to those whose remain in the study, we can either anticipate any bias or remain confident that our results are valid.

10. Table 12.5 summarizes these calculations. For example, the incidence of smoking among nonsmokers is $(50/2,000) \times 1,000 = 25$ per 1,000 subjects, or $(50/18,000) \times 1,000 = 2.8$ per 1,000 person-years. Those with <1 packs/day years of exposure have an incidence rate of $(70/1,000) \times 1,000 = 70$ per 1,000 subjects, and $(70/7,000) \times 1,000 = 10.0$ per 1,000 person- years. The relative risk using incidence rates and incidence density would be $70/25 = 2.8$ and $10/2.8 = 3.6$, respectively. Note that the nonsmokers are the control group in these calculations.

TABLE 12.5. ACTIVE SMOKING AND CORONARY HEART DISEASE

Exposure	No. Subjects	Incidence	Person-Years	Incidence Rate (per 1,000 subjects)	Incidence Density (per 1,000 yrs)	Relative Risk (per 1,000 subjects)	Relative Risk (per 1,000 yrs)
Nonsmoker	2,000	50	18,000	25	2.8	—	—
<1 pack/day	1,000	70	7,000	70	10.0	2.8	3.6
1–2 packs/day	500	80	6,000	160	13.3	6.4	4.8
>2 packs/day	500	100	3,000	200	33.3	8.0	11.9

11. Subjects could be classified on the basis of "pack-years of exposure." Such a classification would be preferable to either incidence rates or incidence density in that it allows for changes in exposure over time.

12. There is a dose-response relationship with both approaches. For example, the risk of CHD for smokers compared to nonsmokers increases from 3.6 to 11.9 as the "dose" of smoking increases.

13. The incidence density for smokers would be $(70 + 80 + 100)/(7,000 + 6,000 + 3,000) \times 1,000 = 15.6/1,000$ person-years. The incidence density for nonsmokers would be $50/18,000 \times 1,000 = 2.8/1,000$ person years. The relative risk would be $15.6/2.8 = 5.57$. If 30 percent of the population are smokers, then the attributable fraction would be $[0.30(5.57 - 1)/0.30(5.57 - 1) + 1] \times 100 = 57.8\%$. The interpretation would be that 57.8 percent of CHD in the population can be attributed to smoking.

Case Control and Cohort Studies

In the previous chapter we described how case control studies typically involve the comparison of those with a particular outcome, such as disease (cases), to those without such an outcome (controls) in terms of past exposures. Morabia (1997) describes how subjects in a case control study are ultimately derived from a perhaps much larger "target" population. Such a population consists of four groups, the groups we find in a typical 2 × 2 table: (1) exposed cases, (2) exposed controls, (3) unexposed cases, and (4) non-exposed controls.

When one conducts a case control study using hospitalized cases and controls, for example, these patients ultimately come from the hospital service area, and fall into one of the four categories mentioned above. We can view each of these four categories of subjects, therefore, as being "samples" from larger population groups.

FIGURE 12.7
Relation of
Case Control
and Cohort
Study

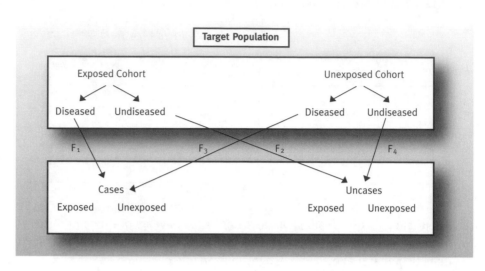

Figure 12.7 illustrates these concepts. The four fractions F_1, F_2, F_3, and F_4 represent the size of the sample from the larger target population. For example, suppose that a statewide cancer registry, such as the Kentucky Cancer Registry, were used to obtain all incident lung cancer cases in Kentucky during 2007. The sample fractions F_1 and F_3 would presumably be 1.00, or 100 percent. If 4,000 controls selected from registered voters in Kentucky represented 1,200 out of 1.2 million smokers and 2,800 out of 2.8 million nonsmokers in the state of Kentucky, then the sampling fractions F_2 and F_4 would be 0.001, or 0.1 percent each.

Morabia (1997) describes how to convert an odds ratio from a case control study to an odds ratio of a cohort study using the following formula. Thus, if the sampling fractions are the same for cases and controls, the odds ratios are also the same. If they differ, such differences represent a form of selection bias.

$$OR_{cohort} = OR_{case\ control}\ [F_2 \times F_3]/[F_1 \times F_4]$$

Case Study 12.4 illustrates how sampling fractions can be used in this way with a study of smoking and prostate cancer.

Case Study 12.4. Smoking and Prostate Cancer

Suppose you conduct a hospital-based case control study to determine if smoking is a risk factor for prostate cancer. You assemble a group of 100 prostate cancer cases from 2004 and 2005 from the University of Kentucky Medical Center and use 500 controls with a diagnosis other than prostate cancer from those same years. You use a survey instrument to measure smoking status. Figure 12.8 summarizes the results.

FIGURE 12.8. SMOKING AND PROSTATE CANCER

		Prostate cancer	
		Yes	No
Smoking status	Yes	60	250
	No	40	250

QUESTIONS

1. What is the odds ratio for the risk of prostate cancer with smoking?
2. You could design a cohort study in the state of Kentucky instead. Suppose that the Kentucky Cancer Registry (a population-based cancer registry) reports 4,000 cases of prostate cancer during 2004 and 2005, 1,200 of whom were smokers. You would like to generalize your results to the target population of males in Kentucky, aged 18 and above, which you estimate to be 1,504,000, of whom 30 percent (451,200) are smokers. What are the sampling fractions for exposed and unexposed cases?
3. What are the sampling fractions for exposed and unexposed controls?
4. Does the hospital-based sample include proportionately more or less exposed subjects than the general population?
5. If we were to conduct a cohort study using the population of males, 18 and above, in the state of Kentucky, what should the odds ratio be?
6. Interpret these results.

ANSWERS

1. The odds ratio would be $(60 \times 250)/(250 \times 40) = 1.5$.

2. The sampling fraction of exposed cases (F_1) would be $[60/(1{,}200)] = 0.05$. The sampling fraction of unexposed cases (F_3) would be $[40/(4{,}000 - 1{,}200)] = 0.0143$.

3. The sampling fraction of exposed controls (F_2) would be $250/451{,}200 = 0.00055$. The sampling fraction of unexposed controls (F_4) would be $[250/(1{,}504{,}000 - 451{,}200)] = 0.00024$.

4. The hospital-based sample contains 52 percent smokers, and the general population contains 30 percent smokers.

5. We can use the sampling fractions to estimate the odds ratio from this cohort study as follows: $OR_{cohort} = OR_{case\ control} [F_2 \times F_3]/[F_1 \times F_4] = 1.5 \times (0.00055 \times 0.0143)/(0.05 \times 0.00024) = 0.975$.

6. The case control study showed that smokers had a 1.5 increased odds of developing prostate cancer. However, the substantial selection bias favoring smokers, particularly among prostate cancer patients, overestimated the risk of cancer among smokers as evidenced by the odds ratio estimate for a population-based cohort study. Were we to calculate a confidence interval around the OR_{cohort} estimate of 0.975, we would probably find the estimate not statistically significantly different from 1.0.

Survey Methodology

Surveys are used to sample populations in a variety of ways. These include opinion polls, marketing surveys, and the U.S. Census (intended, so far, to be a 100 percent sample). Surveys may be used for epidemiologic purposes, one of which is to support cohort studies.

Selection of a cohort through use of a questionnaire is a *specialized survey*. Members of a population or of a sample of a population may be sent a questionnaire asking them to submit information in support of a study. In the Finnish Twin Cohort study, participants were members of the Twin Cohort who responded to a mailed questionnaire "that included items on physical activity, occupation, body weight, height, alcohol use, smoking, and physician-diagnosed diseases" (Kujala et al. 1998, 440). In a study of smoking and risk of hip fracture, women were mailed a questionnaire biennially over a period of up to 12 years (Cornuz et al. 1999). When survey methodology is used in this way, either as a 100 percent sample or as a smaller random sample of a cohort, it is critical that there be a high response rate. Failure to collect data for nonresponders may bias the results of the study.

Another use of surveys is the regular assessment of the health and risk factor status of a population by interviewing a random sample of the population. The Centers for Disease Control and Prevention works with each state to conduct a regular survey of the state's population through the Behavioral Risk Factor Surveillance System Coordinators (1998). This is a random-digit-dialing survey of all adults in the United States who have telephones, sampled by state. Information is obtained about a variety of indicators of health status, risk factors such as smoking, and preventive behavior such as immunizations. Annually or biennially the survey is repeated using a new random sample of the state. It provides useful data for public health management on progress within states and comparisons between states.

Advantages and Disadvantages

The cohort study has a number of advantages over the case-control study. While the case control design "inherently acknowledges time," the cohort study "explicitly incorporates the passage of time" (Samet and Muñoz 1998, 1). Moreover, one can calculate incidence and relative risk directly rather than by estimate. Determining causality is less of an issue in a cohort study since exposures precede the onset of disease by virtue of the study design. Misclassification bias, particularly recall bias, is less of a problem since exposures are systematically and regularly documented during follow-up activities. Finally, the cohort design can be used to study multiple outcomes, such as diseases, or multiple exposures, as long as these variables are measured.

On the other hand, the cohort study is expensive, time consuming, and potentially biased by attrition, as subjects are lost to follow-up. Moreover, it may be difficult to model changes in exposure(s) over time or crossovers (subjects who give up smoking, for instance). With the cohort study, it is nearly impossible to study rare diseases.

Summary

Cohort studies begin with a defined population (cohort), measure baseline information about exposures (personal characteristics, health status, behavior, and risk factors), may measure interim modifications of these exposures, and measure outcomes of interest (morbidity and mortality).

Although typically the cohort is followed prospectively, the cohort may be defined and the exposures measured retrospectively, with outcomes measured in the present. Retrospective cohort studies are different from case control studies. In the former, the study begins with measurement of exposures and traces the cohort forward in time until outcomes occur. In the latter, the study begins by choosing cases on the basis of outcomes, and controls with different outcomes, and traces backward in time to measure past exposures of the cases and controls. The prospective cohort study is usually the most elegant study and allows extremely detailed and exact measurement of exposures, but it is usually expensive in terms of resources and time required. Case control studies and retrospective cohort studies may provide a more efficient, less expensive way to obtain tentative conclusions.

Both case control studies and all forms of cohort studies can show an association between exposure and disease, but they do not establish a causal relationship. To determine a causal relationship between exposure and disease, one must use an experimental study design such as a randomized clinical trial, which is the topic of Chapter 13.

References

The American Heritage Dictionary, 2nd College Edition. 1985. Boston: Houghton Mifflin.

Behavioral Risk Factor Surveillance System Coordinators. 1998. "Influenza and Pneumococcal Vaccination Levels Among Adults Aged >65 Years—United States, 1997." *Morbidity and Mortality Weekly Reports* 47: 797–802.

Colditz, G. A, J. E. Manson, and S. E. Hankinson. 1997. "The Nurses' Health Study: 20-Year Contribution to the Understanding of Health Among Women." *Journal of Womens Health* 6: 49–62.

Cornuz, J., D. Feskanich, W. C. Willett, and G. A. Colditz. 1999. "Smoking, Smoking Cessation, and the Risk of Hip Fracture in Women." *American Journal of Medicine* 106: 311–14.

Delzell, E., C. Louik, J. N. Lewis, and R. R. Monson. 1981. "Mortality and Cancer Morbidity Among Workers in the Rubber Tire Industry." *American Journal of Industrial Medicine* 2: 209–16.

Gann, P. H., C. H. Hennekens, and M. J. Stampfer. 1995. "A Prospective Evaluation of Plasma Prostate-Specific Antigen for Detection of Prostatic Cancer." *Journal of the American Medical Association* 273 (4): 289–94.

Great Britain Parliament. 1998. *Report on the Loss of the S.S. Titanic*. New York: St. Martin's.

Haider, A. W., M. G. Larson, C. J. O'Donnell, J. C. Evans, P. W. F. Wilson, and D. Levy. 1999. "The Association of Chronic Cough with the Risk of Myocardial Infarction: The Framingham Heart Study." *American Journal of Medicine* 106: 279–84.

Hennekens, C. H., F. E. Speizer, B. Rosner, C. J. Bain, C. Belanger, and R. Peto. 1979. "Use of Permanent Hair Dyes and Cancer Among Registered Nurses." *Lancet* 1 (8131): 1390–93.

Hu, F. B., M. J. Stampfer, E. B. Rimm, J. E. Manson, A. Ascherio, G. A. Colditz, B. A. Rosner, D. Spiegelman, F. E. Speizer, F. M. Sacks, C. H. Hennekens, and W. C. Willett. 1999. "A Prospective Study of Egg Consumption and Risk of Cardiovascular Disease in Men and Women." *Journal of the American Medical Association* 281 (15): 1387–94.

Johansson, J.-E., L. Holmberg, S. Johansson, R. Bergström, and H.-O.

Adami. 1997. "Fifteen-Year Survival in Prostate Cancer. A Prospective, Population-Based Study in Sweden." *Journal of the American Medical Association* 277 (6): 467–71.

Klein, R., B. E. K. Klein, and S. E. Moss. 1998. "Relation of Smoking to the Incidence of Age-Related Maculopathy, the Beaver Dam Eye Study." *American Journal of Epidemiology* 147 (2): 103–10.

Kujala, U. M., J. Kaprio, S. Sarna, and M. Koskenvuo. 1998. "Relationship of Leisure-Time Physical Activity and Mortality." *Journal of the American Medical Association* 279 (6): 440–44.

Lewis, J. N. 1975. Unpublished study of Massachusetts workplaces.

Mantel, N. 1973. "Synthetic Retrospective Studies and Related Topics." *Biometrics* 29: 479–86.

Morabia, A. 1997. "Case-Control Studies in Clinical Research: Mechanism and Prevention of Selection Bias." *Preventive Medicine* 26 (5, Pt. 1): 674–77.

Rodríguez, C., E. E. Calle, H. L. Miracle-McMahill, L. M. Tatham, P. A. Wingo, M. J. Thun, and C. W. Heath, Jr. 1997. "Family History and Risk of Fatal Prostate Cancer." *Epidemiology* 8 (6): 653–57.

Samet, J. M., and A. Muñoz. 1998. "Evolution of the Cohort Study." *Epidemiologic Reviews* 20 (1): 1–14.

Schull, W. J. 1995. *Effects of Atomic Radiation: A Half-Century of Studies from Hiroshima and Nagasaki.* New York: Wiley-Liss.

Steering Committee of the Physicians' Health Study Research Group. 1989. "Final Report on the Aspirin Component of the Ongoing Physicians' Health Study." *New England Journal of Medicine* 321: 29–35.

To, T., M. Agha, P. T. Dick, and W. Feldman. 1998. "Cohort Study on Circumcision of Newborn Boys and Subsequent Risk of Urinary-Tract Infection." *Lancet* 352: 1813–16.

Todd, S., M. Woodward, H. Tunstall-Pedoe, and C. Bolton-Smith. 1999. "Dietary Antioxidant Vitamins and Fiber in the Etiology of Cardiovascular Disease and All-Causes Mortality: Results from the Scottish Heart Health Study." *American Journal of Epidemiology* 150 (10): 1073–80.

Truett, J., J. Cornfield, and W. Kannel. 1967. "A Multivariate Analysis of the Risk of Coronary Heart Disease in Framingham." *Journal of Chronic Diseases* 20: 511–24.

White, E., J. R. Hunt, and D. Casso. 1998. "Exposure Measurement in Cohort Studies: The Challenges of Prospective Data Collection." *Epidemiologic Reviews* 20 (1): 43–56.

Willett, W. C., M. J. Stampfer, J. E. Manson, G. A. Colditz, B. A. Rosner, F. E. Speizer, and C. H. Hennekens. 1996. "Coffee Consumption and Coronary Heart Disease in Women." *Journal of the American Medical Association* 275: 458–62.

13

RANDOMIZED CLINICAL TRIALS

Steven T. Fleming

> " 'Please test your servants for ten days, and let us be given some vegetables to eat and water to drink. Then let our appearance be observed in your presence and the appearance of the youths who are eating the king's choice food; and deal with your servants according to what you see.' So he listened to them in this matter and tested them for ten days. At the end of ten days their appearance seemed better and they were fatter than all the youths who had been eating the king's choice food." Daniel 1:12–15, New American Standard Bible

The gold standard of epidemiological research is the *randomized clinical trial* (RCT), also referred to as the *randomized controlled trial.* The RCT is a true experimental study design, in the sense that the researcher can maintain some control over the conditions of the study and, more important, over the assignment of subjects to experimental and control groups. The random assignment of subjects to experimental (i.e., treatment) and control groups is the critical structure of the RCT study design, the purpose of which is to ensure that the two groups are alike in all characteristics other than the treatment under study. With observational studies, such as the case control study, one must make inferences based on a comparison of two groups of patients who may differ in important ways, other than whether they receive a particular treatment. Moreover, the RCT usually follows a formally articulated protocol, with stated objectives and specific procedures for selecting patients, executing treatments, and measuring outcomes. This chapter examines the importance of the randomization process, the various types of RCTs, methods associated with RCTs, and problems and issues related to RCTs.

In Chapter 11, we mentioned that most epidemiological studies compare one group to another to determine the effect of risk factors (i.e., exposures) or treatments (i.e., interventions) on the incidence or course of disease. The studies are classified according to when the disease is identified, when the exposure or treatment is recognized, and when the analysis is conducted.

Figure 13.1 illustrates this paradigm for the randomized controlled trial. Subjects are randomly assigned to either the experimental or control groups in the present. The experimental group will receive some kind of exposure; the control group will not. The two groups will be followed prospectively over a defined time interval and observed.

At some point in the future, the researcher will classify subjects in each group into two or more outcome categories. For example, suppose one

FIGURE 13.1
Schematic for
Randomized
Clinical Trials

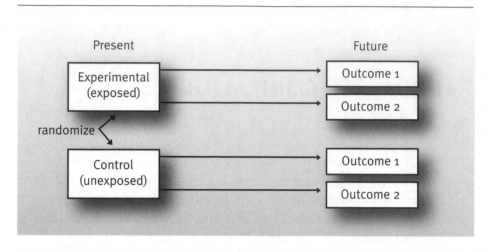

is examining whether tamoxifen can prevent recurrence of breast cancer (Early Breast Cancer Trialists' Collaborative Group 1992). Patients would be randomly assigned to either the experimental group (which receives tamoxifen) or control group (which does not receive tamoxifen). The two groups would be followed prospectively, and at some designated time patients in each group would be classified as having suffered a recurrence of breast cancer (outcome 1) or not (outcome 2).

Lilienfeld and Stolley (1994) distinguish between three types of RCTs: therapeutic trials, intervention trials, and preventive trials. With *therapeutic trials*, a particular agent or procedure is purported to change the disease process in terms of survival, severity, or cure. With *intervention trials*, one is attempting to prevent the onset of disease, typically through the manipulation of risk factors. *Preventive trials* involve agents or procedures, such as vaccines, that can prevent disease from occurring.

The medical literature is full of studies that test the efficacy of therapeutic agents or procedures, such as high-dose chemotherapy for breast cancer (Gradishar, Tallman, and Abrams 1996), zidovudine for HIV infection (Ioannidis et al. 1995), or angioplasty versus thrombolytic therapy for acute myocardial infarction (Weaver et al. 1997).

We can turn to the health services research literature for examples of intervention trials—for example, whether vouchers improve breast cancer screening rates (Stoner et al. 1998), if capitation affects the health of the chronically mentally ill (Lurie et al. 1992), or if comprehensive geriatric assessment affects survival and functional status in the elderly (Reuben et al. 1995).

Preventive trials may include agents such as vaccines, or preventive strategies such as education, each of which is focused typically on primary prevention—curtailing the onset of disease. Intervention and therapeutic trials deal primarily with secondary or tertiary prevention. For example, mammography screening is a secondary prevention intervention designed to detect early-stage breast cancer; lumpectomy or simple mastectomy, on the other hand, is a tertiary prevention intervention designed to halt the spread of the disease.

Randomization

Randomized clinical trials are designed to determine whether particular agents or interventions work. To isolate the effect of an intervention from all other factors (one or more of which may affect the outcome as well), the experimental and control groups should be virtually the same in all respects. In other words, the groups should not differ in ways that may affect the outcome of the study. Randomization is the process used to avoid confounding (refer to the discussion of confounding in Chapter 11). If the two groups are not identical in all respects, the effect of a particular intervention cannot be distinguished from the effects of other factors or characteristics of the group. In short, the results of the study become confounded or difficult to disentangle and interpret. Moreover, the results of the study may be biased if the degree to which the intervention is efficacious is either under- or overestimated.

The underlying premise behind the theory of random assignment to experimental and control groups is that subjects cannot be given a choice of treatment or control because selection into these two groups would then be based on physical, medical, social, and/or cultural characteristics that could affect the outcomes of the study, apart from the treatment or intervention being evaluated.

Suppose, for example, that seriously ill subjects (or their physicians) would be more likely to choose experimental treatment if they had a choice and were not randomly assigned to either treatment or control groups. Their selection into the experimental treatment group might be based on a preference for aggressive treatment as a last hope to improve chances of survival. If the experimental treatment did indeed improve survival, this effect would be underestimated inasmuch as the more seriously ill patients would be more likely to die with or without the treatment. The experimental group would have proportionately more seriously ill patients.

Alternatively, the seriously ill patients might be less likely to choose experimental therapy if it is not well tolerated. In this case, the proportion of healthier patients getting the experimental treatment would be greater, which would cause the treatment effect to be overestimated, with improved survival attributable both to treatment and to healthier patients. In short, the results would be confounded and difficult to disentangle.

Randomization avoids these problems by preventing the selection of patients into treatment and control groups based on characteristics (such as severity of illness) that might affect the outcomes.

The unit of randomization depends on the study design and may be the individual patient, group practice, or geographic area such as zip code or census district. For example, Lurie, Christianson, and Moscovice (1994) randomly assign "elderly Medicaid beneficiaries," Wood and colleagues (1998) define the unit of analysis as "mother-infant pairs," and Palmer and colleagues (1996) define the unit of analysis as "four experimental group practices."

A number of different techniques may be used to implement randomization. Suppose you have a list of 90 subjects eligible to participate in a study, and you want treatment and control groups of ten each. Randomization assumes that each subject in the sample has an equal probability of being selected. Thus, you could not simply select the first ten for the treatment group and the last ten for the controls. Nor could you select every other subject, since those at the top of the list would more likely be selected. Those at the top of the list might be healthier, or smarter, or live next to a toxic waste dump—and the sample would be biased. One simple approach is with a random number table. Table 13.1 was generated from an SAS random number function (also refer to the random number table in Chapter 10).

To use the table, simply look at the number of digits corresponding to the size of the eligible universe of subjects. Since there are 90 eligible subjects in the universe, only the last two digits of each random number need to be examined. Move either vertically or horizontally across the table to select the samples. In this case, the treatment group would consist of the following ten subjects on the list: 68, 25, 2, 23, 66, 18, 61, 83, 15, 59. (Notice that 13 random numbers were examined to select the ten subjects, because subjects 95 and 96 were not on the list. If a subject is repeated, another random number is examined.)

One must also define the universe of subjects eligible for participation in the randomization process. This means that one must clearly define the hypotheses regarding the individuals, physician groups, hospitals, or other units of randomization on whom the treatment or agent is supposed to have an effect.

For example, in a study by DeBusk and colleagues (1994), the question was whether coronary risk factors could be modified by a case management system. The eligible universe of subjects in this case was patients who had suffered an acute myocardial infarction. Other studies may involve

TABLE 13.1
Table of
Random
Numbers

782468	934325	708702	134495	436096
274523	789866	307818	878496	488261
016483	954515	942359	617472	171822
234612	487090	070291	562403	364472
872116	843552	954017	758833	144873

only patients with breast cancer, for example (Early Breast Cancer Trialists' Collaborative Group 1992), or lung cancer (Pritchard and Anthony 1996).

There may be other organizational or geographic constraints that limit the parameters of a study to a particular state or county, or set of hospitals, clinics, or group practices. For example, Pilote and colleagues (1992) define the universe of eligible patients as follows: "from 31 July 1987 to 31 December 1989, 902 patients hospitalized for an acute myocardial infarction were assessed for eligibility. These patients were treated in the coronary care units of four San Francisco Bay area Kaiser-Foundation Medical Centers." Therefore, the universe is limited to (a) hospitalized patients, (b) during a particular time frame, (c) with a defined medical condition, (d) assigned to a coronary care unit, and (e) in one of four specific hospitals.

As mentioned earlier, the concept of randomization is based on probability theory, with each subject in the eligible universe having an equal probability of selection into either the treatment or control group. Elwood (1998) points out the benefits and limitations of this approach. Presumably, randomization of a large number of subjects (say, 100 in each group) will ensure that treatment and control groups will be similar in terms of known (and unknown) characteristics that may be potential confounders. The probability of significant differences being present in any of these characteristics (attributable to chance alone) increases with a smaller sample size.

It is common practice for researchers to describe the characteristics of each group to ensure the reader that the process of randomization did indeed result in groups with similar characteristics. For example, Stoner and colleagues (1998) studied whether vouchers for free mammograms improved cancer screening rates. They compared treatment and control groups in terms of potentially confounding characteristics, such as the subject's perceived risk of breast cancer, family history of breast cancer, and distance to the nearest mammography unit (each of which could independently affect cancer screening rates, apart from the "treatment" of receiving a voucher).

Historical Controls and Crossover Studies

Under some circumstances, it is inappropriate to assign a group of patients to conventional therapy, particularly if the usual therapy is ineffective. In this case, a group of patients from the past with the same disease serves as historical controls. Although this type of study may seem to be in the best interest of the patient, it is not a particularly strong design; that is, the results may be disputed.

The crossover study, a more rigorous approach to using historical controls, has become an important part of pharmaceutical research (Senn 1995). With this type of study, patients are randomly assigned to treatment and control groups, but at some point in time they switch groups. In other words, controls are given the experimental intervention and vice versa. Measurements are taken at the end of each phase. There are obvious limitations with this approach: the residual effects of treatment may persist even after patients switch from one group to the other, in which case the treatment is "contaminated." This is clearly the case with surgical interventions (one cannot undo a surgical operation), and it may be true of many pharmaceuticals as well. "In short, crossover studies should not be abandoned; they should be used intelligently" (Senn 1995).

Methods of Randomized Clinical Trials

The purpose of conducting a randomized clinical trial is to determine whether a particular treatment, agent, or program has a significant effect on the onset of the disease, course of illness, or, in the case of health services research, other outcomes, such as utilization of services. The change in measurable outcome between the treatment and control groups is referred to as the *treatment effect*.

In the medical literature, treatment effects typically include survival (Fisher et al. 1995; Pritchard and Anthony 1996), general health or functional status (Lurie, Christianson, and Moscovice 1994), or some change in the course of illness. Ioannidis and colleagues (1995), for instance, in their analysis of ten studies that examined the effect of zidovudine on AIDS, used specific clinical "endpoints" defined in each study, obviously related to the progression of the disease. Other treatment effects include mammography screening rates (Stoner et al. 1998) and immunization rates (Wood et al. 1998).

A variety of statistical techniques can be used to assess whether the treatment effect is statistically significant. One can determine if a statistically significant difference is found in survival curves (Rosselli-Del-Turco et al. 1994), for instance. There is also a test for calculating the statistical significance of differences in proportions, such as smoking cessation (DeBusk et al. 1994); immunization rates (Wood et al. 1998); or amounts, such as average total charges (Simmer et al. 1991). The size of the treatment effect is another factor. The effect may be statistically significant, but not practically or clinically significant.

Some studies, for instance, report the odds ratio (Early Breast Cancer Trialists' Collaborative Group 1995; Weaver et al. 1997) or relative risk, which quantifies the number of times more likely a particular outcome is probable, given exposure to the treatment. Other studies simply report the difference between outcomes and whether the difference is statistically significant (Lurie, Christianson, and Moscovice 1994), or they report reduction in the odds of an undesirable outcome, such as death (Early Breast Cancer Trialists' Collaborative Group 1995).

Sample Size

One of the more difficult decisions to make when designing an RCT is how big the trial sample should be. These studies are the most expensive type of epidemiological inquiry, and the cost is directly dependent on the size of the sample. However, the precision with which one can discern a difference between treatment and control groups that is statistically significant depends on sample size. One can detect smaller differences with a larger sample. Therein lies the trade-off between cost and precision.

The concepts of type I and type II error, statistical power, and determination of sample size are discussed next.

Figure 13.2, adapted from Lilienfeld and Stolley (1994), illustrates the concept of type I and type II error by a simple typology. Randomized clinical trails are designed to conclude that a treatment is either effective or not effective in terms of its ability to delay the onset or progression of disease, improve survival, increase utilization, or whatever. The conclusion is based on the size of the sample and the size of the treatment effect. In fact, we can never know whether the treatment truly works, but the RCT is the best and most sophisticated attempt that we have to discern reality.

Suppose the results of the RCT suggest that the treatment, agent, or program—collectively referred to as the *exposure*—is effective, and, in fact, it is. This means that reality and the study are congruent. If the study proves that the treatment is not effective, and it truly is not, then reality and study are also congruent. Both of these scenarios deserve our heartfelt celebration, although one can never know for sure—ponder the prolonged debate over whether smoking causes lung cancer, for instance.

If the study suggests that the treatment is effective when it really is not, this is referred to as type I or α-error. It is called a false positive, because

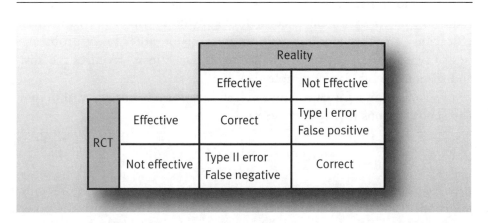

FIGURE 13.2
Conclusions of an RCT Versus Reality

		Reality	
		Effective	Not Effective
RCT	Effective	Correct	Type I error False positive
	Not effective	Type II error False negative	Correct

SOURCE: Adapted from Lilienfeld and Stolley (1994). Used with permission of Oxford University Press.

we have incorrectly asserted that a treatment is efficacious. If the study leads to the conclusion that the treatment is not effective when, in fact, it is effective, this is referred to as type II or β-error. It is a false negative because we have incorrectly concluded that the treatment is not effective, when it actually is.

Types I and II error are inversely related. As the likelihood of reporting a false positive result increases, the likelihood of reporting a false negative decreases, and vice versa (assuming the sample size remains the same).

Clearly one would want to minimize both type I and type II error. Each type of error can have negative consequences on the medical community. False negatives may thwart the future investigation of potentially promising drugs or procedures—or the results of the study may not even be published. False positives may result in the premature dissemination of a technology or agent that simply is not efficacious. There are only two ways to decrease both types I and II error, and thus to improve the validity with which one can make inferences based on randomized trials: increase the sample size or increase the minimum effect size.

Typically, researchers want the probability of type I error (p_1) to be 5 percent or less, which means a 5 percent probability or less that the conclusion that the treatment was effective was false and due to chance alone. The probability of type II error (p_2) should be 20 percent or less. The power of the study is $1 - p_2$. Thus if the probability of type II error is 20 percent, the power of the study is 80 percent, meaning that there is an 80 percent probability that the finding of "no effect" is, in fact, accurate.

The minimum sample size needed for a particular study can be estimated by using a different formula for RCT, cohort, and case control studies (Elwood 1998). In general, the size depends on (1) the minimum types I and II error that the researcher is willing to accept and (2) the minimum treatment effect. Sample size decreases if one is willing to tolerate proportionately more false positive and negative results. Size also decreases if one requires a larger treatment effect before concluding that the treatment is efficacious. In other words, precision, in terms of either lower probabilities of types I and II error or smaller treatment effects, requires the cost and magnitude of a larger sample size.

The formula for calculating sample size for a cohort or trial design with equal groups is (Elwood 1998):

$$n = (p_1 q_1 + p_2 q_2) \times K/(p_1 - p_2)^2$$

where p_1 and p_2 are the proportion of patients with a particular outcome in groups 1 and 2, q_1 and q_2 are the proportion of patients with the other outcome in groups 1 and 2, and K is a constant that is calculated and reflects the types I and II error that the researcher is willing to tolerate (see Elwood 1998). For instance, $K = 6.2$ when the type I error = 5 percent (one-sided, which means that we know that the chance of error is only on one side, e.g., p_1 will definitely be higher than p_2, or vice versa) and the type II error is 20 percent (power = 80 percent), whereas $K = 17.8$ with a type I error = 1 percent and a power = 95 percent.

A decade ago, clodronate was found to have a dramatic effect on reducing new metastases in breast cancer (Diel et al. 1998). The rate of new metastases was 13 percent for women who took the drug and 29 percent for those who did not. If a researcher wanted to replicate the study and hoped to get the same kind of effect, how big should the sample size be? The p_1 and p_2 values will be set at 0.13 and 0.29, respectively, and q_1 and $q_2 = 0.87$ and 0.71. Assume a one-sided type I error = 5 percent and a power of 80 percent, so $K = 6.2$.

$$n = (0.13 \times 0.87 + 0.29 \times 0.71) \times 6.2/(0.13 - 0.29)^2$$
$$n = 77$$

Sample size, n, should be at least 77 in each group. Note that with a lower tolerance for error, say type I = 1 percent and power = 95 percent, $K = 17.8$ and the sample size should be at least 222 subjects in each group.

$$n = (0.13 \times 0.87 + 0.29 \times 0.71) \times 17.8/(0.13 - 0.29)^2$$
$$n = 222$$

Duration and Masking

Since all RCTs are prospective by design, subjects are followed over time to determine the effect of treatment on specific identified outcomes, such as mortality. The length of time necessary to make valid inferences from the study depends on the particular hypothesis in question and on the size of the expected treatment effect.

One concern is the lapse in time and the extent to which the exposure in question will have an effect in that time on measurable outcomes. Some exposures, particularly in preventive trials or in those involving risk factor modification, may demonstrate a beneficial effect on outcomes many years in the future. Although the initial RCT design may have to be lengthened (or shortened) after the commencement of the study, constraints—such as cost and the recruitment of eligible subjects—may be problematic.

The purpose of randomization is to allocate subjects into treatment and control groups in a fashion that selection bias is not introduced, since subjects with risk factors or other confounding characteristics may be more likely to self-select into one group or the other. Furthermore, many clinical trials do not make the patient or others involved with the study aware of group assignment. This is also referred to as *blinding* or *masking*. The concept of masking is based on the premise that patients, clinicians, and researchers ought not to be aware of whether a patient is receiving an experimental agent, treatment, or program, because that awareness could change behaviors in a way that would bias outcomes.

Single masking means that subjects (i.e., patients) are not told whether they are receiving an experimental treatment (although they consented to participation in the study). This requires that the researcher design bogus or placebo exposures. With drugs, for instance, it is convenient to give control subjects pills devoid of pharmacological benefit (placebo). This becomes more difficult if side effects to the medication are anticipated. A fully executed informed consent would require making subjects aware of potential side effects should they be assigned to the treatment group. The onset of side effects could easily unravel single masking.

The idea behind single masking is that subjects may change behaviors in a way that could compromise the study if they are aware of group assignment. For example, control subjects may seek alternative therapies or modify risk factors if they know that they are not receiving an experimental treatment. If this behavior has a favorable effect on outcomes, the observed treatment effect of the drug or procedure being studied will be underestimated. It is somewhat more difficult or even impossible, of course, to develop bogus options for surgical procedures or programs.

Double masking refers to blinding both the subject and the subject's observer with regard to group assignment. The observer is anyone who is measuring outcomes, such as a clinician performing a physical exam or an interviewer supervising an oral or written interview. Double masking is necessary to prevent the observer from changing the structure or thoroughness of the observation in a way that could bias the measured outcome. Byar and colleagues (1990) exemplify this point in a discussion of the utility of blinding in AIDS trials:

> Blinding is especially desirable when subjective end points, such as pain, functional status, or quality of life, are studied, because such evaluations are open to substantial bias. Likewise, without blinding, evaluation of the incidence of opportunistic infections may be biased, because knowledge of the treatment could affect the frequency or thoroughness of surveillance.

With *triple blinding*, the subject, observer, and reviewer of the data are not aware of group assignment. Triple blinding assumes that the researchers or statistical analysts can introduce bias into the process of manipulating or interpreting the data to the extent that they have preconceived notions about the efficacy of the treatment.

Integrity of the Randomization

Given a sufficient number of subjects, randomization increases the like-lihood, more than any other type of study, that both known and unknown characteristics are equally distributed into treatment and control groups. This doesn't always work, though, and the researchers should report whether the difference in each measurable characteristic is statistically significant. In cases with a statistically significant difference between the treatment and control group, stratification of the analyses may be appro-priate, since it allows for a comparison of the treatment effects for the characteristic (e.g., gender) between the groups. Another alternative is to block-randomize at the very beginning of the study. *Block-random-izing* means to randomize within subgroups (gender, age, race) of the eligible population to ensure that the treatment and control groups are identical.

Even when randomization is successful, sometimes the composition of the treatment and control groups changes during the design and exe-cution of the study in such a way that the integrity of the study is jeopard-ized. Eligible subjects may refuse to participate in the study or drop out at some point in time, or they may cross over to the other study group. These refusals, dropouts, or crossovers may bias the results of the study.

Eligible subjects may refuse to participate in the study before they are randomized, in which case the randomized group of subjects may no longer be representative of some universe of patients. Suppose the more seriously ill patients refuse to be involved in a study because of transporta-tion problems. The randomized group of subjects would be somewhat healthier, but unrepresentative, of the true population.

A somewhat thornier problem exists if subjects refuse to participate after they are randomized to either the treatment or control group (although blinding patients to group assignment should reduce the likelihood of this happening). When this happens, the composition of the treatment and con-trol group may be dissimilar to the extent that the refusals are nonrandom, related to patient characteristics, and based on patient preferences for exper-imental treatment or conventional therapy. For example, suppose in an unblinded randomized study, proportionately more seriously ill patients refuse conventional therapy; the result would be a "control" group of some-what less seriously ill patients. If the outcome that is measured (e.g., mor-tality) is related to severity of illness, the treatment effect may be underes-timated, because the group receiving the experimental treatment is composed of more seriously ill patients. The researcher may decide to reduce the like-lihood of refusals by enlisting volunteers. This policy is not without risk, however, because volunteers may differ in significant ways from the pop-ulation they are intended to represent. For example, they may be health-ier, smarter, or more motivated.

Dropouts pose similar problems. Some subjects are simply lost to follow-up, while others choose to discontinue, perhaps because they cannot tolerate the side effects of the experimental medication. The loss of subjects in a study may be nonrandom if dropouts from the experimental and control groups have different characteristics. For example, suppose dropouts from the experimental group tend to be somewhat sicker, and they drop out because they cannot tolerate the medication, while the control group dropouts tend to be somewhat healthier, and they drop out because they are not well-motivated to continue in the study. The result would be experimental and control groups that differ on the basis of severity of illness. The effect of the treatment being studied would probably be underestimated, since the experimental group might now be composed of patients for whom the treatment may not be as efficacious (i.e., if intolerance is related to efficacy). The burden of proof is on the researcher to demonstrate that neither refusals nor dropouts differ from the study participants in terms of characteristics or factors that may influence the outcomes of the study.

Another troubling problem occurs when patients cross over or change from the experimental treatment group to the control or conventional therapy group, or vice versa. This may occur, for instance, if patients cannot tolerate the side effects of the new treatment, or if the more seriously ill patients in the control group require the experimental intervention. The critical question is not necessarily whether to allow patients to cross over—clinical judgment should supercede the purity of experimental design—but how to classify these patients once they have changed treatment.

The classic example of this crossover problem involves studies that have compared medical versus surgical treatment for heart disease. The surgical intervention is typically coronary artery bypass graft surgery. Some of the larger studies have reported crossover rates that range from 25 percent to 38 percent (Weinstein and Levin 1989), which means that a substantial number of subjects originally assigned to the medical control group had to undergo surgical intervention. Should these patients continue to participate in the study, and if so, how? Weinstein and Levin (1989) summarize the possibilities: (1) drop the crossovers, (2) switch the crossover group assignment at the time of the crossover, (3) use the "intention to treat" principle, or (4) discard the study. The first two possibilities would clearly change the composition of the two groups to the extent that control patients who cross over to the surgical intervention group are typically more seriously ill. Regardless of whether the crossovers are dropped or whether they change groups, the presumed similarity of the treatment and control groups brought about by randomization is destroyed. The intention to treat principle preserves the original classification despite crossover to a different treatment. Although the original composition of the two groups is maintained with this approach, the purity of treatment received by each group is contaminated. The crossovers are receiving a different kind of treatment than the other patients in the control group.

The crossover problem may also arise if preliminary results of the study indicate an extremely promising treatment effect, as, for instance, in some of the studies of antiretroviral therapy for HIV infection (Volberding and Graham 1994). In one study, patients were assigned to either "immediate" or "deferred" treatment with zidovudine (an antiretroviral drug), with the deferred group supposedly not receiving the drug until the onset of symptoms. One-third of this group, however, crossed over and received the drug prematurely.

The integrity of randomization is also compromised if the character of the treatment(s) changes. In part, this is an issue of compliance. Subjects in a study may fail to comply with the treatment (e.g., they do not take the pills or take only some of the pills). To avoid (or at least measure) this problem, researchers may provide patients with too many pills and ask them to return the unused ones. Lack of compliance, or partial compliance, changes the character of the treatment and affects the outcomes of the study.

The treatment may also be affected by *dilution* or *contamination*. This means some subjects in the control group are "influenced" by their participation in the study even though they are not assigned to receive the intervention. Elwood (1998) discusses this phenomenon in his mention of the Multiple Risk Factor Intervention Trial Research Group (1982), where subjects were randomized to receive a special intervention to reduce risk factors for coronary artery disease. The control group reduced risk factors as well (although not as much), despite not receiving the special intervention. Presumably, control subjects were influenced by being participants in the study and adjusted their risk factors as a result of feedback from their physicians. In effect, an alternative (and only somewhat inferior) treatment was configured ad hoc by control subjects and their physicians. This resulted in a dilution or contamination of the original study design.

Ethical Considerations

The special relationship between patients and physicians is grounded in trust, based on a long history of physician dedication to the care of individual patients, and guided by the Hippocratic oath to "first do no harm." Despite this sacred trust, physicians regularly face ethical dilemmas, such as when their view of what is best for the patient is challenged by others (third-party payers, for instance). The randomized clinical trial leads them into a particularly difficult ethical quagmire. Physicians are called on to engage their patients in a process that may provide less than optimal treatment in the interest of some larger social good—the advancement of knowledge. Hellman and Hellman (1991) reflect on this dilemma:

The randomized clinical trial routinely asks physicians to sacrifice the interests of their particular patients for the sake of the study and that of the information that it will make available for the benefit of society. This practice is ethically problematic.... If the physician has no preference for either treatment (is in a state of equipose), then randomization is acceptable. If, however, he or she believes that the new treatment may be either more or less successful or more or less toxic, the use of randomization is not consistent with fidelity to the patient.

The legal doctrine of informed consent requires that patients be made aware of the risks and benefits of treatment and that they provide formal consent. However, the principles of randomization and masking, discussed earlier, make informed consent somewhat more difficult. Patients are not given the choice, or perhaps even the knowledge, of which strategy of care they are receiving—experimental treatment, conventional treatment, or no treatment. The experimental treatment may carry some unknown risks with the promise of additional benefits. The calculus of weighing benefits and costs makes it unlikely that both patient and clinician are neutral to the choice of experimental or conventional treatment. Baum (1993) gives a cogent summary of this argument:

One of the wittiest and most scholarly men that I know once explained to me, with irrefutable logic, that randomised controlled trials are ethically impossible. For a patient to be recruited, the clinician must be in perfect equipose about either of the two treatments being evaluated, and that has to be a rare event. Moreover, the patient, having been provided with and understanding perfect information about the trial, must also express perfect equipose—another extremely rare event. The likelihood of these rarities coexisting reaches an astronomically small probability number.

A tension exists between wanting to use the RCT to demonstrate therapeutic benefit and knowing when it is ethically unacceptable to randomly assign some patients to inferior care. No rational patient would choose less than optimal treatment in the interest of science, particularly when no alternatives exist. The double-blind placebo-controlled study of the efficacy of AZT in the treatment of patients with AIDS and AIDS-related complex is a classic example (Fischl et al. 1987). No other conventional therapy for AIDS existed at that time. The study had to be ended prematurely once a significant difference in mortality was demonstrated.

In some instances, uncontrolled clinical trials may be the recommended study design if patients with a poor prognosis have no other alternatives and the experimental treatment is expected to have no significant side effects (Byar et al. 1990).

It may be difficult to justify an RCT to support a growing body of evidence from other less-sophisticated studies when the preponderance of evidence supports a causal relationship between a particular exposure and outcome. For instance, some would argue that we have not conclusively proven that smoking causes cancer, yet few would be willing to support a randomized clinical trial in which subjects were randomly assigned to smoking and nonsmoking groups and followed over a lifetime.

Case Study 13.1 summarizes the landmark RAND Health Insurance Experiment.

Case Study 13.1. The RAND Health Insurance Experiment

The RAND Health Insurance Experiment was probably the largest controlled trial designed to improve health financing policy, particularly with regard to the issue of cost sharing (Newhouse 1991). Between November 1974 and February 1977, 7,691 families were enrolled in the study at six different sites: Dayton, Ohio; Seattle, Washington; Fitchburg/Leominster, Massachusetts; Charleston, South Carolina; Franklin County, Massachusetts; and Georgetown County, South Carolina. The sites were supposed to represent the major census regions; northern and southern rural sites; and a range in city sizes, waiting times to appointments, and physicians per capita.

Each family was randomly assigned to one of 14 different fee-for-service plans or a prepaid group practice—Group Health Cooperative (GHC) in Seattle. A comparison group of patients from GHC was also evaluated (Fischl et al. 1987; Friedman, Furberg, and DeMets 1996). The plans varied by coinsurance rate (0, 25 percent, 50 percent, or 95 percent) and by maximum dollar expenditure (MDE), with an MDE of $1,000 for most families, but 5, 10, or 15 percent of income (or $1,000, whichever was less) for low-income families. The families were followed for either three or five years.

The number of total visits for each of the plans (0, 25 percent, 50 percent, 95 percent coinsurance) was 4.55, 3.33, 3.03, and 2.73 visits, respectively. The number of face-to-face visits for each of these four types of plans was 4.2, 3.5, 2.9, and 3.3, respectively. The number of preventive visits for each of the plans was 0.41, 0.32, 0.29, and 0.27, respectively.

With regard to hospitalization, the results are as follows: The number of hospital admissions for each of the four groups was 0.128, 0.105, 0.092, and 0.099 admissions, respectively. The hospital admission rate across each of the four insurance groups was 13.8, 10.0, 10.5, and 8.8 admissions per 100 persons, respectively. Hospital days were 83, 87, 46, and 28 days per 100 persons for each of the four groups, respectively. Expenses for each of these four groups were $340, $260, $224, and $204, respectively, for outpatient expenses, and $409, $373, $450, and $315 for hospital expenses.

QUESTIONS

1. What kinds of factors is the randomization process likely to control for in this study?

2. How do you interpret the results of this study with regard to the effect of cost sharing on utilization?
3. Was it possible to use blinding in this study? Why or why not?
4. Describe any ethical concerns with this study.
5. Why would this RCT design be better than a cohort study of groups with different coinsurance rates?

ANSWERS

1. There are a variety of reasons why people "choose" health insurance plans, such as their preference for health, aversion to risk, socioeconomic status, anticipated medical expenditures, and so on. Randomization ensures that the different health insurance groups are very similar across these and many other dimensions.
2. As the amount of cost sharing increased, the number of visits, outpatient expenses, the number of hospital admissions and expenses, and hospitalization rates and hospital days all decreased. In summary, as cost sharing increased, utilization decreased.
3. Subjects were obviously not blinded to their cost-sharing group inasmuch as they had to share the financial burden of a portion of their medical care.
4. One could argue that the people who were randomly assigned to very high cost-sharing groups were forced to eliminate or postpone necessary care due to financial constraints. To the extent that this behavior resulted in serious consequences, for example, lack of screening leading to late-stage cancer, it may be considered unethical to assign patients to these treatment groups.
5. If we were to allow subjects to "self-select" into the various cost-sharing groups (cohort study), the characteristics of subjects in these groups would certainly be different, as explained in question 1. For example, sicker patients may elect plans with lower cost sharing because they anticipate high medical expenses and do not want to share in the cost burden.

Factorial Design

One way to reduce the cost of studies is to conduct two experiments simultaneously on the same group of subjects, a design that is referred to as the *factorial design* (Gordis 2004). Suppose you wanted to test the effects of two different drugs, with two very different effects, such as a cancer drug and a cardiovascular disease drug. If the modes of action are independent, and the outcomes are distinct and measurable, you can randomize subjects into four groups as indicated in Figure 13.3: (1) both treatments A and B, (2) treatment A only, (3) treatment B only, and (4) neither treatment A nor B.

FIGURE 13.3
Factorial
Design

		Treatment B	
		Yes	No
Treatment A	Yes	A and B (cell a)	Only A (cell b)
	No	Only B (cell c)	Neither A nor B (cell d)

If the modes of action are independent, the calculation of treatment effect is done separately for treatments A and B by comparing the relevant cells in Figure 13.3. Subjects in cells a and b received treatment A, whereas those in cells c and d did not. Therefore, the treatment effect for treatment A is calculated by comparing the combined outcomes of cells a and b to the combined outcomes of cells c and d. If the outcome is mortality, for instance, we must calculate the combined mortality rate for cells a and b and for cells c and d. The treatment effect—risk difference in this case—would be the former subtracted from the latter. Subjects in cells a and c received treatment B, whereas those in cells b and d did not. The treatment effect for treatment B is calculated as the difference between the combined outcome of cells b and d minus the combined outcome of cells a and c.

The modes of action may not always be independent; that is, treatment A is less effective (antagonistic) or more effective (synergistic) when the patient also receives treatment B, and vice versa. In such cases, one would compare the outcomes of either cell b (for treatment A) or cell c (for treatment B) to cell d. Case Study 13.2 uses a factorial design to test the effects of both vitamin E and n-3 polyunsaturated fatty acids on patients with acute myocardial infarction.

Case Study 13.2. Vitamin E and n-3 Polyunsaturated Fatty Acids After Myocardial Infarction

The GISSI Prevenzione Investigators (1999) conducted a factorial-designed randomized trial to determine the effects of vitamin E and/or n-3 polyunsaturated fatty acids (PUFA) on patients who had recently suffered an acute myocardial infarction (heart attack). Of the 11,324 patients who were randomized, 2,830 received both vitamin E and PUFA, 2,836 received PUFA alone, 2,830 received vitamin E alone, and 2,828 received neither. Table 13.2 reports the incidence of three kinds of adverse outcomes following myocardial infarction (MI).

TABLE 13.2. VITAMIN E, N-3 PUFA, AFTER MYOCARDIAL INFARCTION

| | Death, Nonfatal MI, Nonfatal Stroke | | Cardiovascular Death Only | | Sudden Death Only | |
| | Vitamin E | | Vitamin E | | Vitamin E | |
	Yes	No	Yes	No	Yes	No
PUFA—yes	359	356	155	136	67	55
PUFA—no	371	414	155	193	65	99

SOURCE: Some data from GISSI Prevenzione Investigators (1999).

QUESTIONS

1. Calculate the adverse outcome rate for each cell of the table.
2. Assume there is no interaction between vitamin E and n-3 PUFA, in terms of the effects on post-MI outcomes. Which combined rates need to be calculated now?
3. Calculate the risk difference for each of the three adverse outcomes for (a) those with PUFA (compared to those without PUFA) and (b) those with vitamin E (compared to those without vitamin E).
4. Using the combined rates from question 2, how might we calculate the relative risk of each of the three adverse outcomes for (a) those with PUFA (compared to those without PUFA) and (b) those with vitamin E (compared to those without vitamin E)?
5. Interpret the results from question 4.
6. If one cannot rule out the possibility of an interaction between the two agents (vitamin E and PUFA), then it would be appropriate to compare cells b to d for PUFA, cells c to d for vitamin E, and cells a to d for both vitamin E and PUFA. Calculate relative risks for these comparisons for each adverse outcome and interpret the results.
7. The authors report that some tests for the interaction between PUFA and vitamin E were not significant. Consider the following comparisons and comment. The use of PUFA is associated with a 10 percent lower risk of death, nonfatal MI, and nonfatal stroke when comparing cells a + b to cells c + d, but a 15 percent lower risk when comparing cell a to cell d. Use of PUFA alone is associated with a 45 percent lower risk of sudden death. Use of vitamin E alone is associated with a 35 percent lower risk of sudden death. Use of both PUFA and vitamin E is associated with a 33 percent lower risk.

ANSWERS

1. The adverse outcomes rates are calculated in Table 13.3.

TABLE 13.3. VITAMIN E, N-3 PUFA, AFTER MYOCARDIAL INFARCTION, ADVERSE OUTCOME RATES

PUFA	Death, Nonfatal MI, Nonfatal Stroke		Cardiovascular Death		Sudden Death	
	Vitamin E		Vitamin E		Vitamin E	
	Yes	No	Yes	No	Yes	No
Yes	359/2,830 = 12.7%	356/2,836 = 12.6%	155/2,830 = 5.5%	136/2,836 = 4.8%	67/2,830 = 2.4%	55/2,836 = 1.9%
No	371/2,830 = 13.1%	414/2,828 = 14.6%	155/2,830 = 5.5%	193/2,828 – 6.8%	65/2,830 = 2.3%	99/2,828 = 3.5%

SOURCE: Some data from GISSI Prevenzione Investigators (1999).

2. It is necessary to calculate row and column combined rates, i.e., the combined rate for each outcome for cells a + b, c + d, a + c, and b + d. These rates are summarized below in Table 13.4.

TABLE 13.4. VITAMIN E, N-3 PUFA, AFTER MYOCARDIAL INFARCTION, CELL, COLUMN RATES

	Death, Nonfatal MI, Nonfatal Stroke	Cardiovascular Death	Sudden Death
PUFA (cells a + b)	715/5,666 = 12.6%	291/5,666 = 5.1%	122/5,666 = 2.2%
No PUFA (cells c + d)	785/5,658 = 13.9%	348/5,658 = 6.2%	164/5,658 = 2.9%
Vitamin E (cells a + c)	730/5,660 = 12.9%	310/5,660 = 5.5%	132/5,660 = 2.3%
No Vitamin E (cells b + d)	770/5,664 = 13.6%	329/5,664 = 5.8%	154/5,664 = 2.7%

SOURCE: Some data from GISSI Prevenzione Investigators (1999).

3. The risk difference for PUFA would be (no PUFA rate – PUFA rate), or 13.9 – 12.6 = 1.3, 6.2 – 5.1 = 1.1, and 2.9 – 2.2 = 0.7 for each of the three adverse outcomes, respectively. The risk difference for vitamin E would be (no vitamin E rate – vitamin E rate), or 13.6 – 12.9 = 0.7, 5.8 – 5.5 = 0.3, and 2.7 – 2.3 = 0.4 for each of the three adverse outcomes, respectively. For example, one could interpret these results to mean that the rate of death, nonfatal MI, and nonfatal stroke for those who take PUFA is 1.3 percentage points lower than the rate of those who do not take PUFA.

4. One simply divides the two rates (PUFA/no PUFA) and (vitamin E/no vitamin E) for each of the three adverse outcomes as follows: (a) For PUFA, 12.6/13.9 = 0.91,* 5.1/6.2 = 0.82,* 2.2/2.9 = 0.76;* (b) for vitamin E; 12.9/13.6 = 0.95, 5.5/5.8 = 0.95, 2.3/2.7 = 0.85. Asterisks indicate whether the relative risks are statistically significantly different from 1.0.

5. It would appear that PUFA is associated with a 9 percent lower risk of death, nonfatal MI, or nonfatal stroke following acute myocardial infection, an 18 percent lower risk of cardiovascular death, and a 24 percent lower risk of sudden death. It would also appear that vitamin E is not associated with a decreased risk of any of these outcomes.

6. For PUFA versus control, the relative risks would be 12.6/14.6 = 0.86, 4.8/6.8 = 0.71, 1.9/3.5 = 0.54. For vitamin E versus control, the relative risks would be 13.1/14.6 = 0.90 (not significant), 5.5/6.8 = 0.81, 2.3/3.5 = 0.66. For vitamin E and PUFA versus control, the relative risks would be 12.7/14.6 = 0.87, 5.5/6.8 = 0.81, 2.4/3.5 = 0.69. All relative risks (except one) were statistically significantly different from 1.0, using the 95 percent confidence interval. It would appear that PUFA is associated with a lower risk of each of the adverse events. With these analyses, vitamin E is associated with a 19 percent lower risk of cardiovascular death and a 34 percent lower risk of sudden death.

7. The difference in relative risk for death, nonfatal MI, and nonfatal stroke between the two comparisons would suggest a possible interaction between the two agents, although tests for interaction were not statistically significant. Moreover, for sudden death, the risk reduction is less for both agents than for either agent alone, and is certainly not additive, as one might expect of two agents with "independent" effects, suggesting a possible interaction between the two agents.

Randomized Clinical Trials and Hospital Firms

One efficient method of conducting a randomized clinical trial is through the use of hospital firms. According to Neuhauser (1991), the three underlying concepts of firm research are (1) parallel providers, (2) ongoing random assignment, and (3) continuous/efficient evaluation and improvement.

Basically, hospitals configure parallel and presumably similar systems of care (called "firms") to which patients are randomly assigned and the outcomes of which can be routinely evaluated and improved. Hospital firms become de facto laboratories for controlled trial research, inasmuch as patients can be randomly assigned to the parallel firms as either the experimental intervention group or the control group. The hospital firm is an attractive idea, to the extent that these organizations are interested in being sites for clinical research. The costly and cumbersome process of developing an approach and a structure for randomization is present and ongoing in hospital firms.

A number of hospitals have developed firms since the 1980s, including MetroHealth Medical Center (MCC) in Cleveland, Ohio (Cebul 1991). In MCC, the large department of medicine was split into three parallel group practices. Faculty are randomly assigned to one of three groups, stratified by subspecialty. Residents are randomly assigned when they enter the training program. Nurses, paramedical staff, and clerical staff are dedicated solely to each firm, which is assigned a specific inpatient unit. Patients are assigned to firms using block randomization, which basically means patients are distributed in randomized blocks of three. With block 231, for instance, the first patient would be assigned to firm 2, the next to firm 3, and the third to firm 1.

The MetroHealth firm system was used in a study (Curley, McEachern, and Speroff 1998) to test the efficacy of interdisciplinary hospital rounds as compared to traditional rounds (MDs only). The interdisciplinary rounds, which brought together the MDs, RN, pharmacist, nutritionist, and social worker, were associated with a shorter mean length of stay, lower mean total charges, and similar outcomes in terms of hospital mortality rates.

Firms are specifically designed to accommodate at least three types of controlled trials: (1) clinical trials, (2) education trials, and (3) health services or quality improvement (QI) research (Cebul 1991). With clinical trials, the firms are randomly assigned to the new treatment modality or conventional therapy. Education trials can be designed to compare different teaching approaches, with one or more firms assigned to receive the special intervention. Hospital firms are ideally configured to conduct health services research or QI research, where the issues are modes of delivery, treatment strategies, and outcomes of care.

The design and execution of firm research are not without some concerns (Cebul 1991). The randomization process cannot guarantee that each firm will have patients and providers with similar characteristics. The randomization protocol within firms should prevent clever schemes to circumvent the process, such as allowing residents to choose "interesting" patients (Dawson 1991). The burden is on the researcher to demonstrate the equivalence of each firm at the beginning of the controlled trial. Indeed, the definition of equivalence may vary depending on the research (Cebul 1991).

There is also the question of unit of analysis: patient, provider, or some larger group. The threat of contamination may be even more of a concern with hospital firms than with other kinds of controlled trials, given the "proximity" of competing units, particularly if providers are not blinded (Cebul 1991). Finally, one must face the ethical issues that emerge from placing patients in an "experimental" environment in which they might be exposed to some risks. According to Goldberg and McGough (1991):

> In a sense, firm-system patients are not simply being asked to participate in this or that class of research activity, but rather whether or not they are interested in joining a clinical community whose routine practice has been redefined to include some level of minimal-risk experimentation.

Case Study 13.3 used hospital firms to study inpatient staffing at Henry Ford Hospital in Detroit, Michigan.

Case Study 13.3. Inpatient Staffing at Henry Ford Hospital

Simmer and colleagues (1991) reported on a randomized controlled trial at Henry Ford Hospital in Detroit, Michigan, that compared clinical and financial outcomes on two different inpatient staffing models. The General Internal Medicine inpatient nursing unit was the site of the study in which 1,151 patients were randomly assigned to either a resident (teaching) or staff (nonteaching) service. The resident service provided patient care with the more traditional resident team consisting of a supervising resident, two interns, and a number of third- and fourth-year medical students. The staff service consisted of two senior-level physicians, a physician assistant, and a medical assistant. All patients had an attending physician. Table 13.5 (Simmer et al. 1991, from tables 3 and 4) summarizes the results of the study.

QUESTIONS

1. Exactly what is the experimental "treatment" here?
2. How might differences in the composition of the two services be expected to affect outcomes?
3. Describe the differences in resource use and outcomes between the two services.
4. What other factors might explain the significant differences in financial and clinical outcomes?
5. Describe the integrity of the randomization process and the potential for bias in this study.

TABLE 13.5. CLINICAL AND FINANCIAL OUTCOMES FOR TWO STAFFING MODELS

	Staff	Resident	Significance
Length of stay	7.58	9.21	p < 0.005
Total charges	$6,908	$8,588	p < 0.010
Laboratory charges	$820	$1,170	p < 0.001
Pharmacy	$592	$814	p < 0.005
Radiology	$495	$479	NS
Readmissions within 15 days	7.8%	6.8%	NS
In-hospital mortality	5.2%	8.2%	p < 0.54
8-month mortality	12.5%	14.0%	NS

NOTE: NS = not significant.

SOURCE: Simmer, T. L., D. R. Nuuu, W. M. Rutt, C. S. Newcomb, and D. W. Benfer. 1991. "A Randomized, Controlled Trial of an Attending Staff Service in General Internal Medicine." *Medical Care* 29 (7, Suppl.): JS31–JS40.

ANSWERS

1. The staff service consisting of two senior-level physicians, a physician assistant, and a medical assistant would be considered the experimental treatment here, with the more traditional resident service serving as the "control."
2. The traditional service consists of more traditional "students" who are learning the process of patient care. They would be expected to behave like students, for example they might order more laboratory work. The staff service consists of more seasoned physicians. We might expect a more parsimonious use of resources, and better outcomes of care to reflect their experience with taking care of patients.
3. Patients treated by the resident service had, on average, a longer length of stay and higher charges than patients treated by the staff service, and the differences were statistically significant. The higher in-hospital and eight-month mortality rates and lower readmission rate were not statistically significant.
4. There were other differences between the two groups besides experience; for example, the staff service spent fewer hours on the unit because of additional clinic, research, and teaching responsibilities. The random assignment of patients to one of the two services should have resulted in two very similar groups of patients. It is unlikely that patient differences were responsible for these results.

5. The authors argue for the integrity of the randomization process by assuring that there was no violation of random assignment, no patients reassigned due to "influence of the treatment teams," and no crossovers to the other service. Therefore selection bias should have been minimal. There is no reason to suspect misclassification bias of outcomes due to the length of stay, cost, mortality, or readmission.

Meta-Analysis

Frequently, a review of the literature will reveal a number of studies, some randomized, some not, that have examined the efficacy of a particular treatment or agent. Many of these studies are based on small samples, with low statistical power, and nonsignificant or conflicting treatment effects. Researchers, clinicians, and other decision makers then face the challenge of making sense out of the many worthy efforts that have already taken place, perhaps before a large-scale and more conclusive RCT can be funded. The term *meta-analysis* refers to a set of complex statistical techniques that have been developed to pool the results of multiple studies and to derive aggregate treatment effects.

Meta-analysis is supposed to answer four fundamental questions (Lau and Ioannidis 1998): (1) Do different studies have similar results? (2) What is the best estimate of the treatment effect? (3) To what extent is this estimate precise and robust? (4) Why are there differences among the studies? The purpose of meta-analysis is to increase statistical power, resolve disagreements among multiple studies, improve "effect size" estimates, and pose new questions (Sacks et al. 1987).

Horwitz (1995) compares meta-analysis to the single center and multicenter RCT. With the single center RCT, data are collected from multiple subjects according to an established protocol for selecting and randomizing patients, administering treatments, and measuring outcomes. In a multicenter RCT, researchers use the same protocol at different sites. One might be tempted to draw a methodologic analogy between meta-analysis and the multicenter RCT, in the sense that the purpose of both is to combine the results from multiple and somewhat independent sources of inquiry. The major difference, however, is the lack of a common protocol, which leads to heterogeneity—different patients, different treatments, and sometimes different outcomes.

The first challenge with meta-analysis is to identify which studies to include. This involves the difficult chore of searching the literature (both published and unpublished) for relevant studies, while recognizing that a publication bias exists against small studies and those without a statistically significant treatment effect. Even more difficult, perhaps, is determining the degree of heterogeneity that can be tolerated in terms of different kinds of patients, protocols, treatments, and outcomes. "Apples" and "oranges" should not be combined, but one might derive meaningful results by combining "McIntosh" and "Rome" apples.

The actual statistical techniques that have been formulated to combine the results of multiple studies are beyond the scope of this book. By way of summary, the simplest approach is to calculate an average effect size (ES), where the ES for each study is the difference between the means of the control group and treatment group divided by the standard deviation of the control group (Wortman 1983). The ES is weighted by the degree of uncertainty associated with the results. Other sophisticated approaches have been developed when treatment effects are reported as a risk ratio, odds ratio, risk difference, or incidence rate.

Consider Weaver and colleagues (1997), for example, who were interested in comparing primary coronary angioplasty (PTCA) with intravenous thrombolytic therapy ("Lytic") for acute myocardial infarction. They identified ten randomized studies that met the criteria for inclusion in the meta-analysis. The measured outcome is mortality, and the treatment effect is measured in terms of an odds ratio: the increased (or decreased) odds of death when treated with PTCA versus thrombolytics. Confidence intervals are presented around each estimate, indicating the degree of uncertainty, and a total treatment effect is estimated using meta-analytical techniques.

Although meta-analysis provides a reasonable and quantitative approach to aggregating the fruit of scientific inquiry, it is not without problems, limitations, and severe criticism (Spitzer 1995). Generally, meta-analysis should not be used to contrive statistical significance from a collection of small, insignificant studies, although there may be occasions when this is appropriate, particularly when small treatment effects are relevant (Victor 1995). Meta-analysis is a reasonable approach for dealing with contradictory studies, for reaching urgent consensus, or when the opportunity to conduct a large-scale RCT is gone (Friedman, Furberg, and DeMets 1996).

Heterogeneity is the Achilles' heel of meta-analysis, the vulnerable underbelly at which most critics take aim. Clearly, the credibility of aggregating multiple studies into one large pool depends on demonstrating that all of the studies are reasonably similar in terms of protocol. Some would argue that this is the exception rather than the rule or that, in fact, the observed differences among these "somewhat" similar studies may be clinically relevant. In other words, the process of combining results to obtain some global effect may obscure meaningful differences among the studies related to patients or protocol (Horwitz 1995). Feinstein (1995) goes so far as to describe meta-analysis as "statistical alchemy for the 21st century," which uses a "mixed salad principle" (i.e., combining apples with oranges) to try to get something from nothing "while simultaneously ignoring established scientific principles."

While the jury may still be out regarding the conceptual validity of the meta-analytic approach, it should be justified empirically as well. This may be difficult; for example, Lelorier and colleagues (1997) compared 19 meta-analyses with 12 large and subsequently randomized controlled trials and reported a large measure of disagreement. The authors concluded that "the meta-analysis would have led to the adoption of an inefficient treatment in 32 percent of cases...and to the rejection of a useful treatment in 33 percent of cases."

Community Trials

It may be appropriate for certain kinds of interventions to increase the unit of analysis from the individual subject or patient to a larger "community" unit, such as city, town, region, or census tract. These studies are referred to in the literature as *community trials*, and they may or may not be randomized designs. This kind of study is especially appropriate for interventions that are easier or less costly to deliver through some common venue—such as over the radio or television or in the water supply—or when it may be difficult to prevent treatment "contamination" as discussed earlier.

The design of a community trial is similar in many ways to the more traditional randomized controlled trial. A protocol should be articulated that specifies the procedures for recruiting and selecting communities, delivering the experimental intervention, and measuring the specific effects. Sample size may be even more of a constraint due to the cost and logistics of recruiting multiple communities. If possible, the communities should be similar in terms of size, economies, and ethnicities (Lilienfeld and Stolley 1994), with stable populations and medical care systems that are self-contained (Kessler and Levin 1972).

The execution of the community trial is also similar to the more traditional RCT. The process of recruiting communities to participate in the study is analogous to obtaining informed consent. Local community leaders and elected officials must be convinced of the merit of participating in the study and must formally consent as representatives of the residents who will be affected by the intervention. Baseline measurements of the outcome(s) that should be affected by the intervention (e.g., neonatal mortality rates) are collected for each of the eligible communities that have agreed to participate. The communities are then randomly assigned to either treatment or control groups and followed for a defined period. The difference between end-of-study and baseline outcome(s) is calculated and compared for treatment and control communities to determine if the treatment effect is statistically significant.

Two examples of community trials are the Stanford Five City Project (Farquhar et al. 1985, 1990) and the Minnesota Heart Health Program

(Luepker et al. 1996). Both studies involved individual and community-wide health education efforts, and both used a relatively small number of communities (five for Stanford and six for Minnesota). Both were designed to decrease the rate of cardiovascular disease through prevention. The Stanford study measured physiological risk factors such as blood pressure, weight, and cholesterol, whereas the Minnesota study was aimed at the incidence of coronary heart disease and stroke.

With other studies, the unit of analysis may be smaller. In one study, for instance, 450 Indonesian villages were randomized into a vitamin A treatment group and a control group that did not get the supplementation (Abdeljaber et al. 1991). In another, an AIDS education program was tested in Tanzania, where 18 public primary schools were randomly assigned to an educational intervention designed to promote risk reduction (Klepp et al. 1997). In a third, 296 households in Tecumseh, Michigan, were stratified by size and randomized into a treatment group that received virucidal nasal tissues and a group that did not (Longini and Monto 1988). (The question was whether these tissues were effective in reducing the transmission of influenza across family members.)

The choice of whether to design a community trial vis-à-vis the more traditional RCT depends on the nature and complexity of the intervention, as well as the size of the population on which the intervention must focus (Blackburn 1983; Kottke et al. 1985; Farquhar et al. 1990; Lilienfeld and Stolley 1994). Interventions dealing with risk factor modification and behavioral change, for instance, may be delivered more effectively through some community vehicle, such as education programs in the mass media (Syme 1978). In addition, in cases involving complex interventions, it may be easier to adjust and manipulate the environment with a community trial. If the targeted disease is highly prevalent in certain communities, or if the population to be studied must be necessarily large, it may be more efficient to orchestrate a community trial rather than to incur the expense of recruiting many individual subjects (Lilienfeld and Stolley 1994).

Summary

Neuhauser (1991) pointed to the biblical account of Daniel (before his deliverance from the lion's den) as one of the first clinical trials. The question was whether a diet of vegetables was as efficacious as Babylonian cuisine in terms of "countenance." The conclusion reached after a ten-day trial period was that "their countenances appeared fairer and fatter in flesh than all the children which did eat the portion of the king's meat" (Daniel 1:15, King James Version). This was an interesting observation, though the study was clearly not randomized, nor was it free of confounding factors, given the history of divine intervention on the part of the Lord God of Israel. The randomized clinical trial of today has enjoyed the reputation of being the exalted, gold standard of research to which all other modes of inquiry must bow. Clearly this distinction rests on the laurels of the randomization, as it should, since potentially confounding factors should be equally allocated to treatment and control groups. The authority of the noble RCT can be challenged, however, by threats to validity in the form of refusals, dropouts, crossovers, and contaminated treatments. The RCT is an elegant research design, but not a flawless one.

References

Abdeljaber, M. H., A. S. Monto, R. L. Tilden, M. A. Schork, and I. Tarwotojo. 1991. "The Impact of Vitamin A Supplementation on Morbidity: A Randomized Community Intervention Trial." *American Journal of Public Health* 81 (12): 1654–56.

Baum, M. 1993. "New Approach for Recruitment into Randomised Controlled Trials." [Comment.] *Lancet* 341 (8848): 812–13.

Blackburn, H. 1983. "Research and Demonstration Projects in Community Cardiovascular Disease Prevention." *Journal of Public Health Policy* 4 (4): 398–421.

Byar, D. P., D. A. Schoenfeld, S. B. Green, D. A. Amato, R. Davis, V. DeGruttola, D. M. Finkelstein, C. Gutsonis, R. D. Gelber, S. Lagakos, M. Lefkopoulou, A. A. Tsiatis, M. Zelen, J. Peto, L. S. Freedman, M. Gail, R. Simon, S. S. Ellenberg, J. R. Anderson, R. Collins, R. Peto, and F. Peto. 1990. "Design Considerations for AIDS Trials." *New England Journal of Medicine* 323 (19): 1343–48.

Cebul, R. D. 1991. "Randomized, Controlled Trials Using the Metro Firm System." *Medical Care* 29 (7, Suppl.): JS9–JS18.

Curley, C., J. E. McEachern, and T. Speroff. 1998. "A Firm Trial of Interdisciplinary Rounds on the Inpatient Medical Wards: An Intervention Designed Using Continuous Quality Improvement." *Medical Care* 36 (8, Suppl.): AS4–AS12.

Dawson, N. V. 1991. "Organizing the Metro Firm System for Research." *Medical Care* 29 (7, Suppl.): JS19–JS25.

DeBusk, R. F., N. H. Miller, H. R. Superko, C. A. Dennis, R. J. Thomas, H. T. Lew, W. E. Berger, R. S. Heller, J. Rompf, D. Gee, H. C. Kraemer, A. Bandura, G. Ghandour, M. Clark, R. V. Shah, L. Fisher, and B. Taylor. 1994. "A Case-Management System for Coronary Risk Factor Modification After Acute Myocardial Infarction." *Annals of Internal Medicine* 120 (9): 721–29.

Diel, I. J., E. Solomayer, S. D. Costa, C. Gollan, R. Goerner, D. Wallwiener, M. Kaufmann, and G. Bastert. 1998. "Reduction in New Metastases in Breast Cancer with Adjuvant Clodronate Treatment." *New England*

Journal of Medicine 339 (6): 357–63.

Early Breast Cancer Trialists' Collaborative Group. 1992. "Systemic Treatment of Early Breast Cancer by Hormonal, Cytotoxic, or Immune Therapy." *Lancet* 339 (8785): 71–85.

———. 1995. "Effects of Radiotherapy and Surgery in Early Breast Cancer: An Overview of the Randomized Trials." *New England Journal of Medicine* 333 (22): 1444–55.

Elwood, M. 1998. *Critical Appraisal of Epidemiological Studies and Clinical Trials.* New York: Oxford University Press.

Farquhar, J. W., S. P. Fortmann, J. A. Flora, C. B. Taylor, W. L. Haskell, P. J. Williams, N. Maccoby, and P. D. Wood. 1990. "Effects of Communitywide Education on Cardiovascular Disease Risk Factors: The Stanford Five-City Project." *Journal of the American Medical Association* 264 (3): 359–65.

Farquhar, J. W., S. P. Fortmann, N. Maccoby, W. L. Haskell, P. T. Williams, J. A. Flora, C. B. Taylor, B. W. Brown, Jr., D. S. Solomon, and S. B. Holley. 1985. "The Stanford Five-City Project: Design and Methods." *American Journal of Epidemiology* 264: 359–65.

Feinstein, A. R. 1995. "Meta-Analysis: Statistical Alchemy for the 21st Century." *Journal of Clinical Epidemiology* 48 (1): 71–79.

Fischl, M. A., D. D. Richman, M. H. Grieco, M. S. Gottlieb, P. A. Volberling, O. L. Laskin, J. M. Leedom, J. E. Groopman, D. Mildvan, and R. T. Schooley. 1987. "The Efficacy of Azidothymidine (AZT) in the Treatment of Patients with AIDS and AIDS-Related Complex." *New England Journal of Medicine* 317 (4): 185–91.

Fisher, B., S. Anderson, C. K. Redmond, N. Wolmark, D. L. Wickerham, and W. M. Cronin. 1995. "Reanalysis and Results After 12 Years of Follow-up in a Randomized Clinical Trial Comparing Total Mastectomy with Lumpectomy With or Without Irradiation in the Treatment of Breast Cancer." *New England Journal of Medicine* 333 (22): 1456–61.

Friedman, L. M., C. D. Furberg, and D. L. DeMets. 1996. *Fundamentals of Clinical Trials.* St. Louis, MO: Mosby.

GISSI Prevenzione Investigators. 1999. "Dietary Supplementation with n-3 Polyunsaturated Fatty Acids and Vitamin E After Myocardial Infarction: Results of the GISSI-Prevenzione Trial." *Lancet* 354 (9177): 447–55.

Goldberg, H. I., and H. McGough. 1991. "The Ethics of Ongoing Randomization Trials." *Medical Care* 29 (7, Suppl.): JS41–JS48.

Gordis, L. 2004. *Epidemiology,* 3rd ed. Philadelphia, PA: W. B. Saunders.

Gradishar, W. J., M. S. Tallman, and J. S. Abrams. 1996. "High-Dose Chemotherapy for Breast Cancer." [Comment.] *Annals of Internal Medicine* 125 (7): 599–604.

Hellman, S., and D. S. Hellman. 1991. "Of Mice but Not Men: Problems of the Randomized Clinical Trial." [Comment.] *New England Journal of Medicine* 324 (22): 1585–89.

Horwitz, R. I. 1995. "Large-Scale Randomized Evidence: Large Simple Trials and Overviews of Trials. Discussion: A Clinician's Perspective on Meta-Analysis." *Journal of Clinical Epidemiology* 48 (1): 41–44.

Ioannidis, J. P., J. C. Cappelleri, J. Lau, P. R. Skolnik, B. Melville, T. C. Chalmers, and H. S. Sacks. 1995. "Early or Deferred Zidovudine Therapy in HIV-Infected Patients Without an AIDS-Defining Illness." *Annals of Internal Medicine* 122 (11): 856–66.

Kessler, I. I., and M. L. Levin. 1972. *The Community as an Epidemiological Laboratory.* Baltimore, MD: Johns Hopkins University Press.

Klepp, K. I., S. S. Ndeki, M. T. Leshabari, P. J. Hannan, and B. A. Lyimo. 1997. "AIDS Education in Tanzania: Promoting Risk Reduction Among Primary School Children." *American Journal of Public Health* 87 (12): 1931–36.

Kottke, T. E., P. Puska, J. T. Salonen, J. Tuomilehto, and A. Nissinen. 1985. "Projected Effects of High-Risk Versus Population-Based Prevention Strategies in Coronary Heart Disease." *American Journal of Epidemiology* 121 (5): 697–704.

Lau, J., and J. P. A. Ioannidis. 1998. "Quantitative Synthesis in Systemic Reviews." In *Systemic Reviews: Synthesis of Best Evidence for Health Care Decisions,* 91–101. Philadelphia, PA: American College of Physicians.

LeLorier, J., G. Grégoire, A. Benhaddad, J. Lapierre, and F. Derderian. 1997. "Discrepancies Between Meta-Analyses and Subsequent Large Randomized, Controlled Trials." *New England Journal of Medicine* 337 (8): 536–42.

Lilienfeld, D. E., and P. D. Stolley. 1994. *Foundations of Epidemiology.* New York: Oxford University Press.

Longini, I. M., and A. S. Monto. 1988. "Efficacy of Virucidal Nasal Tissues in Interrupting Familial Transmission of Respiratory Agents: A Field Trial in Tecumseh, Michigan." *American Journal of Epidemiology* 128 (3): 639–44.

Luepker, R. V., L. Rastam, P. J. Hannan, D. M. Murray, C. Gray, W. L. Baker, R. Crow, D. R. Jackobs, Jr., P. L. Pirie, S. R. Mascioli, M. B. Mittelmark, and H. Blackburn. 1996. "Community Education for Cardiovascular Disease Prevention: Morbidity and Mortality Results from the Minnesota Heart Health Program." *American Journal of Epidemiology* 144 (4): 351–62.

Lurie, N., J. Christianson, and I. Moscovice. 1994. "The Effects of Capitation on Health and Functional Status of the Medicaid Elderly: A." *Annals of Internal Medicine* 120 (6): 506–11.

Lurie, N., I. S. Moscovice, M. Finch, and J. B. Christianson. 1992. "Does Capitation Affect the Health of the Chronically Mentally Ill? Results from A." *Journal of the American Medical Association* 267 (24): 3300–04.

Multiple Risk Factor Intervention Trial Research Group. 1982. "Multiple Risk Factor Intervention Trial: Risk Factor Changes and Mortality Results." *Journal of the American Medical Association* 248 (12): 1465–77.

Neuhauser, D. 1991. "Parallel Providers, Ongoing Randomization, and Continuous Improvement." *Medical Care* 29 (7, Suppl.): JS5–JS8.

Newhouse, J. P. 1991. "Controlled Experimentation as Research Policy." In *Health Services Research: Key to Health Policy*, edited by E. Ginzberg, 397. Cambridge, MA: Harvard University Press.

Palmer, R. H., T. A. Louis, H. F. Peterson, J. K. Rothrock, R. Strain, and E. A. Wright. 1996. "What Makes Quality Assurance Effective? Results from a Randomized, Controlled Trial in 16 Primary Care Group Practices." *Medical Care* 34 (9, Suppl.): SS29–SS39.

Pilote, L., R. J. Thomas, C. Dennis, P. Goins, N. Houston-Miller, H. Kraemer, C. Leong, W. E. Berger, H. Lew, R. S. Heller, J. Rompf, and R. F. DeBusk. 1992. "Return to Work After Uncomplicated Myocardial Infarction: A Trial of Practice Guidelines in the Community." *Annals of Internal Medicine* 117 (5): 383–89.

Pritchard, R. S., and S. P. Anthony. 1996. "Chemotherapy Plus Radiotherapy Compared with Radiotherapy Alone in the Treatment of Lung Cancer." *Annals of Internal Medicine* 125 (9): 723–29.

Reuben, D. B., G. M. Borok, G. Wolde-Tsadik, D. H. Ershoff, L. K. Fishman, V. L. Ambrosini, Y. Liu, L. Z. Rubenstein, and J. C. Beck. 1995. "A Randomized Trial of Comprehensive Geriatric Assessment in the Care of Hospitalized Patients." *New England Journal of Medicine* 332 (20): 1345–50.

Rosselli-Del-Turco, M., D. Palli, A. Cariddi, S. Ciatto, P. Pacini, and V. Distante. 1994. "Intensive Diagnostic Follow-up, After Treatment of Primary Breast Cancer: A Randomized Trial." *Journal of the American Medical Association* 271 (20): 1593–97.

Sacks, H. S., J. Berrier, D. Reitman, V. A. Ancona-Berk, and T. C. Chalmers. 1987. "Meta-Analysis of Randomized Controlled Trials." *New England Journal of Medicine* 316 (8): 450–55.

Senn, S. 1995. "A Personal View of Some Controversies in Allocating Treatment to Patients in Clinical Trials." *Statistics in Medicine* 14 (24): 2661–74.

Simmer, T. L., D. R. Nerenz, W. M. Rutt, C. S. Newcomb, and D. W. Benfer. 1991. "A Randomized, Controlled Trial of an Attending Staff Service in General Internal Medicine." *Medical Care* 29 (7, Suppl.): JS31–JS40.

Spitzer, W. O. 1995. "The Challenge of Meta-Analysis." *Journal of Clinical Epidemiology* 48 (1): 1–4.

Stoner, T. J., B. Dowd, W. P. Carr, G. Maldonado, T. R. Church, and J. Mandel. 1998. "Do Vouchers Improve Breast Cancer Screening Rates?

Results from a Randomized Trial." *Health Services Research* 33 (1): 11–28.

Syme, S. L. 1978. "Life Style Intervention in Clinic-Based Trials." *American Journal of Epidemiology* 108 (1): 87–91.

Victor, N. 1995. "The Challenge of Meta-Analysis: Discussion, Indications and Contra-indications for Meta-Analysis." *Journal of Clinical Epidemiology* 48 (1): 5–8.

Volberding, P. A., and N. M. Graham. 1994. "Initiation of Antiretroviral Therapy in HIV Infection: A Review of Interstudy Consistencies." *Journal of Acquired Immune Deficiency Syndromes* 7 (Suppl. 2): S12–S23.

Weaver, W. D., R. J. Simes, A. Betriu, C. Grines, F. Zijlstra, E. Garcia, L. Grinfeld, R. Gibbons, E. Ribeiro, M. DeWood, and F. Ribichini. 1997. "Comparison of Primary Coronary Angioplasty and Intravenous Thrombolytic Therapy for Acute Myocardial Infarction: A Quantitative Review." *Journal of the American Medical Association* 278 (23): 2093–98.

Weinstein, G. S., and B. Levin. 1989. "Effect of Crossover on the Statistical Power of Randomized Studies." *Annals of Thoracic Surgery* 48 (4): 490–95.

Wood, D., N. Halfon, C. Donald-Sherbourne, R. M. Mazel, M. Schuster, J. S. Hamlin, M. Pereyra, P. Camp, M. Grabowsky, and N. Duan. 1998. "Increasing Immunization Rates Among Inner-City, African American Children: A Randomized Trial of Case Management." *Journal of the American Medical Association* 279 (1): 29–34.

Wortman, P. M. 1983. "Meta-Analysis: A Validity Perspective." In *Evaluation Studies Review Annual*, edited by R. J. Light, vol. 8, 157–66. Beverly Hills, CA: Sage.

CLINICAL EPIDEMIOLOGY AND DECISION MAKING

Kevin A. Pearce, Steven T. Fleming, F. Douglas Scutchfield

> *"The greater the ignorance, the greater the dogmatism."* Sir William Osler, Canadian physician, 1849–1919

For the purposes of this chapter, *clinical epidemiology* refers to the use of evidence, derived from observational and experimental studies of human illness or risk factors for illness, in medical decision making. Rational and critical synthesis of available information is a prerequisite. Clinical epidemiology differs from population epidemiology in that the denominator is usually a subpopulation of patients who are treated in a healthcare setting.

This chapter addresses the evolving applications of clinical epidemiology in routine medical practice and discusses some areas ripe for expansion of this type of thinking, all from the viewpoint of the practicing generalist physician. Consider these scenarios:

1. You have recently been given the responsibility of coordinating cardiovascular disease screening and prevention services for a small regional managed care organization (MCO). Two of the large local employers that currently offer your health plan to their employees are especially interested in cholesterol screening and treatment as criteria for continued participation. Your MCO contracts with 175 primary care physicians and 12 cardiologists. You decide to query these physicians for suggestions regarding covered services. Their responses range from "screening for high cholesterol is a waste of time, because people won't change their habits anyway, and the medicines do not work very well," to "all enrollees over the age of 30 should have their cholesterol levels checked regularly, and those with high levels should have lifelong medication as a covered benefit." Several respondents cite research findings to support their opinions.

2. You are the manager of a 20-physician family practice/internal medicine group that is shopping for an electronic medical records system. They want to be sure the system will include prompts and evidence-based guidelines to help them optimize preventive services and the medical management of the four most common chronic diseases in their practice, and that they can update the system as new evidence emerges. Your task is to identify the top three vendors in terms of meeting the group's criteria.

3. As the CEO of an MCO, you are subjected to strenuous lobbying by several contracting employers and physicians. They want your MCO to offer a smoking cessation program as a covered benefit, citing the cost savings to be expected from the prevention of tobacco-related diseases.

In all of these scenarios, and in hundreds of similar ones played out each week, American healthcare managers must navigate through a morass of bias, opinions, and even ulterior motives to arrive at the best solution. Assuming the sought-after solution transcends political and fiscal expedience, clinical evidence will have to be understood and weighed in order for the manager to foster the best outcome.

Implicit is the fact that clinical medicine is moving away from practices based on opinion and tradition toward those based on scientific evidence (Dickersin, Straus, and Bero 2007). This paradigm shift represents a true revolution in healthcare. Although much of what most physicians do today lacks solid supporting evidence, the increasing pace of high-quality clinical research coupled with an information management revolution promises sweeping changes in physician decision making.

Indeed, many practicing physicians are already using clinical epidemiology to guide more and more of their opinions and actions. An understanding of the uses, abuses, and pitfalls of clinical epidemiology will strengthen the influence of healthcare managers, and increase their value to physicians and healthcare organizations. That value will ultimately be manifest in improved health for the patients served.

Experience and Tradition in Medical Practice

Consider another scenario. In 1984, a 60-year-old man was admitted from the emergency department to the coronary care unit with a myocardial infarction (MI). His physician knew the first 48 hours after an MI are a time of high risk for severe or fatally abnormal heartbeat rhythms (arrythmias). Following the advice of his past teachers and the custom of his colleagues, the physician ordered the drug lidocaine to prevent such arrythmias (the drug has been proven to suppress these arrythmias once they occur). He also ordered complete bed rest for three days, followed by a strictly graduated exercise program in the hospital over the next ten days. The man was released home on the 11th day.

This physician, lacking reliable clinical evidence to prove or disprove his course of action, relied heavily on experience and tradition. In the light of current scientific evidence, we now know that the lidocaine he prescribed was more likely to cause serious problems in this type of case than to prevent them, and that for most patients there is no need for an expensive ten days of graduated activity in the hospital after an MI.

Although we often think of medicine as a science, clinical practice relies heavily on experience and tradition as handed down from teacher to student and shared among colleagues. Medical education is generally divided into the basic sciences (e.g., anatomy, physiology, biochemistry, and genetics) and the clinical sciences (e.g., physical diagnosis and the behavioral, medical, and surgical disciplines). The science of medicine is firmly rooted in knowledge derived from the basic sciences.

But the complexity of the human body as a whole, multiplied by the intricacies of human experience and a person's interactions with his or her entire environment, makes clinical practice as much an art as a science. Currently, there is simply a lack of scientifically derived information available to inform practitioners as they make many of their clinical decisions (Shaughnessy, Slawson, and Becker 1998). This is especially problematic in situations where lifelong treatment (e.g., new oral medications for diabetes) is considered, because data on long-term outcomes are often lacking.

Thus, practitioners must often rely on their own experience, that of their teachers and colleagues, logic, intuition, and the traditions upheld by generations comprising a lore of unproven concepts so well-worn that they are assumed to be true. This reliance on nonscientific means has its advantages; if physicians insisted on rigid adherence to scientific proof for their treatments, most patients would get no treatment. Instead, many do receive sensible (if unproven) treatments. Furthermore, experience and tradition humanize the application of science to medicine and encourage caution against the wholesale adoption of scientifically "proven" ideas that run counter to experience (Shaughnessy, Slawson, and Becker 1998). The fallibility of science applied to the human experience justifies such caution.

Still, there are obvious dangers associated with medical practices guided by what is presumed to be "best," as opposed to reliance on best practices supported by rigorous scientific evaluation. More scientifically derived information is needed continuously to inform clinical practices.

The Evidence Base of Clinical Practice

In light of the current information explosion, the limitations of the evidence base applied in clinical practice are astonishing. As of 2006, the National Library of Medicine's MEDLINE (www.nlm.nih.gov) database of medical journal articles contained about 15.6 million references, and at least 500,000 new entries are added each year. Billions of dollars in public and private funds are spent on medical research each year. Why, then, is clinical practice not primarily evidence based?

In our opinion, the main reasons are (1) the gap between the kinds of scientific medical evidence produced and the kinds needed to reliably inform best clinical practices, and (2) barriers that prevent practicing physicians from assimilating the rapid changes and expansions of pertinent scientific information. These barriers slow the transfer of new knowledge from the lab to the bedside to the medical office.

Much of medical research is disease oriented and focused on the basic sciences. As such, it advances knowledge about the biophysical mechanisms of disease. This type of new knowledge forms the basis for many of the advances in the clinical sciences that follow.

However, advances in the basic sciences rarely, if ever, address the length or quality of any patient's life and are usually not directly applicable to clinical decision making. An example of a basic science advance is the elucidation of hormonal mechanisms important to the development of high blood pressure (Ferrario 1990). This advance had to be translated into drug development and extensive clinical trials to influence medical practice (Maggioni 2006).

Clinical research may be *disease oriented* or *patient oriented*. The latter refers to new knowledge that directly addresses length or quality of life, and it is relatively rare. Only a small portion of all medical research published each year produces patient-oriented evidence that can be relied on to improve clinical practices (Slawson, Shaughnessy, and Bennett 1994; Ebell et al. 1999).

An example of a disease-oriented advance in clinical science is the demonstration that a certain class of drug (called statins) lowers cholesterol without negative biochemical side effects (Davignon et al. 1994; Nawrocki et al. 1995). This research has led to patient-oriented studies that show this type of medication to actually prevent heart attacks without serious negative side effects (Grundy et al. 2004). These studies lasted four to five years, so the question remains about whether lifelong treatment with statins is good for people at high risk of heart attack.

Rarely is clinical practice informed by proof from patient-oriented research. Rather, evidence is compiled from multiple sources and weighed. Evidence that most strongly influences clinical practice satisfies the criteria for causality (see box), first proposed by Koch for acute infectious diseases and since revised to be applicable to chronic diseases as well (Evans 1978). These criteria can be applied to evidence about the causes of disease, disease prevention, screening, diagnosis, or treatment of disease. In addition to addressing these criteria, high-quality evidence must be based on valid measurements and must be as free as possible from bias and error. Furthermore, to be applied confidently by clinicians, the evidence must be generalizable from the group of people studied to the patients whom the physician actually sees.

Clinical evidence is derived from observational and experimental studies. It is generally held that well-controlled clinical experiments (i.e., randomized controlled trials, or RCTs) provide a higher quality of evidence than do observational studies (i.e., case reports, cohort or case control studies).

This is because observational studies are more prone to bias than are well-controlled experiments. In practice, experimental investigations usually follow observational studies as a way to confirm hypotheses generated by the observations. The results of these clinical experiments can be used to guide medical practices in a process called *evidence-based clinical decision making*.

CRITERIA FOR CAUSALITY

Strength of association: Exposure is strongly associated with disease; treatment is strongly associated with improvement.

Consistency of association: The apparent relationship between exposure and disease is consistent from study to study and/or population to population.

Temporality of relationship: Hypothesized cause precedes hypothesized effect; that is, exposure precedes disease, or treatment precedes improvement.

Specificity of effect: Exposure always causes only one disease, and is the sole cause for that disease; treatment brings about specific improvement (this criterion often is not applicable in multifactorial diseases).

Dose-response gradient: The duration and/or intensity of exposure are associated with more severe or frequent disease; more treatment is associated with more improvement (obvious toxicity limitations on the latter).

Biological plausibility: Basic scientific evidence supports the cause-effect relationship between exposure and disease or treatment and improvement.

Experimental confirmation: Controlled experiments confirm the hypothesized cause-effect relationship (preferably in real patients when ethically feasible).

As an example of applying these rules of evidence to a clinical problem, let us revisit the scenario in which you are the CEO of an MCO who is being pressured to offer a smoking cessation program as a covered benefit. Believing short-term political expedience to be insufficient for your decision, you ask the medical director of your MCO to help you look at the evidence that such programs can be expected to actually improve enrollees' health. The medical director convinces you to focus on the most common (heart disease) and most feared (lung cancer) diseases associated with smoking in an examination of the evidence.

Always the open-minded skeptic, you want to review the evidence base related to these questions:

1. Does cigarette smoking really cause heart disease and lung cancer?
2. Does quitting smoking reduce the risk of these diseases?
3. Are smoking cessation programs effective?

Question 1: Does cigarette smoking really cause heart disease and lung cancer?

A review of the published evidence shows a strong and consistent association between smoking and lung cancer (tenfold increase in risk) and a moderate and consistent association with heart disease (two- to threefold risk). Furthermore, prospective observational studies have established causal temporality by showing that smoking preceded the onset of disease. The same studies have shown that the duration and intensity (packs per day) of cigarette smoking is positively associated with the risk of developing lung cancer or heart disease. Laboratory studies on cigarette smoke and experiments involving short-term smoking by human volunteers have demonstrated multiple biological mechanisms that plausibly explain a causal link between smoking and these diseases (U.S. Department of Health and Human Services [USDHHS] 1989; U.S. Preventive Services Task Force 2007; Ockene and Miller 1997).

Most of the criteria for causality are fulfilled, but there are two gaps: (1) cigarette smoking is neither the sole specific cause of lung cancer or heart disease, nor does it always lead to either disease (contrast this with the HIV virus and AIDS); and (2) although animal experiments have partially confirmed the causal link, there are not (and never will be) fully controlled human experiments confirming that smoking causes these diseases.

Question 2: Does quitting smoking reduce the risk of lung cancer and heart disease?

Once again, observational studies show a strong and consistent association between smoking cessation and dramatic reductions in the risk of lung cancer and heart disease that almost reach the magnitude of the increased risk associated with smoking in the first place. The temporality criterion is fulfilled as prospective observational studies consistently show that ex-smokers develop lung cancer or heart disease at lower rates than those who continue to smoke. Biological plausibility related to quitting is fulfilled by laboratory studies of cigarette smoke combined with observational studies of biochemical, cellular, and physiological changes in humans who quit smoking (USDHHS 1989; U.S. Preventive Services Task Force 2007; Ockene and Miller 1997). In this case, intensity of the exposure (quitting) is not applicable, but the relative risks of lung cancer and heart disease, compared to those for continuing smokers, keep falling for 5 to 15 years after quitting.

The shortfalls in proving causality are, again, (1) smoking cessation does not specifically guarantee prevention of these diseases, nor is it the only thing that protects against them; and (2) there are not (and will probably never be) well-controlled experiments of the long-term health effects of actual smoking cessation. There is, however, limited experimental evidence that shows long-term beneficial health effects of smoking cessation programs (U.S. Preventive Services Task Force 2007; Ockene and Miller 1997).

Question 3: Are smoking cessation programs effective (i.e., do smoking cessation programs cause smokers to quit)?

In this case, there is more experimental confirmation than observational evidence. In multiple controlled experiments in which smokers were randomly assigned to receive a smoking cessation program versus no special treatment, there has been a consistent, though usually modest, effect of smoking cessation programs on quitting rates after one year. Temporality is not an issue in these experimental data (only current smokers were exposed to the interventions). Most of these programs used either individual or group counseling; some used only brief individual advice from a physician; some combined nicotine replacement therapy or other drug therapy with advice or counseling. Intensity and duration of the program were not clearly associated with success rates, but a dose-response effect of nicotine replacement was observed. Biological plausibility was fulfilled through animal and human experiments on nicotine addiction.

Specificity of effect is lacking in this evidence base, and strength of association is, at best, moderate. Smoking cessation programs do not always cause people to quit, and many people quit without a program. In fact, programs without nicotine replacement or other medication increase quit rates by about 6 percent above the "background" rate of 3 percent to 5 percent, and those incorporating nicotine replacement and/or other medication accomplish 12-month abstinence rates of 15 percent to 35 percent (U.S. Preventive Services Task Force 2007).

For each question, you must weigh the evidence to arrive at an answer. Do the strengths of the evidence base for each question outweigh the shortfalls enough for you to answer each in the affirmative and move on from the decision whether to provide the service to how to provide it?

Suppose you conclude that the evidence is sufficient to answer "yes" to each of your three questions about smoking. Your work is not yet completed, because you have to consider potential confounding factors that could limit the application of these findings to the people covered by your health plan.

Did the smokers included in these studies have important similarities or differences compared with your health plan enrollees? Factors such as general health, age, education, motivation, employment, and social support might be important in terms of the health effects of smoking and the effectiveness of smoking cessation programs. Also, were the study circumstances surrounding the smoking cessation programs significantly different than they would be for your enrollees? Where were the programs offered? What prompted people to use the programs? In short, decision makers must bear in mind that a body of high-quality evidence that adequately fulfills criteria for causality is not necessarily applicable to all individuals or all groups. In practice, thoughtful consideration should be employed to decide if the evidence base applies to the people, setting, and circumstances under your scrutiny.

The Clinical Encounter

To better understand how physicians use (or could use) clinical epidemiology, let us examine what happens when a patient visits a physician. First, consider common types of questions that patients bring with them:

• What is wrong with me?
• What are my options now? What would I experience with each option?
• Can I get rid of this illness? If so, what do I have to go through, and how long will it take?
• I know what I need...can I convince the doctor to prescribe it?
• How am I doing with my chronic problems?
• How can I stay as healthy as possible for as long as possible?

Next, consider the same questions as they are posed by the physician:

• What is this patient's diagnosis?
• What are the treatment options?
• What is the prognosis (including potential adverse effects) for this individual for each treatment option (including no treatment)?
• Has the patient been educated according to the available pertinent medical evidence?
• Are the current and future effects of this patient's chronic problems being minimized?
• What should be done to maximize this person's health, and to prevent disability and disease for as long as possible?

Let us also consider potential areas of synergy and conflict for the physician in terms of providing the best medical care to each individual as opposed to promoting the best possible care for an entire patient population:

- What, if anything, should limit the amount of medical resources used for any one of my patients?
- What should my staff and I do to have the most positive impact on all of my patients?

These questions translate to issues of diagnosis, treatment, prevention, and cost-effectiveness, all of which can be informed by the use of clinical epidemiology by the physician. Conversely, the physician can approach them through reliance on experience, tradition, intuition, or all three, with little attention to clinical epidemiology. The availability of reliable clinical evidence will often determine the physician's approach to any problem, but knowledge of, and comfort with, clinical epidemiology is obviously critical.

We will use two hypothetical primary care physicians to illustrate the ends of the spectrum between barely using clinical epidemiology (Dr. Lore) versus heavy reliance on it (Dr. Skeptic). Case Study 14.1 considers the diagnostic decision-making process, while Case Study 14.2 examines the therapeutic decision-making process.

Please note: All case studies in this chapter are for educational purposes only and not intended to guide clinical decision making.

Case Study 14.1. Making a Diagnosis for a Patient Presenting with Chest Pain

Bob Brown is a 50-year-old insurance salesman who comes to the doctor complaining of chest pain that usually occurs in the middle of the night, lasts for about an hour, and goes away. These symptoms have been present for eight to ten months and are gradually worsening. Mr. Brown reports general good health and takes no medicine; he almost never goes to the doctor. He quit smoking ten years ago. His father had a heart attack at age 65. His physical exam is normal except that he is 30 pounds overweight and his blood pressure is mildly elevated. His total serum cholesterol level is moderately high. His resting electrocardiogram is normal. Dr. Lore and Dr. Skeptic go through the same steps in pursuing a diagnosis, as they:

1. make a mental list of plausible diagnoses based on their education and experience;
2. think about the consequences of missing any diagnosis or of pursuing treatment for the wrong diagnosis; and
3. decide which tests will aid them in making the correct diagnosis.

On the basis of experience, they both rank three plausible diagnoses for his chest pain: (1) gastroesophageal reflux disease (GERD, or "heartburn"),

(2) coronary heart disease (angina), and (3) chest wall pain. They agree that the pain is not typical for coronary disease, and the normal physical exam argues against chest wall pain.

Dr. Lore recalls his cardiology teachers' admonitions—never miss a case of coronary disease because you may next see the patient in the morgue—and he remembers certain past patients with this atypical sort of chest pain who ended up having coronary disease more vividly than he remembers those who had something less serious.

Dr. Lore tells Mr. Brown that he should have a heart catheterization procedure (dye injected through a long tube threaded into the heart) as soon as possible, and immediately refers him for this test. He tells the patient that if the catheterization is normal, he should have some tests done on his throat (esophagus) and stomach to determine if he has GERD.

Mr. Brown's heart catheterization is normal. Dr. Lore refers Mr. Brown for a fiber-optic exam of his stomach and esophagus (endoscopy), plus 24-hour monitoring for acid in the esophagus. GERD is the diagnosis. Also noting that Mr. Brown's blood pressure is still high, Dr. Lore adds the diagnosis of hypertension.

Dr. Skeptic has a different approach as he thinks about the evidence base that can help him rank the probabilities of the three hypothesized diagnoses, help gauge the short- and long-term risks of misdiagnosis, and help him weigh the accuracy of diagnostic tests against their risks and costs. His experience and the results of observational studies on the incidence, prevalence, and natural history of the diagnoses in question tell him that:

1. In this type of practice setting, about 15 percent of patients who gave a history of chest pain unrelated to exercise had coronary disease, 19 percent had GERD, and 36 percent had chest wall pain (Klinkman, Stevens, and Gorenflow 1994).
2. About 4 percent of men this age in the general population have heart-related chest pain (angina), and about 3 percent report new-onset angina each year (Rosamond et al. 2007).
3. According to his heart disease risk factors, this patient has about a 1.4 percent per year risk (which means a 13.2 percent risk over the next ten years) of having a heart attack (MI), and there are effective treatments to prevent MI (Wilson et al. 1998; Grundy et al. 2004).
4. According to studies of men referred for exercise treadmill testing, Mr. Brown's chance of having coronary disease of sufficient severity to require bypass surgery or other invasive treatment is 10 to 15 percent (Pryor et al. 1991).
5. GERD is common and uncomfortable but not very dangerous; it can rarely lead to esophageal cancer after being present with uncontrolled symptoms for many years (exact risk unknown). Treatment often requires long-term use of prescription medicines to control symptoms, but treatment may not reduce the risk of cancer (Moayyedi and Talley 2006).
6. Chest wall pain with no obvious etiology based on history and physical exam poses no significant health risk, and it usually resolves on its own,

but it can be treated with a short course of an over-the-counter analgesic such as aspirin.

Dr. Skeptic also concludes that coronary heart disease would be the most important diagnosis not to miss. However, the evidence suggests that Mr. Brown has less than a 15 percent chance of having coronary disease and that the risk of a fatal or nonfatal MI occurring within the next few weeks is very low. Given that the pain is unlikely to be from his chest wall (according to his physical exam), it is more likely that Mr. Brown has symptomatic GERD, which is treatable but usually not dangerous. Therefore, Dr. Skeptic feels that there is time to carefully consider the next diagnostic steps.

Studies on the risks and accuracy of potentially useful tests reveal that:

1. The risk of a serious complication from heart catheterization is about ten times higher than the risk from an exercise treadmill test (Scanlon et al. 1999; Gibbons et al. 2002).
2. The accuracy of exercise testing for the detection of clinically significant coronary disease is close to that of heart catheterization (the gold standard). With a pretest probability of 15 percent, the negative predictive value of treadmill testing is 90–95 percent (that of heart catheterization is 100 percent by definition). By the same calculus, the positive predictive value of exercise testing is about 35 percent (Gibbons et al. 2002). (The concepts of sensitivity and specificity, and of positive and negative predictive value, are discussed in Chapter 3.)
3. Heart catheterization costs about 20 times as much as exercise testing.
4. A fiber-optic exam of the stomach and monitoring the esophagus for acid reflux are useful for patients with suspected GERD who do not respond to therapy, but they are less cost-effective than an empirical trial of anti-reflux medication (Fass et al. 1998; Sonnenberg, Delco, and El-Serag 1998; Moayyedi and Talley 2006).

A positive exercise test will still lead to a heart catheterization, but for this patient the odds strongly favor a negative (normal) exercise test as the outcome. Therefore, Dr. Skeptic concludes that the modest gain in accuracy of ruling out significant coronary disease by starting with heart catheterization does not outweigh its risks and costs. Dr. Skeptic schedules an exercise test instead. If it is normal, he will explain to the patient the options of further testing for GERD versus a trial of medication.

Mr. Brown completes the exercise treadmill test with no sign of coronary disease, but his resting blood pressure is still elevated, and it goes up with exercise much more than normal. On the basis of all this information, Dr. Skeptic diagnoses hypertension and recommends a two-week trial of medication for GERD. This results in almost complete resolution of Mr. Brown's chest pain symptoms.

Dr. Lore and Dr. Skeptic each arrived at the probable diagnosis of GERD by different paths. Dr. Lore's path was more risky and expensive than Dr. Skeptic's. Our attention now turns to treatment.

Case Study 14.2. Treatment Options for a Patient Diagnosed with GERD

Dr. Lore prescribes an anti-GERD medication that has been used with some success for many years, as is his habit in these cases. His experience with a newer, more expensive medication is still limited, so he tends to avoid prescribing it.

In contrast, Dr. Skeptic again thinks about the evidence base regarding medications for GERD. He considers the older medicine but reviews the evidence comparing the older medicine to the newer one (Thomson et al. 1998; Revicki et al. 1999; Moayyedi and Talley 2006). Because of the newer drug's pharmacology, biological plausibility supports the idea that it may better control GERD. In fact, there is evidence, from several head-to-head randomized comparisons of the older versus the new medicine, that shows the newer medicine controls symptoms better. However, the newer medication costs about four times as much. The comparison literature includes cost-effectiveness studies favoring the newer medication. Finally, Dr. Skeptic notes that the newer medication now has more than 12 years of reported studies about its efficacy and safety, and he is satisfied that it has a low risk of serious side effects. From the evidence available to him, Dr. Skeptic concludes that the newer medication should be prescribed.

Both doctors have also diagnosed hypertension in Mr. Brown. From basic medical knowledge and experience, they both know that hypertension increases the risk of heart attack and stroke and that the standard of care is to treat hypertension with medication along with advice to cut down on salt, exercise more, and lose weight.

Currently, more than 75 different drugs for the treatment of hypertension are available on the U.S. market. Dr. Lore likes to prescribe a newer antihypertensive medication (we'll call it Newpress) because it is heavily advertised to keep blood pressure down with a low incidence of side effects, and his favorite cardiologist has touted Newpress as a great drug. Like many newer drugs for high blood pressure, it costs five to ten times as much as older, off-patent antihypertensives. Dr. Lore tells Mr. Brown that he is at high risk for heart attack, stroke, and kidney failure because of his high blood pressure. He prescribes Newpress and explains that such medication will probably be required for the rest of Mr. Brown's life. Mr. Brown reluctantly accepts this fate, which Dr. Lore tells him he must if he wants to avoid a heart attack, stroke, or kidney failure.

Dr. Skeptic is gratified that for hypertension treatment, there is an extensive body of evidence that can guide his treatment recommendations for Mr. Brown. He considers the following:

1. On the basis of multiple observational studies and clinical trials involving thousands of patients with high blood pressure, Dr. Skeptic can estimate Mr. Brown's combined risk of heart attack or stroke to be 10 percent to 15 percent

over the next ten years. Treating his hypertension can be expected to reduce this risk by about one-fifth (Pearce et al. 1998). His risk of kidney failure in the next ten years is less than 0.3 percent (Klag et al. 1996), and treatment has not been proven to push that risk even lower in patients with normal kidney function (Jaimes, Galceran, and Raij 1996).

2. Reducing salt intake, avoiding alcohol, exercising, and losing weight may lower Mr. Brown's blood pressure to the high-normal range, but probably will not get it down to a level at which it poses no risk (Chobanian et al. 2003).

3. Five types of older, inexpensive antihypertensive drugs have been proven to prevent heart attacks and strokes without serious side effects (Chobanian et al. 2003), but Newpress has not been tested in this manner.

4. When compared directly with each other in RCTs, six major classes of antihypertensive drugs share similar rates of side effects (Neaton et al. 1993). Newpress belongs to one of those classes, but Newpress has never been directly compared in controlled clinical trials with other antihypertensives.

On the basis of this information, Dr. Skeptic advises Mr. Brown that it is acceptably safe to spend a few months trying to get his blood pressure under control through changes in lifestyle, but that he may still need antihypertensive medication. The current evidence strongly favors the drugs known as thiazides, ACE-inhibitors, and beta-blockers because they have been proven to improve health (not just lower blood pressure). Therefore, Dr. Skeptic will prescribe one of these proven drugs if Mr. Brown's blood pressure is still elevated after a few months of trying lifestyle modifications. He will see Mr. Brown every few weeks, adjusting the treatment regimen until his blood pressure is controlled without unacceptable side effects.

Prevention

Rational efforts to prevent disease and disability are rooted solidly in clinical epidemiology. In fact, preventive practices not supported by clinical epidemiologic evidence may be dangerous, costly, or both. Physicians, patients, and healthcare managers interested in prevention are presented with an almost endless array of possibilities. Time and money resources are always limited. How should they be allocated to the myriad health maladies that could possibly be prevented?

Experience and tradition have led in the past to numerous practices of questionable value, such as obtaining multiple "routine" tests, including chest x-rays, extensive blood test profiles, electrocardiograms, spine x-rays, body computed tomography scans, and urine tests on all adults. Results of some of these screening tests can lead to more invasive or expensive tests and treatments with little or no demonstrable benefit to patients.

Over the past two decades, clinical epidemiology has been applied to define more rational preventive practices (U.S. Preventive Services Task Force 2007). Epidemiology is critical to our understanding of the prevalence of any disease and its natural history, and thus the burden of suffering from it. It is also used to elucidate the etiology of diseases and, therefore, their risk factors. Finally, clinical epidemiology is used to evaluate the effect of preventive interventions. For any health problem and potential preventive strategy, the following questions should be posed:

1. Is the burden of suffering sufficient to justify the preventive effort under consideration?
2. How good is the evidence to support the potential effectiveness of early intervention?
3. How practical is the preventive strategy for use with the targeted population in the targeted settings?

As discussed in Chapter 2, prevention can be conceptualized to occur on three levels:

- *Primary prevention* aims to keep disease or injury from ever occurring—for example, using condoms to prevent infections that cause cervical cancer.
- *Secondary prevention* aims to stop disease before it becomes symptomatic—for example, using Pap smears to detect cervical cancer at early, asymptomatic stages that are highly curable.
- *Tertiary prevention* refers to medical treatments used to limit the disability caused by symptomatic or advanced disease—for example, performing a hysterectomy for invasive cervical cancer in an attempt to save the patient's life.

Most primary prevention occurs without much physician involvement; it relies mainly on personal health practices, public health initiatives, laws, and governmental actions. Highway design, water treatment, pesticide use, work safety programs, and food handling/preparation all involve primary prevention. Physicians' practices usually involve secondary and tertiary prevention, although they often advise their patients on lifestyle issues pertinent to primary prevention.

Because one health problem can lead to another, the distinctions between the three levels of prevention can blur. For instance, treatment of high blood pressure can be thought of as secondary prevention of hypertension or primary prevention of stroke. With that caveat in mind, we concentrate here on secondary prevention, noting that tertiary prevention can be thought of as treatment of symptomatic disease.

In clinical practice, secondary prevention usually starts with screening for a disease or its modifiable risk factors (or precursors). The disease should meet the foregoing criteria listed in terms of commonness, severity, effectiveness of early intervention, and practicality of the screening test. Since screening for the presence of a disease does nothing by itself to prevent illness or death, screening must be linked to effective and acceptable treatment or to limitation of the spread of the disease to others. The setting, population, and availability of post-screening medical services are all key factors.

For example, using chest radiography to screen for lung cancer among homeless adults in America cannot be recommended because (1) there are major obstacles to the delivery of that screening service in that setting; (2) by the time lung cancer is visible on a screening chest x-ray, it is usually no more curable than when it becomes symptomatic (U.S. Preventive Services Task Force 2007); and (3) even if early detection were helpful, the needed post-screening services are often not available to that population.

Case Study 14.3 considers prevention options for Mr. Brown.

Case Study 14.3. Prevention and Control Strategies

Bob Brown's adventures with chest pain have prompted him to become concerned about his overall health. He tells his doctor that he wants to get completely "checked out" to be sure that there are no other health problems he needs to worry about. Dr. Lore and Dr. Skeptic are still on the case in their parallel universes.

Recognizing Bob's new-found anxiety about his health, Dr. Lore recommends a full "executive health evaluation," amounting to a comprehensive battery of screening tests. In addition to the physical exam and tests already done, these tests include blood and urine tests to screen for anemia, kidney disease, liver disease, thyroid trouble, diabetes, and prostate cancer. They also include a chest x-ray to screen for lung cancer, emphysema, and tuberculosis. Spine x-rays are scheduled to screen for arthritis and osteoporosis. An examination of the colon with a six-foot flexible scope is scheduled to screen for colon cancer.

Everything comes back normal except that there are a few blood cells in the urine, the prostate blood test (prostate-specific antigen, or PSA) is at the 98th percentile for his age, his cholesterol levels are still elevated, and his serum calcium level is 2 percent over the upper limit of normal.

Dr. Lore orders a parathyroid blood test because of the slightly high calcium level, and special kidney x-rays with intravenous dye injected because of the blood cells in the urine. In addition, he refers Bob to a urologist for a prostate biopsy and to have a scope passed into his bladder to look for bladder cancer.

Bob complies with all test recommendations. His health fears escalate as he anxiously awaits each round of results. To his relief, the results of each subsequent test and examination are normal, but a nagging fear that he has cancer remains. He actually feels less healthy than before he got his checkup.

Dr. Lore next addresses Mr. Brown's high cholesterol levels. He advises him that high cholesterol increases the risk of heart attack and that diet can help some, but that he should take cholesterol-lowering medicine indefinitely to really get the levels down. He tells him that both his experience and published studies have shown that the medicine he prescribes does a good job of lowering cholesterol levels, and he prescribes his favorite anticholesterol medicine. Dr. Lore does not address whether lowering cholesterol with medicine is likely to actually prevent a heart attack.

Dr. Skeptic has a different approach to secondary prevention. He questions which screening tests really do more good than harm, which ones are worth the resources spent on them, and what needs to be done to make a firm diagnosis in response to a suggestive screening test result.

He recognizes that the "normal" range for many tests is defined by the values seen in 95 percent of those tested. Therefore, the "normal" range typically excludes the 5 percent of people who happen to be at the ends of the spectrum, most of whom have no health problem related to the test result. Therefore, "chasing down" the significance of test results that are just outside the normal range in asymptomatic people often leads to discomfort, anxiety, and expense without improving or protecting health. For some tests, abnormal results in asymptomatic people indicate a high enough risk of a related and treatable disease to warrant further investigation.

So Dr. Skeptic applies rational criteria in his choice of screening tests. For any potential screening strategy, he looks for high-quality, patient-oriented evidence that helps fulfill the criteria for effective screening and prevention discussed at the beginning of this section. He finds this evidence in the form of observational epidemiologic studies and in controlled clinical trials.

For 50-year-old men, the available evidence argues against using blood tests to screen for nonspecific metabolic problems, anemia, kidney disease, liver disease, and thyroid disease. It also argues against the urine test, chest x-ray, and spine x-rays ordered by Dr. Lore. The evidence is mixed on the value of the PSA prostate test and using the six-foot scope for colon cancer screening; studies are needed to resolve these controversies. The only screening tests in this scenario that are well supported by patient-oriented evidence are the blood sugar and blood cholesterol tests (U.S. Preventive Services Task Force 2007).

Dr. Skeptic focuses on Mr. Brown's cholesterol test results. The fact that the evidence supports such screening means that effective and acceptable treatment of high cholesterol is available. But first, before making a diagnosis of high cholesterol, Dr. Skeptic recommends confirmation of the high cholesterol levels by repeat testing. Thus confirmed, he moves on to treatment.

In Dr. Skeptic's view, "effective treatment" means one that should preserve or improve health, not simply lower the cholesterol level on a blood test. Weighing the potential risks and costs against the benefits of preventive treatments prescribed to asymptomatic people is of paramount importance. Dr. Skeptic's review of the available evidence shows that:

1. There is consistent, high-quality evidence that lowering serum cholesterol prevents coronary disease (Grundy et al. 2004); the evidence suggests that it also prevents stroke (Hebert et al. 1997).

2. Dietary advice/counseling leads to, on average, a 3 to 6 percent reduction in total and LDL cholesterol levels (Tang et al. 1998).
3. The most effective cholesterol-lowering drugs (statins) lower total and LDL cholesterol by 20 to 50 percent. In the major studies looking at heart attacks in middle-aged men, these drugs lowered cholesterol by an average of 30 percent and reduced the rate of heart attack by about 40 percent without serious side effects (Grundy et al. 2004). Most of these studies lasted about five years. Long-term safety and efficacy of this type of medication have not been proven. But this type of drug has been marketed in the United States for almost 20 years, and provided that appropriate monitoring and avoidance of risky drug combinations are respected, major safety concerns have not come to light.
4. As already mentioned, Bob Brown's risk of heart attack is about 13.2 percent over the next ten years. Given his normal exercise test, his risk may be lower.
5. Every 1 percent drop in total cholesterol level results in a 1 to 2 percent drop in a person's risk of heart attack (Wilson et al. 1998; Grundy et al. 2004). Thus, a 30 percent reduction in Bob's total cholesterol level, accomplished with medication that must be continued indefinitely, would lower his ten-year risk from about 13.2 percent to between 5.3 percent and 9.2 percent. Low-fat dieting alone can be expected (at best) to bring Bob's ten-year risk down to 12.4 percent. Combined control of his hypertension and high cholesterol would lower his ten-year risk to about 6 percent.
6. The cost of the type of cholesterol-lowering medicine proven to prevent heart attacks is $35 to $100 per month. Related to other preventive treatments, this is considered to be cost-effective (Huse et al. 1998).

Presented with this information about preventing heart attack by controlling high cholesterol, Bob opts for trying a low-fat diet first. If that does not lower his cholesterol enough, he wants to try the medicine. This approach is fine with Dr. Skeptic, given the short-term and long-term absolute risks of heart attack calculated from the epidemiologic evidence.

Cost-Effectiveness and the Number Needed to Treat

The cost-effectiveness of healthcare services for prevention and treatment of disease is getting increasingly more attention. This is not surprising: our options for spending healthcare resources are growing much faster than the resources themselves. The importance of cost-effectiveness in medical decision making has been implied in the foregoing case studies, but it has not been formally addressed.

Excellent overviews of cost-effectiveness analysis in medicine have been published (Drummond et al. 1993; Russell et al. 1996). The monetary costs to prevent one illness, disability, or death can be compared across treatment options, conditions, or outcomes. Such figures are sometimes reported as a dollar amount spent per year of life saved. Standards do not yet exist for what constitutes minimal cost-effectiveness, but many accepted screening and treatment regimens cost from $10,000 to $100,000 per year of life saved. Although practicing physicians probably envision complex economic models of cost-effectiveness only rarely, they are becoming more sophisticated about the costs to achieve a desired clinical outcome. Cost-effectiveness is usually expressed as the cost to prevent one unwanted outcome, or the cost per year of life saved, if applicable.

A relatively simple concept that is growing in use among physicians is the *number-needed-to-treat* (NNT). The NNT, multiplied by the unit cost of a procedure or prescription, can help physicians compare the cost-effectiveness of medical options. Mathematically, the NNT is the inverse of the risk difference (RD) (Laupacis, Sackett, and Roberts 1988). The RD is the difference between the rate of outcomes in a group receiving a certain service or treatment and the rate among those receiving a comparative treatment (or no treatment).

For example, if the rate of heart attack among those receiving a new treatment is 20 per 1,000 patients per year, and the rate of those receiving standard treatment is 30 per 1,000 per year, the RD will be 10 heart attacks per 1,000 patients, or 10/1,000. The NNT would thus be 1,000/10, which means that 100 patients would need to get the new treatment for a year in order to prevent one heart attack.

When addressing chronic disease, the NNT is often expressed in person-years of treatment. An NNT of 100 person-years could mean that 100 people have to be treated for one year, or 10 people for 10 years, and so on. The actual underlying pathophysiology and clinical database must be understood to appropriately understand any NNT that includes a time factor.

Case Study 14.4 considers family history and numbers-needed-to-treat for Mr. Brown and his sister.

Case Study 14.4. Family History and Number Needed to Treat

Mr. Brown has a younger sister, Mary O'Connell, who is 33 years old. Mr. Brown asks her to see his doctor to have her cholesterol checked.

Drs. Lore and Skeptic both find her to be generally healthy with no known cardiovascular risk factors except that her father has heart disease. They each opt to check her serum cholesterol levels, which turn out to be just like her older brother's. Dr. Lore gives her the same advice he gave her brother and prescribes his favorite anticholesterol medicine, which costs $65 per month.

Dr. Skeptic was prepared to prescribe cholesterol-lowering medicine to her brother, but he thinks about potential differences in efficacy (and cost-effectiveness) for this treatment between these siblings. First, he notes that women of Mrs. O'Connell's age were not included in the clinical trials that demonstrated that such medication reduces heart attack rates. But he decides to give such treatment the benefit of doubt, in the assumption that the medicine will have the same positive effect in young women that it shows in middle-aged men.

On the basis of that assumption, Dr. Skeptic looks at the NNT. He finds that for a woman with Mrs. O'Connell's heart attack risk profile, the five-year NNT would be about 1,000 (Wilson et al. 1998; Robson 1997). That is, to prevent one heart attack using the best type of cholesterol medicine available, one would have to treat 1,000 women like Mrs. O'Connell for five years. At $35 to $100 per month for medicine, the drug cost alone would be $2 million to $6 million to prevent one heart attack. That does not include the costs of blood tests and doctor visits for follow-up. By contrast, the five-year NNT for her brother was approximately 35 (Shepherd et al. 1995; Downs et al. 1998), with an associated medication cost to prevent one heart attack of about $74,000 to $210,000. Major differences in cost-effectiveness, attributable to differences in risk, are revealed by this simple calculation. The excessive cost to those who pool their funds for healthcare, plus the lack of proof that this medicine actually works in women in their thirties, leads Dr. Skeptic to advise against medication at this juncture, and to recommend diet and exercise.

The Future

The growing evidence base for best clinical practices, especially pertaining to preventive services, has not begun to achieve its potential to improve the quality and cost-effectiveness of medical care. This is not from lack of interest or a dull market response to these concepts. For example, effective preventive services such as disease screening, immunizations, and clinical counseling are not performed as often as either patients or their physicians desire. One can think of a variety of reasons for this, but probably the most important are the lack of appropriate information systems to facilitate the incorporation of the current and growing evidence base into practice (Scutchfield 1992), and a healthcare financing structure that fails to reward evidence-based practice.

Our Dr. Skeptic is an example of somewhat wishful thinking about a primary care physician who regularly applies clinical epidemiology in the examination room. He has overcome significant barriers to accomplish this. Without sophisticated information systems, most physicians, at best, are able to have a good grasp of the evidence base related to only a portion of the medical care they provide. The problem of "keeping up" with a constantly

evolving and growing body of pertinent medical knowledge is roughly pro-
portional to the breadth of health problems that a given physician deals
with. This magnifies the challenge for primary care practitioners. Added
to that is the significant problem of remembering—and finding the time
during patient visits—to provide comprehensive, evidence-based preventive services to people who do not specifically request them during their
visits to the physician.

Current reimbursement systems for physicians rest almost entirely
on volume (production-based models), rather than outcomes (quality-based
models). Generally, physicians in the United States earn more money by
treating more patients, not by demonstrating quality in the prevention,
evaluation, and treatment services they provide.

Most visits to primary care physicians last 10 to 20 minutes. How
can the physician assess the patient's needs, desires, and preferences, then
apply the latest patient-oriented evidence to treatment and prevention?
In general, the current approach is twofold: (1) pursue independent
study/reading outside of patient care time to try to keep up with the evidence base, and (2) use multiple visits with a patient over time to provide evidence-based, tailored treatments together with comprehensive
preventive services. This approach is problematic. Its success depends on
a constant high level of personal discipline by busy physicians. It is also
expensive because of multiple patient visits, and requires a lot of energy
spent by office staff, physicians, and patients to keep prevention and treatment services optimal for each patient. The economic necessity of serving large volumes of patients each day discourages setting aside special
time to make high-quality, evidence-based practice a high priority.

Healthcare managers can play a major role in solving this dilemma,
because of the potential power of sophisticated medical office management
systems and medical informatics. In terms of office management, a team
approach to consistently providing a high level of patient-oriented, evidence-
based care is critical. This requires buy-in and active participation by all personnel, from the receptionists to the medical director. Improved methods
of patient education, patient empowerment, and doctor-patient communication—all of which increase physicians' time efficiency—require attention.
Practical approaches to continuous quality improvement, motivated by tan-
gible and intangible rewards for all involved, are integral to success.

Medical informatics holds great promise for letting physicians bring
a growing and ever-changing evidence base to the point of care. This means
providing the clinician with rapid access to high-quality information that
is directly applicable to medical decision making for the individual patient
during the visit.

For example, if Dr. Lore had had such a system when he considered Bob Brown's possible diagnosis of GERD, a few keystrokes could
have gained him access to all of the key evidence needed to conclude

that the most cost-effective approach would be an empirical trial of a certain type of medication. He would not have felt a need to order uncomfortable and expensive tests, and would have avoided prescribing less effective medicine.

Appropriate information systems will also include computerized tracking and reminder systems that will improve the timely delivery of proven preventive services, often forgotten because they address health-care without the motivation of symptoms to be alleviated. For example, Dr. Lore could have routinely seen a list of the screening and preventive services shown to be worthwhile for a man of Mr. Brown's age (as the computer automatically accessed demographic information entered when Mr. Brown registered as a new patient in the practice). Furthermore, the system could automatically notify this individual patient by mail of any preventive services that are past due, accompanied by instructions on how to get them done. Likewise, receptionists and nurses can be prompted to remind the patient to ask the doctor about certain services when the patient shows up for any visit.

Appropriate billing, keyed to supporting documentation, will be automated, as will health plan formulary and referral restriction notifica-tions, at the point of care. Patients will be able to interact with health pro-fessionals over the Internet, provided reimbursement structures support this. Finally, sophisticated information systems will decrease the time physi-cians spend on finding and processing clinical information about individ-ual patients, such as consultation and test reports.

Such clinical information systems are already in operation in many healthcare facilities across the country, with a growing competitive market for them. However, few (if any) yet have the ability to bring the latest high-quality evidence to the point of care and effectively track chronic disease management and preventive services. Furthermore, many of these infor-mation systems are too cumbersome to achieve their desired outcomes of improved quality at reduced long-term cost.

Optimal medical informatics and systems management remain great challenges, but powerful economic forces will continue to push their devel-opment. Patients, physicians, employers, and insurers will all exert increas-ing pressures on the marketplace to deliver the most cost-effective, high-quality healthcare obtainable. Those who fail to respond to the explosion of information available to these parties as they select health plans, providers, and practice settings will likely disappear from the healthcare field.

Healthcare managers will have a major role to play in this arena. Their success will depend on their abilities to keep the quality of medical care and its associated outcomes of primary importance as they work to maximize revenue and control costs. Healthcare managers and their fam-ilies will have to depend on the healthcare system they help to build.

Case Study 14.5 is an exercise in clinical decision making.

Case Study 14.5. Clinical Decision-Making Toolbox

Clinical decisions can be improved by combining the strengths of epidemiology and decision-making theory. A *probability* is simply a number between 0 and 1 that represents the chance that an event will occur. For example, a mortality rate or a prevalence rate, if expressed in terms of proportions, can represent the chance that a patient will die, or the chance that a patient with a set of symptoms has a particular disease. The odds of an event is simply the probability that the event will occur divided by the probability that it will not occur.

Hunink and Glasziou (2001) have written an elegant text that expostulates a number of specific ways in which the marriage of epidemiology and decision-making theory can quantify, and thus facilitate, many of the types of decisions clinicians make.

Diagnostic Decision Making

The *likelihood ratio* (LR) is a measure of test performance and can be used to improve clinical decision making. It is the probability of a particular test result (e.g., test positive) for those with disease divided by the probability of a particular test result (e.g., test positive) for those without disease. For example, if the probability of testing positive is 0.50 (or 50 percent) if you have the disease and 0.25 (or 25 percent) if you don't have the disease, then the LR is 0.50/0.25, or 2.

Let LR+ be the likelihood ratio of a positive test result, and LR− be the likelihood ratio of a negative test result. For a test with only two results (the test result is either positive or negative) the two likelihood ratios can be calculated as follows:

$$LR+ = \text{sensitivity}/(1 - \text{specificity})$$
$$LR- = (1 - \text{sensitivity})/\text{specificity}$$

Suppose that we want to have Bob Brown complete the treadmill test. Let us assume a sensitivity of 70 percent and a specificity of 90 percent for this test.

The pretest probability of disease is either the prevalence of disease in the population or the prevalence of disease for patients with particular symptoms. Mr. Brown goes to the office of Dr. Skeptic, and without doing any tests at all, Dr. Skeptic's best guess at the pretest probability of heart disease is 0.15 (15 percent). The purpose of the treadmill test is to revise "upward" or "downward" the pretest probability of disease. The likelihood ratio is used for this purpose. You can convert a pretest probability to a "post-test" probability with the following three steps:

- Convert pretest probability into pretest odds
  Pretest odds = pretest probability/(1 − pretest probability)
- Convert pretest odds to post-test odds with likelihood ratio
  Post-test odds (positive-test) = pretest odds × LR+ (for a positive test)
  Post-test odds (negative test) = pretest odds × LR− (for a negative test)
- Convert post-test odds to post-test probability
  Post-test probability = post-test odds/(1 + post-test odds)

QUESTIONS

1. What are the positive (LR+) and negative (LR−) likelihood ratios associated with this test?
2. What are the pretest odds that Bob Brown has heart disease?
3. What are the post-test odds that Bob Brown has heart disease with a positive treadmill test? With a negative treadmill test?
4. What is the post-test probability that Bob Brown has heart disease given a positive treadmill test? With a negative treadmill test?
5. How does this test help Dr. Skeptic make his diagnosis?

ANSWERS

1. LR+ = 0.70/0.10 − 7 and LR− = 0.30/0.9 = 0.333.
2. Pretest odds that Bob Brown has heart disease = 0.15/(1 − 0.15) = 0.1765.
3a. Post-test odds (positive test) = 0.1765 × 7 = 1.24.
3b. Post-test odds (negative test) = 0.1765 × 0.333 = 0.059.
4a. Post-test probability (positive test) = 1.24/(1 + 1.24) = 0.55.
4b. Post-test probability (negative test) = 0.059/(1 + 0.059) = 0.056.
5. Dr. Skeptic's best guess at the chance that Bob Brown has heart disease is 15 percent before the test, 55 percent if he tests positive, and 5.6 percent if he tests negative.

Treatment Choices

Suppose Bob Brown arrives at the emergency room (ER) instead of the physician's office with chest pain. The physician needs to decide whether to give him immediate thrombolytic therapy or wait and see whether symptoms progress. How could probability theory be used to improve this decision?

Assume that 20 percent of such men who present at the ER with chest pain have an acute myocardial infarction (AMI, or heart attack). Therefore, the probability of that patient having an AMI is 0.20, which means that the probability that he does not have an AMI is 0.80.

The physician goes to the literature and obtains the following mortality rates: (1) 8 percent mortality rate for those who get thrombolytic therapy and do have an AMI; (2) 0.4 percent mortality (presumably from intracranial bleeding) for those who get thrombolytic therapy but do not have an AMI; 9 percent mortality for those who do not get thrombolytic therapy but suffer an AMI; o percent mortality for those who do not get thrombolytic therapy and do not suffer an AMI.

QUESTIONS

1. A decision tree illustrates and quantifies the decisions that need to be made in this context. What would the decision tree look like for this situation?
2. What is the probability that the patient will die if you start thrombolytic therapy immediately? What is the probability that the patient will die if you wait?
3. Which is the preferred choice in this situation?

ANSWERS

1. Notice that the decision tree (Figure 14.1) shows decision(s) that need to be made (thrombolytic therapy or "wait"). These are called *decision nodes* (the little squares). The tree also has *chance nodes*, which reflect information about which we are not entirely certain (the little circles). We estimate the prevalence of AMI among patients with these symptoms, and estimate the mortality rates as stated above. These estimates are represented by probabilities. In the decision tree, we have the decision node first, then the diagnostic uncertainty chance node (0.20 with AMI, 0.80 without). Each of these chance nodes is then followed by the outcome chance nodes. The 8 percent mortality rate associated with thrombolytic therapy means that 92 percent survive. Notice that the associated probabilities must add up to 1 (0.08 + 0.92 = 1.0).

2. If you start immediate thrombolytic treatment, the probability of dying is calculated by working from left to right across the decision tree. Note that the top four probabilities to the right of the decision tree are associated with the four groups of patients who get thrombolytic therapy, and the bottom four probabilities are associated with the four groups of patients who *do not* get thrombolytic therapy. The four probabilities associated with each of the two groups add up to 100 percent. For example, $0.2 \times 0.08 = 0.016$ or 1.6 percent of those who get thrombolytic therapy will suffer an AMI and die; $0.92 \times 0.2 = 0.184$ or 18.4 percent of those who get thrombolytic therapy will suffer an AMI but live; 0.3 percent of this group will not suffer an AMI but die anyway (due to the thrombolytic treatment); and 79.7 percent of the group will not suffer an AMI and live. To calculate the total mortality associated with a particular decision (thrombolytic treatment or wait) one simply adds up the probabilities of mortality associated with each choice: (a) $0.016 + 0.003 = 0.019$ for the thrombolytics; (b) $0.018 + 0 = 0.018$ for waiting.

3. The probability of death associated with thrombolytics is 0.019 (1.9 percent mortality). The probability of death associated with waiting is 0.018 (1.8 percent mortality). Waiting is the preferred choice here. In real life, the probabilities in the decision tree will depend on other clinical factors such as the results of an electrocardiogram.

FIGURE 14.1. DECISION TREE FOR TREATMENT OPTIONS FOR ACUTE MYOCARDIAL INFARCTION

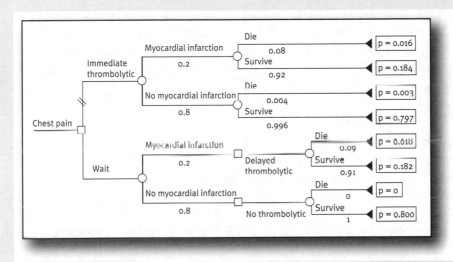

SOURCE: Hunink and Glasziou (2001). Reprinted with permission of Cambridge University Press.

Treatment Threshold

Let us define the *benefit* of treatment as the difference in outcome for diseased patients who receive treatment compared to those who do not. For the above example, patients with an AMI suffer an 8 percent mortality rate if treated (i.e., given thrombolytics), and a 9 percent mortality rate if untreated. Thus, the benefit of treatment is 9% – 8% or 1% (0.01).

The *harm* of treatment is the difference in outcome for patients without the disease who receive treatment compared with those who do not. With the example, patients without an AMI suffer a 0.4 percent mortality rate with thrombolytics and a 0 percent mortality rate without this treatment. Thus, the harm of treatment is 0.4 percent – 0 percent or 0.4 percent mortality.

The benefit typically measures the outcome advantage of treatment, whereas the harm measures the "risk(s)" associated with treatment. The *treatment threshold* is defined as the prevalence of disease around which the decision to treat pivots, based on the risks and benefits associated with treatment. It can be calculated as follows:

Treatment threshold = harm/(harm + benefit)

QUESTIONS

1. If the benefit associated with thrombolytic therapy is 1 percent and the harm is 0.4 percent, what is the treatment threshold?
2. What does this treatment threshold mean?

ANSWERS

1. Threshold = 0.004/(0.004 + 0.01) = 0.286.
2. If the prevalence of AMI is less than 28.6 percent, the risks associated with treatment outweigh the benefits, and treatment should be withheld. If the prevalence is greater than 28.6 percent, the risks associated with a possible AMI outweigh the risks of treatment, and treatment should be provided.

Deciding When to Test

The purpose of a diagnostic test is to provide information that will change at least one clinical decision, with risks to the patient that are less than the expected benefit to be gained by changing that decision. Testing is not helpful in two situations: (1) the disease is so prevalent that false negatives might dissuade the physician from recommending treatment; (2) the disease is so "rare" that false positives might persuade the physician to recommend unnecessary treatment.

Figure 14.2 illustrates these concepts with three regions of disease prevalence: (1) the "do not treat–do not test" region; (2) the "test" region; and (3) the "treat and do not test" region. The "no treat–test threshold" is the prevalence of disease at which we are indifferent between testing and withholding treatment. The "test–treat" threshold is the prevalence of disease at which we are indifferent between testing and treating without the test. Both of these thresholds depend on the characteristics of the test and are defined as follows:

$$\text{No treat–test threshold} = \frac{\text{harm} \times (1-\text{specificity})}{\text{harm} \times (1-\text{specificity}) + \text{benefit} \times \text{sensitivity}}$$

$$\text{Test-treat threshold} = \frac{\text{harm} \times (\text{specificity})}{\text{harm} \times \text{specificity} + \text{benefit} \times (1-\text{sensitivity})}$$

QUESTIONS

1. The rapid whole blood assay of Troponin I is a blood test that is a biomarker for AMI. At the time a patient arrives at the ER, this test has a sensitivity of 63 percent and specificity of 92.6 percent. The sensitivity of this test increases to 98 percent four hours after patient arrival (Heeschen et al. 1999). The cost and benefit of thrombolytic therapy versus waiting is 0.004 and 0.01, respectively. Calculate the no treat–test threshold for the Troponin I test given the choice of thrombolytic therapy versus waiting for Bob Brown with the suspected AMI.

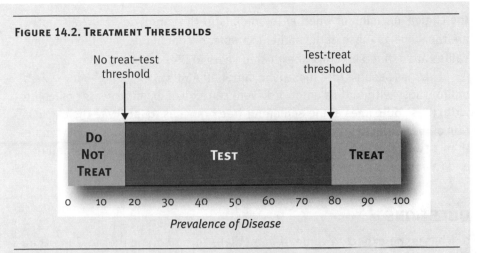

FIGURE 14.2. TREATMENT THRESHOLDS

No treat–test threshold

Test-treat threshold

Do Not Treat

TEST

TREAT

0   10   20   30   40   50   60   70   80   90   100

Prevalence of Disease

SOURCE: Hunink and Glasziou. (2001). Reprinted with permission of Cambridge University Press.

2. Calculate the test-treat threshold for the Troponin I test given the choice of thrombolytic therapy versus waiting for Bob Brown with the suspected AMI.
3. What do these thresholds mean?
4. Suppose there are risks associated with the test itself. Does this change the results?

ANSWERS

1. The no treat–test threshold = $0.004 \times (1 - 0.926)/[0.004(1 - 0.926) + 0.01 \times 0.63] = 0.045$.
2. The test-treat threshold = $0.004 \times 0.926/[(0.004 \times 0.926) + (0.01 \times [1 - 0.63])] = 0.500$.
3. If the prevalence of AMI is less than 4.5 percent, we should withhold testing because the risks associated with a false positive are too high, and thrombolytics may be given unnecessarily. If the prevalence of AMI is greater than 50 percent, thrombolytics should be given without testing because the risk of false negatives may dissuade us from treatment. Within the range of 4.5 percent to 50 percent, testing is useful.
4. Yes, the equations for these thresholds assume that the test has no risks or "toll." If the test has a toll, this must be factored into the calculations. See Hunink and Glasziou (2001) for these formulas.

Prognosis

Decision trees can be used to calculate the difference in survival between two choices of treatment. Bob Brown arrives at the ER with chest pain and prompts the clinical decision of whether to administer thrombolytics. Mortality rates are the same as those of the earlier example, except in this case the outcome values are defined in terms of expected years of life.

Let us assume that those who suffer an AMI can expect ten more years of life. Those without this untoward event can expect 25 more years of life. We write these outcomes at the end of our tree branches to facilitate the calculation of the "expected" value of each choice. The expected value is nothing more than a "weighted average," which takes into account the various probabilities and the outcomes associated with each option.

QUESTIONS

1. What is the expected value of immediate thrombolytic therapy? In other words, on average, how many more years of life can people who present to the ER with AMI symptoms and are treated with thrombolytics expect?
2. What is the expected value of the waiting strategy? In other words, on average, how many more years of life can people who present to the ER with AMI symptoms and do not receive thrombolytics expect, at least initially?
3. Which of the two options is preferred in terms of life expectancy?

FIGURE 14.3. DECISION TREE WITH OUTCOMES FOR TREATMENT OPTIONS OF ACUTE MYOCARDIAL INFARCTION

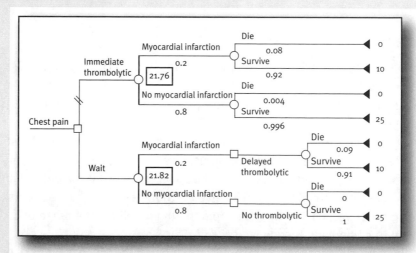

SOURCE: Hunink and Glasziou (2001). Reprinted with permission of Cambridge University Press.

ANSWERS

1. The expected value of immediate thrombolytic treatment is (0.2 × 0.08 × 0) + (0.2 × 0.92 × 10) + (0.8 × 0.004 × 0) + (0.8 × 0.996 × 25) = 21.76 years.

2. The expected value of waiting is (0.2 × 0.09 × 0) + (0.2 × 0.91 × 10) + (0.8 × 0 × 0) + (0.8 × 1 × 25) = 21.82 years.
3. The waiting strategy is preferred because it has the highest life expectancy.

References

Chobanian, A. V., G. L. Bakris, H. R. Black, W. C. Cushman, L. A. Green, J. L. Izzo, Jr, D. W. Jones, B. J. Materson, S. Oparil, J. T. Wright, Jr., E. J. Roccella, National Heart, Lung, and Blood Institute Joint National Committee on Prevention, Detection, Evaluation, and Treatment of High Blood Pressure, and National High Blood Pressure Education Program Coordinating Committee. 2003. "The Seventh Report of the Joint National Committee on Prevention, Detection, Evaluation, and Treatment of High Blood Pressure: The JNC-7 Report." *Journal of the American Medical Association* 289 (19): 2560–72.

Davignon, J., G. Roederer, M. Montigny, M. R. Hayden, M. Tan, P. W. Connelly, R. Hegele, R. McPherson, P. J. Lupien, and C. Gagne. 1994. "Comparative Efficacy and Safety of Pravastatin, Nicotinic Acid and the Two Combined in Patients with Hypercholesterolemia." *American Journal of Cardiology* 73 (5): 339–45.

Dickersin, K., S. E. Straus, and L. A. Bero. 2007. "Evidence-Based Medicine: Increasing, Not Dictating Choice." *British Medical Journal* 334 (Suppl. 1): S10.

Downs, J. R., M. Clearfield, S. Weis, E. Whitney, D. R. Shapiro, P. A. Beere, A. Langendorfer, E. A. Stein, W. Kruyer, and A. M. Gotto, Jr. 1998. "Primary Prevention of Acute Coronary Events with Lovastatin in Men and Women with Average Cholesterol Levels." *Journal of the American Medical Association* 279 (20): 1615–22.

Drummond, M., A. Brandt, B. Luce, and J. Rovira. 1993. "Standardizing Methodologies for Economic Evaluation in Health Care." *International Journal of Technology Assessment in Healthcare* 9 (1): 26–36.

Ebell, M. H., H. C. Barry, D. C. Slawson, and A. F. Shaughnessy. 1999. "Finding POEMS in the Medical Literature." *Journal of Family Practice* 48 (5): 350–55.

Evans, A. S. 1978. "Causation and Disease: A Chronological Journey." *American Journal of Epidemiology* 108 (4): 248–58.

Fass, R., M. B. Fennerty, J. J. Ofman, I. M. Gralnek, C. Johnson, E. Camargo, and R. E. Sampliner. 1998. "The Clinical and Economic Value of a Short Course of Omeprazole in Patients with Noncardiac Chest Pain." *Gastroenterology* 115 (1): 42–49.

Ferrario, C. M. 1990. "Importance of the Renin-Angiotensin-Aldosterone System (RAS) in the Physiology and Pathology of Hypertension." *Drugs* 39 (2): 1–8.

Gibbons, R. J., G. J. Balady, J. T. Bricker, B. R. Chaitman, G. F. Fletcher, V. F. Froelicher, D. B. Mark, B. D. McCallister, A. N. Mooss, M. G. O'Reilly, W. L. Winters, R. J. Gibbons, E. M. Antman, J. S. Alpert, D. P. Faxon, V. Fuster, G. Gregoratos, L. F. Hiratzka, A. K. Jacobs, R. O. Russell, S. C. Smith, and the American College of Cardiology/American Heart Association Task Force on Practice Guidelines Committee to Update the 1997 Exercise Testing Guidelines. 2002. "ACC/AHA 2002 Guideline Update for Exercise Testing: Summary Article. A Report of the American College of Cardiology/American Heart Association Task Force on Practice Guidelines (Committee to Update the 1997 Exercise Testing Guidelines)." *Journal of the American College of Cardiology* 40 (8): 1531–40.

Grundy, S. M., J. I. Cleeman, C. N. Merz, H. B. Brewer, Jr., L. T. Clark, D. B. Hunninghake, R. C. Pasternak, S. C. Smith, Jr., N. J. Stone, and the Coordinating Committee of the National Cholesterol Education Program. 2004. "Implications of Recent Clinical Trials for the National Cholesterol Education Program Adult Treatment Panel III Guidelines." *Journal of the American College of Cardiology* 44 (3): 720–32.

Hebert, P. R., M. Gaziano, K. S. Chan, and C. H. Hennekens. 1997. "Cholesterol Lowering with Statin Drugs, Risk of Stroke, and Total Mortality." *Journal of the American Medical Association* 278 (4): 313–21.

Heeschen, C., B. U. Goldmann, L. Langenbrink, G. Matschuck, and C. W. Hamm. 1999. "Evaluation of a Rapid Whole Blood ELISA for Quantification of Troponin I in Patients with Acute Chest Pain." *Clinical Chemistry* 45 (10): 1789–96.

Hunink, M. G. M., and P. P. Glasziou. 2001. *Decision Making in Health and Medicine: Integrating Evidence and Values.* New York: Cambridge University Press.

Huse, D. M., M. W. Russell, J. D. Miller, D. F. Kraemer, R. B. D'Agostino, R. C. Ellison, and S. C. Hartz. 1998. "Cost-Effectiveness of Statins." *American Journal of Cardiology* 82 (11): 1357–63.

Jaimes, E., J. Galceran, and L. Raij. 1996. "End-Stage Renal Disease: Why Aren't Improvements in Hypertension Treatment Reducing the Risk? Current Opinion." *Cardiology* 11 (5): 471–76.

Klag, M. J., P. K. Whelton, B. L. Randall, J. D. Neaton, F. L. Brancati, C. E. Ford, N. B. Shulman, and J. Stamler. 1996. "Blood Pressure and End-Stage Renal Disease in Men." *New England Journal of Medicine* 334 (1): 13–18.

Klinkman, M. S., D. Stevens, and D. W. Gorenflow. 1994. "Episodes of Care for Chest Pain: A Preliminary Report from MIRNET." *Journal of Family Practice* 38 (4): 345–52.

Laupacis, A., D. L. Sackett, and R. S. Roberts. 1988. "An Assessment of Clinically Useful Measures of the Consequences of Treatment." *New England Journal of Medicine* 381 (20): 1728–33.

Maggioni, A. P. 2006. "Efficacy of Angiotensin Receptor Blockers in Cardiovascular Disease." *Cardiovascular Drugs and Therapy* 20: 295–308.

Moayyedi, P., and N. Talley. 2006. "Gastro-esophageal Reflux Disease." *Lancet* 367 (9528): 2086–100.

Nawrocki, J. W., S. R. Weiss, M. H. Davidson, D. L. Sprecher, S. L. Schwartz, P. J. Lupien, P. H. Jones, H. E. Haber, and D. M. Black. 1995. "Reduction of LDL Cholesterol by 25% to 60% in Patients with Primary Hypercholesterolemia by Atorvastatin, a New HMG-CoA Reductase Inhibitor." *Arteriosclerosis, Thrombosis, and Vascular Biology* 15 (5): 678–82.

Neaton, J. D., R. H. Grimm, Jr., R. J. Prineas, J. Stamler, G. A. Grandits, P. J. Elmer, J. A. Cutler, J. M. Flack, J. A. Schoenberger, and R. McDonald. 1993. "Treatment of Mild Hypertension Study: Final Results." *Journal of the American Medical Association* 270 (6): 713–24.

Ockene, I. S., and N. H. Miller. 1997. "Cigarette Smoking, Cardiovascular Disease, and Stroke." *Circulation* 96 (9): 3243–47.

Pearce, K. A., C. D. Furberg, B. M. Psaty, and J. Kirk. 1998. "Cost-Minimization and the Number Needed to Treat in Uncomplicated Hypertension." *American Journal of Health* 11 (6): 618–29.

Pryor, D. B., L. Shaw, F. E. Harrell, K. L. Lee, M. A. Hlatky, D. B. Mark, L. H. Muhlbaier, and R. M. Califf. 1991. "Estimating the Likelihood of Severe Coronary Artery Disease." *American Journal of Medicine* 90 (5): 553–62.

Revicki, D. A., S. Sorensen, P. N. Maton, and R. C. Orlando. 1999. "Health-Related Quality of Life Outcomes of Omeprazole Versus Ranitidine in Poorly Responsive Symptomatic Gastroesophageal Reflux Disease." *Digestive Diseases* 16 (5): 284–91.

Robson, J. 1997. "Information Needed to Decide About Cardiovascular Treatment in Primary Care." *British Medical Journal* 314: 277.

Rosamond, W., K. Flegal, G. Friday, K. Furie, A. Go, K. Greenlund, N. Haase, M. Ho, V. Howard, B. Kissela, S. Kittner, D. Lloyd-Jones, M. McDermott, J. Meigs, C. Moy, G. Nichol, C. J. O'Donnell, V. Roger, J. Rumsfeld, P. Sorlie, J. Steinberger, T. Thom, S. Wasserthiel-Smoller, Y. Hong, and the American Heart Association Statistics Committee and Stroke Statistics Subcommittee. 2007. "Heart Disease and Stroke Statistics—2007 Update: A Report from the American Heart Association Statistics Committee and the Stroke Statistics Subcommittee." *Circulation* 115 (5): e69–e171.

Russell, L. B., M. R. Gold, J. E. Siegel, N. Daniels, and M. C. Weinstein. 1996. "The Role of Cost-Effectiveness Analysis in Health and Medicine." *Journal of the American Medical Association* 276 (14): 1172–77.

Scanlon, P. J., D. P. Faxon, A. Audet, B. Carabello, G. J. Dehmer, K. A. Eagle, R. D. Legako, D. F. Leon, J. A. Murray, S. E. Nissen, C. J. Pepine, R. M. Watson, J. L. Ritchie, R. J. Gibbons, M. D. Cheitlin, T. J. Gardner, A. Garson, Jr., R. O. Russell, Jr., T. J. Ryan, and S. C. Smith, Jr. 1999. "ACC/AHA Guidelines for Coronary Angiography: Executive Summary and Recommendations." *Circulation* 99 (17): 2345–57.

Scutchfield, F. D. 1992. "Clinical Preventive Services: The Patient and the Physician." *Clinical Chemistry* 38 (Suppl.): 1547–51.

Shaughnessy, A. F., D. C. Slawson, and L. Becker. 1998. "Clinical Jazz: Harmonizing Clinical Experience and Evidence-Based Medicine." *Journal of Family Practice* 47 (6): 425–28.

Shepherd, J., S. M. Cobbe, I. Ford, C. G. Isles, A. R. Lorimer, P. W. MacFarlane, J. H. McKillop, and C. J. Packard. 1995. "Prevention of Coronary Heart Disease with Pravastatin in Men with Hypercholesterolemia." *New England Journal of Medicine* 333 (20): 1301–7.

Slawson, D. C., A. F. Shaughnessy, and J. H. Bennett. 1994. "Becoming a Medical Information Master: Feeling Good About Not Knowing Everything." *Journal of Family Practice* 38 (5): 505–13.

Sonnenberg, A., F. Delco, and H. B. El-Serag. 1998. "Empirical Therapy Versus Diagnostic Tests in Gastroesophageal Reflux Disease: A Medical Decision Analysis." *Digestive Diseases and Sciences* 43 (5): 1001–8.

Tang, J. L., J. M. Armitage, T. Lancaster, C. A. Silagy, G. H. Fowler, and A. W. Neil. 1998. "Systematic Review of Dietary Intervention Trials to Lower Blood Total Cholesterol in Free-Living Subjects." *British Medical Journal* 316 (7139): 1213–20.

Thomson, A. B., N. Chiba, D. Armstrong, G. Tougas, and R. H. Hunt. 1998. "The Second Canadian Gastroesophageal Reflux Disease Consensus: Moving Forward to New Concepts." *Canadian Journal of Gastroenterology* 12 (8): 551–56.

U.S. Department of Health and Human Services. 1989. *Reducing the Health Consequences of Smoking: 25 Years of Progress. A Report of the Surgeon General.* Pub. No. DHHS (CDC) 89-8411. Rockville, MD: U.S. Department of Health and Human Services.

U.S. Preventive Services Task Force. 2007. Home page. [Online information; retrieved 2/8/08.] http://www.ahrq.gov/clinic/uspstfix.htm.

Wilson, P. W. F., R. B. D'Agostino, D. Levy, A. M. Belanger, H. Silbershatz, and W. B. Kannel. 1998. "Prediction of Coronary Heart Disease Using Risk Factor Categories." *Circulation* 97 (18): 1837–47.

APPLICATIONS OF EPIDEMIOLOGY TO SPECIFIC DISEASES

The three chapters in this section focus on the application of epidemiologic principles to three major diseases that incur a substantial burden on society, both in terms of human suffering and financial resources. Two of the diseases, cardiovascular disease and dementia, would be classified as chronic diseases. They are caused by a number of different risk factors, some behavioral, some environmental, and some genetic. They tend to afflict the elderly much more than the young. Though some progress has been made in pharmacologic and surgical treatments, perhaps more so for cardiovascular disease than dementia, it seems likely that these two diseases will continue to plague the human race for years to come. The third disease, HIV/AIDS, is relatively new on the disease horizon, tends to afflict a different demographic cohort (the young and healthy), and has elements of both an infectious and chronic disease. It seems clear that the disease is caused by an infectious agent, the human immunodeficiency virus (HIV), but the treatment of the disease by anti-retroviral drug therapy cannot eradicate (i.e., cure) the disease, as is the case with most other infectious diseases. Thus, in some ways, the disease behaves more like a chronic than an acute disease.

The purpose of these three chapters is to present a "capstone" experience for the reader with a focus on these three diseases. At the very least, the healthcare manager should become familiar with these three diseases, as they represent a huge burden to society. Beyond that, however, the reader should be challenged to use these three diseases to review the specific concepts and principles that were presented in previous chapters of this text. Concepts presented earlier in this text, such as mortality and morbidity rates, disease transmission, screening, planning and quality measurement, and cost-effectiveness analysis can be applied to one or more of these diseases with a view toward solidifying the understanding of these concepts through this capstone experience.

CARDIOVASCULAR DISEASE

Steven R. Browning and Steven T. Fleming

> *"Sudden death is more common in those who are naturally fat than in the lean."* Hippocrates

Twenty-five hundred years ago, Hippocrates speculated that there was a link between obesity and sudden death. Although this link has been tested and scientifically affirmed in recent decades, Lavie and Milani (2003) suggest a Hippocrates paradox (or more accurately an "obesity paradox"), where a risk factor that seems so clearly related to disease does not necessarily lead to poorer prognosis; that is, obese patients with cardiovascular disease may actually have a better prognosis than lean patients with the same disease, particularly following surgery.

Nevertheless, cardiovascular disease (CVD) is the leading cause of death in the United States and most developed countries. Despite proven primary and secondary prevention strategies, the global burden of CVD will increase dramatically in the twenty-first century, especially in countries such as China and India (Yusuf et al. 2001). Current projections indicate that CVD will be the leading cause of death in both the developing and developed world (Thorvaldsen et al. 1997; Rosamond et al. 2007).

The epidemic of CVD will continue for years to come due to dramatic increases in obesity and diabetes, especially in the younger generations. The scientific evidence continues to accumulate that most CVD is preventable; however, CVD will represent the major economic burden on the healthcare system, with estimated direct and indirect costs of about $431.8 billion in 2007 in the United States (Rosamond et al. 2007). Health managers will be confronted by challenges in balancing the choices between primary and secondary prevention efforts, as well as disease management strategies and the use of technology, for addressing the burden of CVD.

Research on the epidemiology of CVD began in the 1940s and 1950s with the Framingham Heart Study and other longitudinal investigations (Dawber and Kannel 1958). The essential notion of risk factors developed in these early studies and the well-established risk factors for

CVD—cigarette smoking, hypertension, high serum cholesterol, obesity, and lack of exercise—were confirmed in these early investigations. From an epidemiologic perspective, these cohort studies were "groundbreaking" investigations, as many of the methods currently used in the design and analysis of epidemiologic studies were developed during these investigations.

The term *risk factor* appeared first in a Framingham publication in 1961 (Kannel et al. 1961). The concept of the impact of multiple risk factors, risk stratification, logistic regression, and the development of risk prediction models arose from Framingham and other early studies.

Public health has focused on both primary and secondary prevention activities for reducing the burden of CVD. *Primary prevention* refers to "the prevention of the onset of symptomatic disease in persons without prior symptoms of CVD by means of treatment of risk factors with lifestyle modifications or drugs" (Wilson and Pearson 2005). Primary prevention efforts have targeted smoking cessation, weight loss, exercise, the promotion of a healthier diet, and lipid lowering drugs for reducing the risk of CVD. *Secondary prevention* refers to the prevention of death or recurrence of disease in those who are already symptomatic. Secondary prevention includes medical interventions such as cholesterol reduction therapy (e.g., statins), screening for disease, and therapeutic lifestyle changes (e.g., dietary therapy and exercise).

In contrast to clinical interventions, public health efforts place greater emphasis on *primordial prevention*, which aims to reduce risk factors for CVD (smoking, sedentary lifestyle, high fat diet) to decrease the likelihood of individuals and populations developing the disease.

In this chapter, we focus on the epidemiology of CVD, highlighting the current burden of CVD in the United States and evaluating trends in disease mortality and morbidity. Primary and secondary approaches to the prevention of CVD are discussed. In particular, we focus on the issue of screening for CVD and review aspects of the current debates regarding noninvasive techniques for the screening of CVD and of surgery for obesity, presented in the context of two case studies.

The Epidemiology of CVD

Cardiovascular disease is a term that includes myocardial infarction (MI, heart attack), angina pectoris, atherosclerosis, cerebrovascular diseases (stroke), heart failure, hypertension, and other circulatory outcomes. In accordance with the International Classification of Diseases (ICD-10) system for standardized disease classification, total cardiovascular disease encompasses ICD-10 codes 100–199 and Q20–28. The use of the ICD-10 classification system is presented in Chapter 3. Congenital cardiovascular defects are often included in the definition of total cardiovascular disease (Q20–28). Consequently, total cardiovascular disease is a broad category.

It is estimated that 79.4 million American adults (one in three) have CVD, and 47 percent (37.5 million) of these persons are age 65 years and older (Rosamond et al. 2007). High blood pressure is the most prevalent type of CVD, with 90 percent of those with CVD having high blood pressure. *High blood pressure* (HBP) is defined as a systolic blood pressure of 140 mm Hg or greater and/or a diastolic blood pressure of 90 mm Hg or greater, taking antihypertensive medications, or being told at least twice by a physician or other health professional that one has HBP.

The second most prevalent component of total CVD is coronary heart disease (CHD), with 15.8 million cases in the United States in 2004 (Rosamond et al. 2007). CHD (ICD-10 codes 120–125) includes acute myocardial infarctions, other acute ischemic (coronary) heart disease, angina pectoris, atherosclerotic cardiovascular diseases, and other conditions.

It is important to be familiar with the various types of CVD and with the disease classification systems that organizations such as the American Heart Association (AHA) use for the classification of CVD. In general, statistics compiled by the National Center for Health Statistics and the AHA use standard definitions. The definition of the disease is an important issue in both the design and the analysis of epidemiologic studies, and in the interpretation of the resulting data. For this chapter, our focus will be on CVD, CHD, and stroke.

Trends in CVD Mortality

Since the late 1960s, the mortality rate for CVD in the United States, including deaths from CHD and stroke, has steadily declined (see Figure 15.1) (Cooper et al. 2000). From 1980 to 2000, the age-adjusted death rate for CHD fell from 542.9 to 266.8 deaths per 100,000 population among men and from 263.3 to 134.4 deaths per 100,000 women (Ford et al. 2007). Recent data have suggested that the decline in CHD and stroke mortality has slowed since about 1990. Age-adjusted CHD mortality rates decreased at a rate of greater than 3 percent per year for the 20-year period from 1970 to 1990. However, for the period between 1990 and 1997, CHD mortality declined at a rate of 2.7 percent (Cooper et al. 2000).

In any examination of trends in mortality data, one of the first questions to ask is whether the increase or decline is real. Trends in mortality over time may be due to changes in the prevalence of cardiovascular risk factors in the population (e.g., rates of smoking or high blood pressure), changes

FIGURE 15.1
Death Rates
for Major
Cardiovascular
Diseases in
the United
States from
1900 to 1997

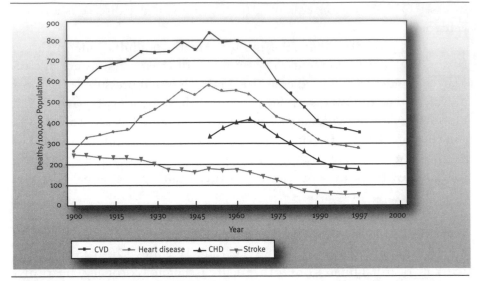

NOTE: Rates are age-adjusted to the 2000 standard.

SOURCE: Cooper, R., J. Cutler, P. Desvigne-Nickens, S. P. Fortmann, L. Friedman, R. Havlik, G. Hogelin, J. Marler, P. McGovern, G. Morosco, L. Mosca, T. Pearson, J. Stamler, D. Stryer, and T. Thom. 2000. "Trends and Disparities in Coronary Heart Disease, Stroke, and Other Cardiovascular Diseases in the United States: Findings of the National Conference on Cardiovascular Disease Prevention." *Circulation* 102 (25): 3137–47. Used with permission.

in the treatment of, and medical therapies for, CVD, or perhaps changes in the collection and recording of mortality data over the period under consideration (e.g., coding of death certificates).

For planning purposes, it is crucial to understand the secular changes in the distribution of disease over time. The development of policies and programs for improving the health status of the population should be, in part, premised on an understanding of these trends. To understand if population-based interventions are effective, analysts need to account for background changes in disease rates, which may be occurring at the same time as their intervention programs. A multitude of factors at both the individual and the population levels can influence rates of disease in a population. For example, population-wide changes in dietary habits may be occurring concurrently with increased use of lipid-lowering medications or changes in smoking patterns.

An appreciation of the magnitude of the decline in CVD mortality in the United States provides an important lesson. In general, upward or downward secular changes in mortality are considered among the most persuasive evidence that CVD is strongly influenced by environmental factors. The declines we have witnessed in CVD mortality in the United States are not evident around the world. High rates of CVD in eastern Europe and Russia, which continue to rise, have been documented (Cooper 1981; Peasey et al. 2006). Bobak and Marmot (2005) provide a thorough review of this unprecedented epidemic of CVD in central and eastern Europe, relating the CVD epidemic, in part, to socioeconomic inequalities and the profound societal transformation that occurred in the late twentieth century with the fall of Communist regimes, which influenced poverty levels, diet, stress, and excess alcohol consumption in this population (Bobak and Marmot 2005).

To make appropriate decisions regarding the allocation of resources to the prevention of CVD, it is necessary to understand how much of the decline in CVD mortality may be attributed to medical interventions, and how much may be attributed to changes in the prevalence of CVD risk factors (e.g., smoking, unhealthy cholesterol levels, and high blood pressure) in the population.

Secondary prevention through medical technology and pharmaceutical treatments has grown rapidly in the last several decades. The use of evidence-based therapies—including thrombolysis, coronary artery bypass grafting, coronary angioplasty and stents, and angiotensin converting enzyme (ACE) inhibitors and statins—has become a standard approach to treatment. It has been argued that a major contributor to the decline in mortality has been the availability of new technology and therapeutics, which have led to substantial (35–50 percent) reductions in the risk of disease (Shaw et al. 2001).

However, others have argued for the primacy of population changes in risk factors for explaining the decline in mortality and have advocated preventive approaches for decreasing CVD in populations (Ford et al. 2007). In a persuasive analysis of the factors that account for the decline in CHD in the United States between 1980 and 2000, Ford and colleagues (2007) examined the respective roles of medical therapies and population-based changes in risk factor levels as predictors of the decline in CHD mortality. The researchers used a previously validated statistical model known as the IMPACT mortality model (Capewell, Morrison, and McMurray 1999; Capewell et al. 2000). In brief, the model incorporates data on major population risk factors for CHD (smoking, high blood pressure, unhealthy cholesterol levels, etc.) and all usual medical and surgical treatments for CHD. The model is based on reasonable epidemiologic assumptions regarding the numbers of deaths that may be prevented or postponed by medical or surgical treatments or by changes in population risk factors. The development of statistical models for making these projections for planning purposes is a common research strategy employed by epidemiologists and medical researchers.

To illustrate the types of "logic" employed by this model, take the following example. Assume that there are 102,280 men in the United States between the ages of 55 and 64 years who are hospitalized with an acute myocardial infarction. Further, assume that the expected mortality reduction, if all of these males are provided with aspirin, is 15 percent (Ford et al. 2007). The age-specific one-year case fatality rate for acute myocardial infarc-

FIGURE 15.2
Percentage of
the Decrease
in Deaths
from Coronary
Heart Disease
Attributed to
Treatments
and Risk
Factor
Changes

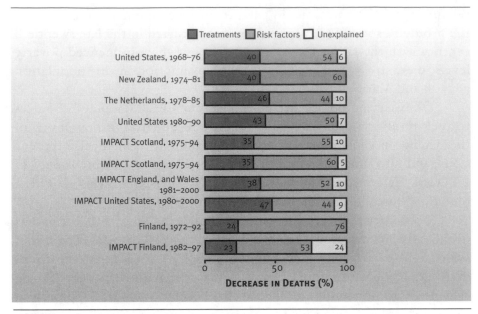

SOURCE: Ford et al (2007).

tion is 5.4 percent. If 84 percent are given aspirin, what number of deaths will be prevented or postponed for at least one year by the use of aspirin among this group of men? The solution is simply to multiply the statistics in a linear combination to calculate the number of deaths prevented:

102,280 population × 0.84 provided with aspirin × 0.15 mortality reduction × 0.054 deaths from acute MI in one year = 696

Ford and colleagues (2007) concluded that "half of the decline in U.S. deaths from coronary heart disease from 1980 to 2000 may be attributable to reductions in major risk factors and approximately half to medical based therapies." In their analysis, they noted that reductions in total cholesterol and reductions in blood pressure were the primary contributors to the changes in risk factors in the population over this period. The model used by these researchers is further strengthened by the concordance of their results with those found in other industrialized countries studied, including England, New Zealand, Scotland, and Finland (see Figure 15.2).

The slowing of the trends in CVD mortality in recent years also appears to be consistent with some general slowing of the trends in the decline of risk factors (smoking and hypertension), as well as the detrimental and well-documented increasing trends in diabetes and body mass index (obesity). The epidemics of obesity and diabetes will require substantial investments in population-based prevention programs if we wish to improve the trends in the incidence of and mortality from CVDs.

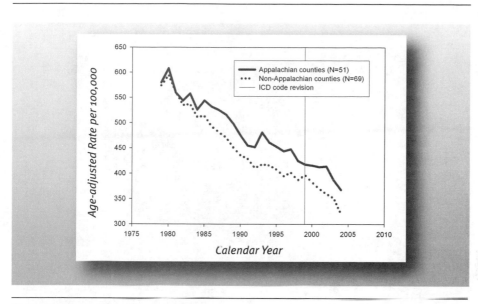

SOURCE: Rugg, Bailey, and Browning (2008).

FIGURE 15.3
Cardiovascular Disease Mortality Rates in Kentucky for All Age, Race, and Gender Groups, Appalachian Versus Non-Appalachian Counties, 1979–2004

Data on more localized trends in CVD can be especially useful for health planners. Mortality data can be easily accessed from government websites such as those at the Centers for Disease Control and Prevention (CDC). *CDC Wonder* is an easily accessible source for mortality data and is available from the CDC website. In addition, current prevalence data on risk factors for CVD in various geographic locations (states, counties) can be obtained from the Behavioral Risk Factor Surveillance System, which also can be accessed over the Internet from the CDC home page (www.cdc.gov). For example, data obtained from *CDC Wonder* are useful for describing trends in CVD mortality in Kentucky and indicate higher rates in the Appalachian region of the state in comparison with the non-Appalachian region (see Figure 15.3).

The Geographic Distribution of CVD

Geographical variations in CVD mortality and prevalence provide further evidence of the relationship between environmental factors and lifestyles and the occurrence of disease. Fundamental to the practice of epidemiology is the observation that the occurrence of disease varies across person, place, and time. The geographic distribution of CVD has been an area of research since Ancel Keys undertook the Seven Countries Study in the mid-1950s, which systematically examined the influence of diet across geographically and culturally distinct populations (Keys et al. 1986; Keys 1997). CHD mortality rates varied widely across countries, from a high rate in East Finland

FIGURE 15.4
Heart Disease
Death Rates
For All Males
Age 35 Years
and Older
From 1991–
1995

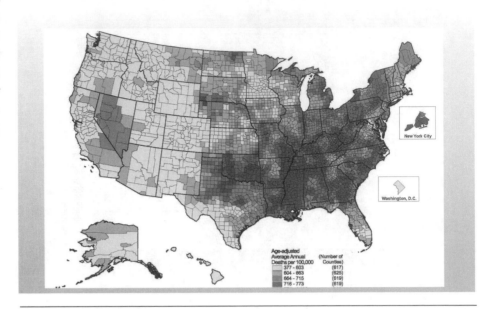

SOURCE: Barnett et. al (2001).

(68/1,000) to a low rate in Japan (7/1,000). It is well understood that historical factors within a geographic region can have a profound influence on the distribution of CVD.

The Japanese–Honolulu–San Francisco Study provided persuasive evidence that changes in lifestyle were related to changes in the incidence of CHD (Robertson et al. 1977). Native Japanese who moved to Honolulu, Hawaii, and then San Francisco adopted the rates of disease of the location to which they immigrated within a generation, presumably reflecting the strong influence of changes in lifestyle in the new location. Similarly, the increasing rates of CVD in areas of the former Soviet Union, following political and social changes in that region in the early 1990s, indicate how quickly social factors can influence the rates of CVD. Besides being of interest to medical geographers and epidemiologists, an understanding of the geographic distribution of disease can play a role in making appropriate decisions regarding the location of health services, in understanding patterns of utilization of those services, and in making predictions regarding future needs within a geographic region.

The use of geographic information systems (GIS) for the creation of maps describing the spatial distribution of disease, as well as the location of health services and care utilization patterns, has been growing in popularity among researchers and health managers. Online databases are becoming increasingly available to analysts and researchers for mapping current health surveillance data to understand the spatial distribution of risk factors, diseases, and other health outcomes. With respect to cardiovascular outcomes, CDC has supported the development of national and regional atlases for heart disease and stroke based on mortality data.

Figure 15.4 shows the map of heart disease mortality for all men age 35 years and older in the United States for the period 1991–1995 (Barnett et al. 2001). The map illustrates the considerable geographic variation in heart disease death rates across states. CHD death rates at the county level ranged from 377 to 1,102 deaths per 100,000 persons. There is a clear east-west gradient in heart disease mortality. The Appalachian region, the Ohio-Mississippi River Valley, the Mississippi Delta, and the eastern Piedmont and coastal regions of Georgia, South Carolina, and North Carolina had many counties in the top two quintiles of the distribution of the rates. Most of the counties in the Pacific Northwest and in the Rocky Mountain region of Colorado were in the lowest quintile.

It is important to note a few of the technical specifics regarding these types of maps. First, the rates of mortality are age-adjusted, with the U.S. population in 1970 (in this case) as the standard. The age adjustment is needed to control for the differing age distributions that exist across regions. The procedure essentially accounts for the confounding influence of age on mortality and makes the rates comparable across regions (see Chapter 6). These rates are also spatially smoothed. This approach is intended to account for some of the instability of the rates at the county level and reduces the distinction between counties to illustrate the broader disease patterns.

The mapping of public health surveillance data can be used to establish public health priorities, to evaluate the impact of programs, and to identify emerging trends. For example, as was apparent in Figure 15.3, the rates of CVD are particularly high in the Appalachian region of Kentucky. The Appalachian region of the state has been particularly vulnerable to high rates of CVDs and other chronic health conditions, in part from its history of economic underdevelopment (Barnett et al. 1998; Barnett et al. 2000). The underdevelopment has contributed to the higher rates of unemployment, poverty, disability, and low adult educational attainment in the region.

A closer look at total CVD mortality rates in the Appalachian region of Kentucky is revealed in Figure 15.5. This graphic shows the rates of total CVDs by county for both genders in Kentucky from 1999 to 2004. The profile is different from the previous figure since the outcome is total CVD and not heart disease, and because the data in the map are not smoothed. Nevertheless, the pattern of high CVD death rates in the eastern, southeastern, and some western counties in the state is evident.

FIGURE 15.5
Age–
Adjusted
Cardiovascular
Disease
Mortality
Rates for
Kentucky,
1999–2004,
Total
Population

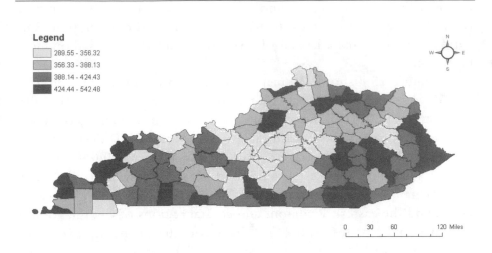

Legend

■ 289.55 – 356.32
■ 356.33 – 388.13
■ 388.14 – 424.43
■ 424.44 – 542.48

0   30   60   120 Miles

SOURCE: Map created by Jeffrey Jones, University of Kentucky, based on data from the Centers for Disease Control.

An understanding of the disease distribution can provide evidence of need for services. Barnett and colleagues (1998) have used data from the American Hospital Association to describe the distribution of medical services in the Appalachian region, employing GIS approaches to mapping medical services. These researchers found that most counties in the Appalachian region of the United States do not have cardiac rehabilitation units (CRUs). Evidence has supported the association between the availability and use of CRUs (secondary prevention) and the improvements in mortality from coronary heart disease. These units provide rehabilitative services to patients who have serious coronary heart disease or who are recovering from heart attacks (MIs). The units are typically located in general hospitals and are supervised by a physician with a team that usually includes a nurse, social worker or psychologist, exercise physiologist, and others. Barnett and colleagues (1998) document the uneven distribution of medical care resources in Appalachia and argue for improved access to facilities and programs for cardiac rehabilitation.

The Biology of CVD and Risk Factors

Before epidemiologic investigation of CVD, it was thought there may be a single etiology (cause) that would differentiate those who had atherosclerotic heart disease from those who did not. However, after more than 50 years of focused research on the issue, it is clear that CVD is a multifactorial disease process and that certain lifestyle habits can promote the development of disease in genetically susceptible persons. That is, the development of CVD is considered a "multifactorial process involving a variety of predisposing risk factors, each of which is best considered as an ingredient of a cardiovascular risk profile" (Kannel, McGee, and Gordon 1976).

This emphasis forces health professionals to look at the whole patient and to seek to understand the cumulative and synergistic nature of the risk factors in making treatment decisions. For total CVD, the risk factors include cigarette smoking, blood lipids (i.e., cholesterol), glucose intolerance (i.e., diabetes), high blood pressure, and left ventricular hypertrophy as assessed by the electrocardiogram. The standard risk factors have been significantly related to CHD risk in cohort investigations such as the Framingham Heart Study.

Approaches to clinical risk assessment have been developed from data based on the Framingham study. The epidemiologic data have established that the assessment of risk based on any single individual risk factor, say a total cholesterol level above 200 mg/dl, can be inefficient and would miss persons with several borderline risk factors who experience most of the cardiovascular events in the population. The Framingham risk equation was developed to estimate the probability that persons with certain characteristics would develop CVD in a specified interval. This equation makes use of measurements of traditional risk factors (age, total cholesterol, smoking status, high-density lipoprotein [HDL] level, and systolic blood pressure) to calculate the probability of a CHD event. Current guidelines in the United States for primary prevention recommend initial clinical assessment and risk stratification of individuals based on the traditional standard risk factors using the Framingham Risk Score (FRS), followed by specific therapies.

Atherosclerosis is responsible for the majority of cases of CHD and many cases of stroke. Atherosclerosis begins to develop early in life and progresses with time; however, the extent of progression varies among individuals. Calcification of the coronary artery (CAC) is part of the development of atherosclerosis. CAC occurs in small amounts in early arterial lesions, but is found more frequently after the third decade of life.

CAC is measured by a technique known as electron beam computed tomography (EBCT). This is a fast computed tomography method for scoring the amount of calcium in the coronary artery; the measurement of coronary artery calcium can be completed in 10–15 minutes. Cardiac computed tomography has been increasingly used in the United States with the intent of identifying patients with obstructive coronary artery disease on the basis of the estimated amount of calcium present (Greenland et al. 2007). CAC scoring can be used to globally indicate a patient's risk of a CHD event given its strong association with the total atherosclerotic disease burden.

Managerial and Economic Considerations with Screening

In the past, clinical researchers often enjoyed considerable freedom in developing new, applied research techniques in the hope of identifying disease and providing treatment to patients with certain conditions and diseases. However, as previously discussed in the text, healthcare spending has continued to increase at rates higher than inflation, and decisions regarding healthcare rationing are increasingly being forced upon practitioners and the public.

Evidence-based medicine is becoming the standard on which decisions regarding clinical appropriateness are made. That is, it is now necessary to generate a "certain amount of evidence" to justify the use of a new procedure or therapeutic intervention. The assessment of coronary artery calcification in asymptomatic individuals provides a case study of the issue of using a relatively expensive screening technology in patients and populations to improve risk prediction, treatment, and outcomes.

Generally, evidence-based medicine relies on data from randomized clinical trials (Chapter 13) for making decisions regarding the appropriateness of and evidence for using new procedures and medications. There have been no clinical trials to evaluate the impact of coronary artery calcium testing in asymptomatic patients on outcomes (such as quality of life or mortality) (Greenland et al. 2007). One study, the St. Francis Heart Study (discussed below), did consider reductions in clinical endpoints. The St. Francis Heart Study was a randomized clinical trial where eligible subjects were screened with coronary EBCT.

Cardiologists and medical researchers have argued that efforts should be directed toward screening the asymptomatic population for coronary artery disease. One argument is that "on average, only 50–60 percent of the variability in the health outcome can be predicted by traditional risk factors, using the Framingham model" (Shaw et al. 2003). The established noninvasive methods for the evaluation of coronary artery disease, such as stress testing, have generally identified only patients with advanced atherosclerotic disease or a myocardial infarction.

One of the principles of CVD prevention is that "the intensity of the intervention for an individual (or population) should be adjusted to the baseline risk" (Greenland et al. 2007). This principle is intended to optimize efficacy, safety, and cost-effectiveness of the intervention; that is, we do not want to apply expensive treatment and high-risk procedures to individuals (or populations) who are at lower absolute risk for the disease of interest. For example, cholesterol and blood pressure guidelines in the United States have tried to achieve a balance between treatment intensity and the severity of a patient's risk (Greenland et al. 2007). The principle suggests that the benefit of a drug or therapy is greater when the patient's risk is high. It has become standard practice to divide patients into risk categories depending on calculated ten-year risk estimates. The National Cholesterol

Education Program guidelines stratify patients in lipid-lowering categories into four risk categories: high risk, moderate high risk, moderate risk, and lower risk.

One of the key issues with CAC screening is that consideration needs to be given to the most appropriate population for screening. *Screening* is the "identification of unrecognized disease or defect by the application of tests, examinations, or other procedures that can be applied rapidly and inexpensively to populations" (Valanis 1999). For patients or populations at low risk, there is limited reason for using an expensive screening technology. The reality is that screening tests often create some problems while trying to solve others. Targeting the screening test to the population that would most benefit is a necessary principle. The requirements for valid screening tests were discussed in Chapter 3.

Screening tests are applied to healthy individuals or populations to identify disease before there are symptoms and to permit early treatment. Diagnostic tests are applied to patients with symptoms with a view toward reaching an accurate diagnosis.

With respect to CAC testing, one of the primary requirements for a screening test is that there must be a high level of evidence that it will improve health outcomes (i.e., a reduction in events, improved survival, or an extended quality of life). As an example, clinical trials have been conducted to assess screening for abdominal aortic aneurysms (Greenland et al. 2007). The results from these trials show favorable support for screening for abdominal aortic aneurysms. Similar studies are not available to support coronary artery calcium measurements for screening for CHD. In the absence of this type of evidence, how does one proceed?

To justify the use of a new screening test, the new test would need to be better than what is currently available as the "gold standard." All clinical tests have limitations, and all techniques have the potential to misclassify or misrepresent the true state of disease. It is often asserted that the sensitivity and specificity of a given test are invariant for that test; they are a test characteristic. However, we know that in practice this is not the case. For screening purposes, the current approach to screening is to use the Framingham Risk Score (FRS). For CHD, the gold standard for diagnosis can be considered coronary angiography. Two questions need to be answered: (1) Is there a strong relationship between measured CAC and CHD events? and (2) Does the measurement of CAC provide incremental information beyond what can be obtained from the FRS?

Analysis of six studies in a meta-analysis reported by Greenland and colleagues (2007) (Figure 15.6) provides some resolution to the first question. The meta-analysis reports the individual and summary relative risks. The relative risks compare individuals at higher risk of events to those at lower risk at different measured levels of coronary artery calcium. The figure reports a summary relative risk of 4.3 (95 percent confidence interval:

FIGURE 15.6
Meta–Analysis
on the
Prognostic
Value of CAC
Screening

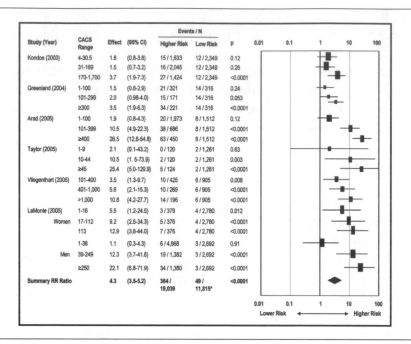

SOURCE: Greenland et al. (2007). Used with permission of the American Heart Association.

3.5–5.2) for any measurable calcium compared to a low-risk CAC. This means that a three- to five-year risk of detectable calcium elevates a patient's CHD risk of an event over fourfold (p <0.0001).

To address the question of whether the measurement of CAC provides information beyond that obtained from the Framingham Risk Score, one can examine an appropriate receiver operating characteristic (ROC) curve. The area under the ROC curve is known as the C-statistic. A ROC analysis plots the sensitivity (fraction of true positives) versus 1 – specificity (fraction of false positives) of a risk factor for predicting events. ROC curves are ideally suited to evaluate the discrimination of a prediction. If a given risk factor or set of risk factors predicted the onset of cardiovascular events perfectly, the curve would reach 100 percent in the upper left corner. The area under the curve would be 100 percent with a C-statistic = 1. A useless predictor would produce a straight line from the origin to the upper right corner with a C-statistic = 0.5. Comparing the C-statistic from a curve based on traditional risk factors to a curve based on the traditional risk factors and CAC would allow one to determine the incremental improvement in using the CAC score in predicting risk. Greenland et al. (2007) did demonstrate that CAC scores were independently predictive of CHD risk beyond the Framingham Risk Score.

The Framingham Risk Score is one of the most widely used algorithms for the prediction of CHD. The Framingham scoring includes the major risk factors like gender, total cholesterol, HDL cholesterol, systolic blood pressure, cigarette smoking, and age. One of the key questions is whether the addition of CAC to the known risk factors in the Framingham model will improve the prediction of CHD. Case Study 15.1 explores screening for CAC using electron bean computed tomography.

Case Study 15.1. Screening for CAC

Initially, electron beam computed tomography (EBCT) had been used for measuring coronary calcium for risk stratification and diagnosis in individuals with symptoms of coronary disease. Recently, however, there have been efforts to promote the use of EBCT for screening in asymptomatic patients.

The definition of the gold standard of the disease classification is needed in any consideration of screening. For the scenario below, we will assume that the gold standard is diagnostic catheterization, and significant coronary disease is indicated by 50–70 percent stenosis by coronary angiography.

Patients underwent coronary angiography following the presentation of clinical signs and symptoms of coronary disease. Using a fast computed tomography instrument, we further assume that the sensitivity of a coronary calcium score of >0 was 95 percent and the specificity was 66 percent.

One of the key considerations in evaluating the use of screening tests in asymptomatic populations is the underlying prevalence of the disease. The predictive value of the screening test will vary depending on this prevalence. Suppose that we decide to use EBCT in a population of low-risk individuals (prevalence of disease = 10 percent).

QUESTIONS

1. Given the sensitivity and specificity for the EBCT above, what would be the positive predictive value (PPV) of the screening test in a population of 1,000 individuals? How many false positives would results from using the test?
2. In using diagnostic technology, it is evident that the sensitivity of the test is highest when the cutpoint for the disease is lowest (e.g., a low CAC score). Increasing the cutpoint of the test will lower the sensitivity of the test but increase the specificity of the test. Let's assume that we change the cutpoint at which we make a decision for a positive test. We now set the CAC score for a positive test at 100, which equates to a sensitivity of 87 percent and a specificity of 79 percent. Assuming a low-risk population with a disease prevalence of 10 percent among 1,000 persons, recalculate the positive predictive value of the test and the number of false positives. How does this scenario compare to the previous one?
3. Let's now assume that the baseline prevalence of disease increases. That is, we are now screening an intermediate risk population (perhaps an older population) that has a baseline disease prevalence of 50 percent. (This

can also be considered the pretest probability of disease—the likelihood that the disease is present before the testing is performed.) Assume a sensitivity of 0.95 and a specificity of 0.66. What is the positive predictive value for this situation?

4. EBCT calcium scores correlate with the extent of atherosclerosis and with the risk of subsequent CHD events (myocardial infarctions or deaths). Suppose you conducted a cohort study of 30,826 persons and obtained the data given in Table 15.1 below. Coronary artery calcium scores were obtained at baseline using EBCT. The cohort study was conducted over a five-year period with follow-up for myocardial infarctions and CHD deaths. Using Table 15.1 below, calculate the relative risk (RR) for each level of CAC compared to the low-risk referent (CAC score = 0). Interpret these results.

TABLE 15.1. COHORT STUDY OF EBCT CALCIUM SCORES

CAC Score	CHD Event (Death or MI)	Total Population
<0 (referent)	45	12,163
1–100	67	9,514
101–400	110	5,209
401–999	182	3,940
Total	404	30,826

SOURCE: Greenland et al. (2007).

ANSWERS

1. Refer to Table 15.2 below to answer the question.

   a. Step 1: If there are 1,000 subjects who are screened with EBCT and the prevalence of disease is 10 percent, then 100 of them will actually have CHD (0.10 × 1,000 = 100).

   b. Step 2: Of the 100 subjects who actually have CHD, 95 of them will test positive with EBCT (sensitivity 0.95 × 100 = 95), and 5 will test negative (100 − 95 = 5).

   c. Step 3: Of the 900 subjects without CHD, 594 of them will test negative if the specificity is 66 percent (0.66 × 900 = 594), and 306 will test positive (900− 594 = 306).

   d. The number of false positives is 306 (they test positive and do not have CHD). The PPV is (95/401) × 100 = 23.7%. That is, only 24 percent of persons who test positive will have CHD. Four-hundred-one persons will test positive under this scenario, and 306 of these persons (76 percent) who test positive will not have the condition and will be false positives.

TABLE 15.2. EBCT TEST CHARACTERISTICS: 95% SENSITIVITY, 66% SPECIFICITY, 10% PREVALENCE

	CHD	No CHD	Total
CAC score >0 (positive test)	95	306	401
CAC score = 0 (negative test)	5	594	599
Total	100	900	1,000

2. Refer to Table 15.3 below to answer the question.

TABLE 15.3. EBCT TEST CHARACTERISTICS: 87% SENSITIVITY, 79% SPECIFICITY, 10% PREVALENCE

	CHD	No CHD	Total
CAC score >0 (positive test)	87	189	276
CAC score = 0 (negative test)	13	711	724
Total	100	900	1,000

a. Step 1: If there are 1,000 subjects who are screened with EBCT and the prevalence of disease is 10 percent, then 100 of them will actually have CHD ($0.10 \times 1,000 = 100$).

b. Step 2: Of the 100 subjects who actually have CHD, 87 of them will test positive with EBCT (sensitivity $0.87 \times 100 = 87$), and 13 will test negative ($100 - 87 = 13$).

c. Step 3: Of the 900 subjects without CHD, 711 of them will test negative if the specificity is 79 percent ($0.79 \times 900 = 711$), and 189 will test positive ($900 - 711 = 189$).

d. The number of false positives is 189 (they test positive and do not have CHD). The PPV is $(87/276) \times 100 = 31.5\%$. That is, only 31.5 percent of people who test positive will have coronary heart disease. Two-hundred-seventy-six persons will test positive under this scenario, and 189 of these persons (68 percent) who test positive will not have the condition and will be false positives. The PPV is improved in this scenario, in comparison to (a) above; there has been an increase in the PPV, and the number of false positives has declined.

3. Refer to Table 15.4 below to answer this question.

a. Step 1: If there are 1,000 subjects who are screened with EBCT and the prevalence of disease is 50 percent, then 500 of them will actually have CHD ($0.50 \times 1,000 = 500$).

TABLE 15.4. EBCT TEST CHARACTERISTICS: 95% SENSITIVITY, 66% SPECIFICITY, 50% PREVALENCE

	CHD	No CHD	Total
CAC score >0 (positive test)	475	170	645
CAC score = 0 (negative test)	25	330	335
Total	500	500	1,000

b. Step 2: Of the 500 subjects who actually have CHD, 475 of them will test positive with EBCT (sensitivity 0.95 × 500 = 475), and 25 will test negative (500 – 475 = 25).

c. Step 3: Of the 500 subjects without CHD, 330 of them will test negative if the specificity is 66 percent (0.66 × 500 = 330), and 170 will test positive (500 – 330 = 170).

d. The number of false positives is 170 (they test positive and do not have CHD). The PPV is (475/645) × 100 = 73.6%. That is, 74 percent of people who test positive will have CHD. Six-hundred-forty-five persons will test positive under this scenario, and 170 of these persons (26.4 percent) who test positive will not have the condition and will be false positives. The PPV is improved in this scenario, in comparison to either (a) or (b) above; there has been an increase in the PPV, and the number of false positives has declined.

4. Calculating from the data given in Table 15.1, the incidence of CHD events (per 1,000 population) for the CAC scores is 3.7 (45/12,163 × 1,000), 7.0 (67/9,514 × 1,000), 21.1 (110/5,209 × 1,000), 46.2 (182/3,940 × 1,000), and 13.1 (404/30,826 × 1,000) for the referent, 1–100, 101–400, 401–999, and total scores, respectively. Relative risks for the three higher levels (1–100, 101–401, and 401–999) and total are calculated as follows: 7.0/3.7 = 1.9 (score 1–100), 21.1/3.7 = 5.7 (score 101–401), 46.2/3.7 = 12.5 (score 401–999), and 13.1/3.7 = 3.5 (total). These results suggest a dose-response relationship in that increasingly higher CAC scores are related to increasingly higher risk of CHD events.

Other Considerations for Screening Tests

When making decisions regarding screening programs, it is important to consider the general principles that constitute the recommendations for screening programs.

As is often stated in introductory texts of epidemiology, "a disease must be detectable during the preclinical phase by some test, and early treatment should convey a benefit over treatment at the time the disease would have come to attention without screening" (Rothman 2002). That is, there is no point in screening if early treatment or intervention does not extend life or improve outcomes.

There are a number of characteristics of CVD, and heart disease in particular, that make it an attractive target for screening. The requirement for an extended preclinical stage is relevant for CVD as the early stages of atherosclerosis become evident in childhood.

In our example of screening using CAC, there have been limited data to suggest that the use of this technology would actually improve patient outcomes. Patients who are screened and have high scores need to receive appropriate and effective interventions to reduce their long-term risk for coronary heart disease. The St. Francis Heart Study provides qualified data to address this issue (Ardehali et al. 2007). Treatment with a cholesterol lowering drug (atorvastatin, 20 mg/dl) reduced the low-density lipoprotein cholesterol by 39–43 percent (p <0.0001) and triglycerides by 11–17 percent (p = 0.02), and reduced clinical endpoints by 30 percent (based on a comparison of 6.9 percent in treated subjects by 9.9 percent in the untreated, p = 0.08). Consideration needs to be given to how effectively such an aggressive intervention could be implemented in a population-based program. A final consideration is safety, acceptability, and cost-effectiveness. We will comment in more detail below on the issue of safety, acceptability, and cost-effectiveness.

Cost-Effectiveness of CAC

Healthcare managers can be challenged in making decisions regarding the use of new technologies for improving healthcare. In the case of evaluating noninvasive screening tests for the detection of CVDs, these decisions require consideration of several factors. The most important principle would be to demonstrate that CAC screening would enhance the quality of life or prolong life. Cost-effectiveness analysis is a typical approach for making this evaluation.

When there are well-conducted randomized clinical trials (RCTs) establishing the efficacy of certain treatments and procedures and the results of these trials are generally in agreement, the decisions are easier. However, randomized trials do not exist for the evaluation of CAC measurements on survival and quality of life in patients. Analysts who undertake cost-effectiveness studies often need to develop their models using simulations, garnering as much information as possible from the medical literature.

Despite the challenges, researchers have undertaken cost-effectiveness analysis of CAC scoring. The incremental cost-effectiveness ratio (ICER) is one measure for reporting the results from these types of studies. This measure compares the differences in both costs and outcomes for two interventions that compete with each other for resources. Results from a study by O'Malley, Greenberg, and Taylor (2004) offered an ICER of $86,752 per life year saved for a 42-year-old subject comparing a person with any CAC score greater than zero to a CAC score equal to zero. Shaw and colleagues (2003) undertook a similar analysis and presented results stratified by the estimated risk of coronary events. For individuals with a risk of less than 0.6 percent per year, the ICER approached $500,000 per life year saved, indicating that it was not cost-effective to use coronary calcium measurements in low-risk individuals. If the estimated event rate was 1 percent per year, the ICER was $42,339 per life year saved; if the event rate was 2 percent per year (high risk), the ICER was estimated as $30,742 per life year saved (Shaw et al. 2003).

However, even if the analysis suggests a beneficial measure of the cost-effectiveness of screening, the realities of budgets often present challenges in the implementation. It was stated by Froelicher and colleagues (1999) that the cost of the equipment necessary to implement this screening method on a widespread basis would be prohibitively high. Only 42 EBCT Machines were available in the United States in 1999, and adding the necessary units at a cost of $1 million to $2 million per machine would be difficult, if not impossible. It was added that the yearly maintenance of these machines would be approximately $150,000 per machine, adding to the expense of this method. The high cost of the equipment itself would make this method impossible for a number of patient populations to access.

In summary, consensus committees have concluded that CAC measurement in patients with a low CHD risk (<10 percent per ten-year risk of estimated CHD events) is not recommended, nor would screening of the general population be recommended. For asymptomatic patients with intermediate CHD risk (10–20 percent per ten-year risk), it has been concluded that it may be reasonable to consider CAC measurements since such patients may be classified into a higher risk category and receive more aggressive management.

In the cost-effectiveness case study below, we consider the issue of gastric bypass for severe obesity, with the resulting conclusion being substantially more convincing than the issue of screening for coronary calcium.

Case Study 15.2. Cost-Effectiveness of Gastric Bypass for Severe Obesity

Craig and Tseng (2002) conducted a cost-effectiveness analysis on gastric bypass surgery by comparing the lifetime costs and outcomes between surgery and no treatment from the payer perspective. They used data from the Framingham Heart Study to estimate life expectancy for a target group of 35–55-year-old men and women who were relatively healthy; that is, they were nonsmokers without CVD, drug addictions, or major psychological disorders, but had a body mass index

(BMI) of between 40 and 50. Craig and Tseng used a decision model that assumed a 1.5 percent mortality rate with surgery, and a 3 percent mortality rate if the patient had a subsequent reversal or revisional surgery. (Note that the authors of the study report slightly different numbers due to rounding.)

QUESTIONS

1. Which costs should be included in this analysis?
2. The authors estimated "health-related quality of life" across age, gender, and BMI, which is summarized in Table 15.5 below. How does quality of life vary across BMI, age, and gender?

TABLE 15.5. HEALTH-RELATED QUALITY OF LIFE, BY SEX, AGE, AND BODY MASS INDEX

Age (Years)

	Men					Women				
BMI	35	45	55	65	75	35	45	55	65	75
25	0.929	0.912	0.886	0.850	0.805	0.908	0.889	0.857	0.813	0.755
30	0.903	0.880	0.853	0.823	0.790	0.875	0.846	0.811	0.770	0.722
35	0.877	0.848	0.821	0.797	0.775	0.842	0.804	0.765	0.727	0.688
40	0.851	0.816	0.789	0.770	0.760	0.809	0.761	0.719	0.684	0.654
45	0.825	0.784	0.756	0.743	0.745	0.775	0.718	0.673	0.641	0.621
50	0.799	0.752	0.724	0.717	0.730	0.742	0.675	0.627	0.598	0.587

SOURCE: Craig and Tseng (2002). Used with permission.

3. Table 15.6 summarizes the life expectancy, quality-adjusted life expectancy, and total costs of gastric bypass compared with no treatment, for men or women with a BMI of 40 or 50 who are 35 years old. How does life expectancy compare for men versus women, and for those with gastric bypass versus those without gastric bypass?
4. Calculate the incremental costs and incremental effectiveness (both in years and in quality-adjusted-life years [QALYs].
5. With the incremental costs, incremental life expectancy, and incremental QALYs, calculate the incremental cost-effectiveness ratios for men and women with BMIs of 40 or 50, using both life expectancy and QALYs as measures of effectiveness. Is gastric bypass cost-effective using both measures of effectiveness? Interpret the ICER for women with a BMI of 40 or 50 in terms of cost/life year.
6. Suppose the case fatality rates for those with gastric bypass surgery, reversals, and revisions were higher than the rates used in the decision model. How would this affect both the numerator (costs) and the denominator (effectiveness) of the ICER?

TABLE 15.6. EFFECTIVENESS AND COSTS IN BASE CASE ESTIMATES, BY RISK SUBGROUP AT AGE 35 YEARS

	Life Expectancy (Years)				QALY				Total Cost ($)			
	Gastric Bypass		No Treatment		Gastric Bypass		No Treatment		Gastric Bypass		No Treatment	
BMI	Men	Women	Men	Women	Men	Women	Men	Women	Men	Women	Men	Women
40	23.00	24.63	22.97	24.72	19.56	19.82	18.51	18.21	68,600	59,000	38,500	35,300
50	22.83	24.46	22.52	24.46	18.87	18.88	16.83	16.03	75,000	64,800	53,200	48,500

SOURCE: Craig and Tseng (2002). Used with permission.

ANSWERS

1. Since the authors conducted the analysis from the payer perspective, they included the costs of initial surgery, treatment of complications, follow-up care, and the costs associated with the treatment of diseases related to obesity, such as coronary heart disease, stroke, type 2 diabetes, hypercholesterolemia, and hypertension.

2. Quality of life decreases with age for both men and women. Women have slightly lower quality of life scores for each age category. Quality of life decreases with increasing BMI, and such decreases are greater for women than men.

3. Men have lower life expectancy than women with and without treatment. Both life expectancy and QALYs increase somewhat with gastric bypass.

4. For those with a BMI of 40, the incremental costs of gastric bypass versus no treatment would be $68,600 – $38,500 = $30,100 for men and $59,000 – 35,300 = $23,700 for women. For those with a BMI of 50, the incremental costs of gastric bypass versus no treatment would be $75,000 – $53,200 = $21,800 for men and $64,800 – 48,500 = $16,300 for women. For those with a BMI of 40, the incremental effectiveness in years of life expectancy would be 23.00 – 22.97 = 0.03 for men and 24.63 – 24.72 = –0.09 for women. For those with a BMI of 50, the incremental effectiveness in years of life expectancy would be 22.83 – 22.52 = 0.31 for men and 24.46 – 24.46 = 0 for women. For those with a BMI of 40, the incremental effectiveness (in QALYs) would be 19.56 – 18.51 = 1.05 for men and 19.82 – 18.21 = 1.61 for women. For those with a BMI of 50, the incremental effectiveness (in QALYs) would be 18.87 – 16.83 = 2.04 for men and 18.88 – 16.03 = 2.85 for women.

5. For those with a BMI of 40, ICERs for men would be $30,100/0.03 = $1,003,333 per life year and $30,100/1.05 = $28,666 per QALY; ICERs for women would be $23,700/–0.09 = indeterminate, and $23,700/1.61 = $14,720 per QALY. Notice that the ICER (life years) for women is "indeterminate," because it implies that there is a cost associated with a "reduc-

tion," rather than an addition to years of life. For those with a BMI of 50, ICERs for men would be $21,800/0.31 = $70,323 per life year and $21,800/2.04 = $10,686 per QALY; ICERs for women would be $16,300/0 = ∞ (the authors report $9,130,000) and $16,300/2.85 = $5,719 per QALY. Remember that our calculations are slightly different than the authors due to rounding (that is, the authors reported a minuscule life expectancy increase for women with a BMI of 50 who got gastric bypass, but it was so small we rounded it to zero for this case study). When effectiveness is measured in QALYs, gastric bypass is clearly cost-effective with the cost per QALY well below the conservative $100,000/QALY threshold. When life expectancy is not adjusted for quality, however, gastric bypass is cost-effective only for men with a BMI of 50. Since women with a BMI of 40 with no treatment lived slightly longer than those with gastric bypass, the ICER was indeterminate, because the procedure was incrementally more costly than no treatment, and produced a negative effectiveness. For women with a BMI of 50, the life expectancy for those with and without gastric surgery was the same, although the ICER of $9,130,000 reported by the authors suggests a very small increase in life expectancy for those with the treatment.

6. Perioperative deaths and complications that precede deaths would increase costs to the gastric bypass surgery patients, but more patient deaths would also result in less future medical costs, which should decrease the overall costs of gastric bypass surgery patients. High case fatality rates for gastric bypass should decrease both life expectancy and quality-adjusted life expectancy, making incremental effectiveness (the denominator) lower. If the costs of perioperative deaths and complications are greater than the future medical cost savings due to premature death, then the incremental cost would be higher with these higher case fatality rates. Higher incremental costs and lower incremental savings should result in a higher ICER.

Strategies for the Prevention of CVD

One of the arguments posed earlier in this chapter was that the disparities in the burden of CVDs are primarily due to environmental variables and include differences in CVD risk factors, lifestyles, and the use of primary and secondary preventive services. The concluding section of this chapter examines how the population-based perspective for addressing issues related to the reduction of CVD morbidity and mortality suggests strategies for achieving these aims that may be different than those usually considered by health managers.

While the declines in CVD mortality in the United States over the past few decades are encouraging, it remains less certain whether there has been a concomitant decline in the incidence of CVDs (Rosamond et al. 1998). CVDs remain the number one cause of death in the United States, and the successful translation of the knowledge of risk factors for CVD into effective public health and medical interventions has a long way to go.

The challenge regarding the prevention of CVD was effectively articulated by Geoffrey Rose, who is considered one of the fathers of cardiovascular epidemiology (Rose 1991, 2001). More than 20 years ago, Rose argued that shifting the distribution curve of a single risk factor such as high blood pressure or total cholesterol by a small amount in the entire population would have a greater impact on mortality rates than treating only persons with a high level for that risk factor.

Rose thus defined two strategies for the prevention of disease: the high-risk strategy and the population strategy. The *high-risk strategy* is the traditional, medical approach to the prevention of disease, which seeks to identify high-risk susceptible individuals, usually through screening, and to offer them some individual "protection" through treatment or medical therapy.

Cardiovascular medicine employs such a strategy when it uses the Framingham Risk Equation to calculate the 10- or 20-year risk of coronary heart disease for a patient (Greenland et al. 2007). The algorithm, as previously mentioned, is based on gender, total cholesterol, HDL cholesterol, systolic blood pressure, cigarette smoking, and age. The focus is on "total risk" rather than simply the elevation of one risk factor. The use of algorithms that employ multiple risk factors better characterizes the "baseline risk" for an event and thus improves the effectiveness and efficacy of any intervention. Consequently, cholesterol lowering drugs (most typically statins) are recommended for everyone with preexisting coronary disease (Manuel et al. 2006).

This approach is effective because it targets the group that accounts for a large proportion of the total population at risk for CHD. One of the strong arguments for this approach is that it is cost-effective given limited resources; one should concentrate limited medical resources and time where the need is greatest.

The *population strategy* for the prevention of disease is fundamentally different. This approach attempts to control the determinants of incidence of disease and to lower the mean level of the risk factors. It is a "radical approach" in the sense that it attempts to alter some of the norms of society—to change the behaviors and the culture of a population. It is traditional public health or, as Rose (1993) refers to it in his text *the strategy of preventive medicine*, as mass behavior change.

Rose (2001) initially argued that "from Framingham data one can compute that a 10 mm Hg lowering of the blood pressure distribution as a whole would correspond to a 30 percent reduction in total attributable mortality." Wald and Law (2003) have argued that a "polypill" of six low doses of a drug (including a statin) given to all men and women over age 55 would reduce coronary heart disease by a remarkable 80 percent, although this recommendation remains controversial.

The future for the prevention of CVD will likely see roles for both high-risk and population strategies and hybrid approaches that make the best use of these ideas. Which strategy is optimal? These issues will continue to be debated. Within the United States and other developed counties, CVD will continue to be the leading cause of death. The strategies for the reduction of burden of risk factors, such as obesity and diabetes, in populations will require knowledge of the evidence base for successful management and intervention programs directed toward primary and secondary prevention of CVD.

In this chapter, we have examined the data on the burden of CVD and have used epidemiologic approaches to examine the trends and the distribution of the disease in populations. Focusing on screening for coronary artery calcium and the use of gastric bypass surgery for the control of severe obesity, we examined the important issues to consider for screening programs and in conducting cost-effectiveness analysis. This chapter underscores the importance of using epidemiologic methods and data for optimizing healthcare decisions.

As we mentioned at the outset of the chapter, the Greek physician Hippocrates observed an association between obesity and sudden death as early as the fifth century B.C. Now, more than 2,000 years later, we enjoy medical advances undreamed of by the Periclean healer. As clinical and public health professionals, we do well to recall his most famous exhortation: *primum non nocere* (first do no harm). The decisions regarding whether to screen for coronary artery calcium in the population or to elect gastric bypass surgery for patients are often complex; however, for cardiovascular diseases, there are well-known risk factors (e.g., smoking, sedentary lifestyle, poor diet, uncontrolled hypertension) that place individuals and populations at increased risk and should always form the basis of our discussions of the prevention of this multifactorial disease.

Acknowledgments

We appreciate the editorial assistance of Teresa Donovan, in the Department of Preventive Medicine and Environmental Health at the University of Kentucky, and constructive comments from Alison Bailey, MD, and Mary R. Tooms. We further recognize the technical expertise of Jeff Jones, PhD, in the development of the map of mortality rates for this chapter.

References

Ardehali, R., K. Nasir, A. Kolandaivelu, M. J. Budoff, and R. S. Blumenthal. 2007. "Screening Patients for Subclinical Atherosclerosis with Non-Contrast Cardiac CT." *Atherosclerosis* 192 (2): 235–42.

Barnett, E., M. Casper, J. A. Halverson, G. A. Elmes, V. E. Braham, Z. A. Majeed, A. S. Bloom, and S. Stanely. 2001. *Men and Heart Disease: An Atlas of Racial and Ethnic Disparities in Mortality.* Atlanta, GA: Office for Social Environment and Health Research, West Virginia University, and National Center for Chronic Disease Prevention and Health Promotion, Centers for Disease Control and Prevention.

Barnett, E., G. Elmes, V. Braham, J. Halverson, J. Lee, and S. Loftus. 1998. *Heart Disease in Appalachia: An Atlas of County Economic Conditions, Mortality and Medical Care Resources.* Morgantown, WV: Office of Social Environment and Health Research, Prevention Research Center, West Virginia University.

Barnett, E., J. A. Halverson, G. A. Elmes, and V. E. Braham. 2000. "Metropolitan and Non-Metropolitan Trends in Coronary Heart Disease Mortality Within Appalachia, 1980–1997." *Annals of Epidemiology* 10 (6): 370–79.

Bobak, M., and M. Marmot. 2005. "Coronary Heart Disease in Central and Eastern Europe and the Former Soviet Union." *Coronary Heart Disease Epidemiology: From Aetiology to Public Health.* New York: Oxford University Press.

Capewell, S., C. E. Morrison, and J. J. McMurray. 1999. "Contribution of Modern Cardiovascular Treatment and Risk Factor Changes to the Decline in Coronary Heart Disease Mortality in Scotland Between 1975 and 1994." *Heart* 81 (4): 380–86.

Capewell, S., R. Beaglehole, M. Seddon, and J. McMurray. 2000. "Explanation for the Decline in Coronary Heart Disease Mortality Rates in Auckland, New Zealand, Between 1982 and 1993." *Circulation* 102 (13): 1511–16.

Cooper, R. 1981. "Rising Death Rates in the Soviet Union: The Impact of Coronary Heart Disease." *New England Journal of Medicine* 304 (21): 1259–65.

Cooper, R., J. Cutler, P. Desvigne-Nickens, S. P. Fortmann, L. Friedman, R. Havlik, G. Hogelin, J. Marler, P. McGovern, G. Morosco, L. Mosca, T. Pearson, J. Stamler, D. Stryer, and T. Thom. 2000. "Trends and Disparities in Coronary Heart Disease, Stroke, and Other Cardiovascular Diseases in the United States: Findings of the National Conference on Cardiovascular Disease Prevention." *Circulation* 102 (25): 3137–47.

Craig, B. M., and D. S. Tseng. 2002. "Cost Effectiveness of Gastric Bypass for Severe Obesity." *American Journal of Medicine* 113: 491–98.

Dawber, T. R., and W. B. Kannel. 1958. "An Epidemiologic Study of Heart

Disease: The Framingham Study." *Nutrition Reviews* 16 (1): 1–4.

Ford, E. S., U. A. Ajani, J. B. Croft, J. A. Critchley, D. R. Labarthe, T. E. Kottke, W. H. Giles, and S. Capewell. 2007. "Explaining the Decrease in U.S. Deaths from Coronary Disease, 1980–2000." *New England Journal of Medicine* 356 (23): 2388–98.

Froelicher, V. F., W. F. Fearon, C. M. Ferguson, A. P. Morise, P. Heidenreich, J. West, and J. E. Atwood. 1999. "Lessons Learned from Studies of the Standard Exercise ECG Test." *Chest* 116 (5): 1442–51.

Greenland, P., R. O. Bonow, B. H. Brundage, M. J. Budoff, M. J. Eisenberg, S. M. Grundy, M. S. Lauer, W. S. Post, P. Raggi, R. F. Redberg, G. P. Rodgers, L. J. Shaw, A. J. Taylor, W. S. Weintraub, and the American College of Cardiology Foundation Clinical Expert Consensus Task Force (ACCF/AHA Writing Committee to Update the 2000 Expert Consensus Document on Electron Beam Computed Tomography), Society of Atherosclerosis Imaging and Prevention, and Society of Cardiovascular Computed Tomography. 2007. "ACCF/AHA 2007 Clinical Expert Consensus Document on Coronary Artery Calcium Scoring by Computed Tomography in Global Cardiovascular Risk Assessment and in Evaluation of Patients with Chest Pain: A Report of the American College of Cardiology Foundation Clinical Expert Consensus Task Force (ACCF/AHA Writing Committee to Update the 2000 Expert Consensus Document on Electron Beam Computed Tomography) Developed in Collaboration with the Society of Atherosclerosis Imaging and Prevention and the Society of Cardiovascular Computed Tomography." *Journal of the American College of Cardiology* 49 (3): 378–402.

Kannel, W. B., D. McGee, and T. Gordon. 1976. "A General Cardiovascular Risk Profile: The Framingham Study." *American Journal of Cardiology* 38 (1): 46–51.

Kannel, W. B., T. R. Dawber, A. Kagan, N. Revotskie, and J. Stokes III. 1961. "Factors of Risk in the Development of Coronary Heart Disease—Six Year Follow-up Experience. The Framingham Study." *Annals of Internal Medicine* 55: 33–50.

Keys, A. 1997. "Coronary Heart Disease in Seven Countries. 1970." *Nutrition* 13 (3): 250–52; discussion, 249, 253.

Keys, A., A. Menotti, M. J. Karvonen, C. Aravanis, H. Blackburn, R. Buzina, B. S. Djordjevic, A. S. Dontas, F. Fidanza, M. H. Keys, et al. 1986. "The Diet and 15-Year Death Rate in the Seven Countries Study." *American Journal of Epidemiology* 124 (6): 903–15.

Lavie, C. J., and R. V. Milani. 2003. "Obesity and Cardiovascular Disease: The Hippocrates Paradox?" *Journal of the American College of Cardiology* 42 (4): 677–79.

Manuel, D. G., J. Lim, P. Tanuseputro, G. M. Anderson, D. A. Alter, A. Laupacis, and C. A. Mustard. 2006. "Revisiting Rose: Strategies for

Reducing Coronary Heart Disease." *British Medical Journal* 332 (7542): 659–62.

O'Malley, P. G., B. A. Greenberg, and A. J. Taylor. 2004. "Cost-Effectiveness of Using Electron Beam Computed Tomography to Identify Patients at Risk for Clinical Coronary Artery Disease." *American Heart Journal* 148 (1): 106–13.

Peasey, A., M. Bobak, R. Kubinova, S. Malyutina, A. Pajak, A. Tamosiunas, H. Pikhart, A. Nicholson, and M. Marmot. 2006. "Determinants of Cardiovascular Disease and Other Non-Communicable Diseases in Central and Eastern Europe: Rationale and Design of the HAPIEE Study." *BMC Public Health* 6: 255.

Robertson, T. L., H. Kato, T. Gordon, A. Kagan, G. G. Rhoads, C. E. Land, R. M. Worth, J. L. Belsky, D. S. Dock, M. Miyanishi, and S. Kawamoto. 1977. "Epidemiologic Studies of Coronary Heart Disease and Stroke in Japanese Men Living in Japan, Hawaii and California. Incidence of Myocardial Infarction and Death from Coronary Heart Disease." *American Journal of Cardiology* 39 (2): 239–43.

Rosamond, W. D., L. E. Chambless, A. R. Folsom, L. S. Cooper, D. E. Conwill, L. Clegg, C. H. Wang, and G. Heiss. 1998. "Trends in the Incidence of Myocardial Infarction and in Mortality Due to Coronary Heart Disease, 1987 to 1994." *New England Journal of Medicine* 339 (13): 861–67.

Rosamond, W., K. Flegal, G. Friday, K. Furie, A. Go, K. Greenlund, N. Haase, M. Ho, V. Howard, B. Kissela, S. Kittner, D. Lloyd-Jones, M. McDermott, J. Meigs, C. Moy, G. Nichol, C. J. O'Donnell, V. Roger, J. Rumsfeld, P. Sorlie, J. Steinberger, T. Thom, S. Wasserthiel-Smoller, Y. Hong, and the American Heart Association Statistics Committee and Stroke Statistics Subcommittee. 2007. "Heart Disease and Stroke Statistics—2007 Update: A Report from the American Heart Association Statistics Committee and the Stroke Statistics Subcommittee. *Circulation* 115 (5): e69–e171.

Rose, G. 1991. "Ancel Keys Lecture." *Circulation* 84 (3): 1405–9.

———. 1993. *The Strategy of Preventive Medicine*. New York: Oxford University Press.

———. 2001. "Sick Individuals and Sick Populations." *International Journal of Epidemiology* 30 (3): 427–32; discussion, 433–34.

Rothman, K. 2002. *Epidemiology: An Introduction*. New York: Oxford University Press.

Rugg, S. S., A. L. Bailey, S. R. Browning. 2008 "Preventing Cardiovascular Disease in Kentucky: Epidemiology, Trends, and Strategies for the Future." *Kentucky Medical Association Journal*. (April): 153-64.

Shaw, L. J., A. E. Iskandrian, R. Hachamovitch, G. Germano, H. C. Lewin, T. M. Bateman, and D. S. Berman. 2001. "Evidence-Based Risk Assessment in Noninvasive Imaging." *Journal of Nuclear Medicine* 42 (9): 1424–36.

Shaw, L. J., P. Raggi, D. S. Berman, and T. Q. Callister. 2003. "Cost

Effectiveness of Screening for Cardiovascular Disease with Measures of Coronary Calcium." *Progress in Cardiovascular Diseases* 46 (2): 171–84.

Shaw, L. J., P. Raggi, E. Schisterman, D. S. Berman, and T. Q. Callister. 2003. "Prognostic Value of Cardiac Risk Factors and Coronary Artery Calcium Screening for All-Cause Mortality." *Radiology* 228 (3): 826–33.

Thorvaldsen, P., K. Kuulasmaa, A. M. Rajakangas, D. Rastenyte, C. Sarti, and L. Wilhelmsen. 1997. "Stroke Trends in the WHO MONICA Project." *Stroke* 28 (3): 500–6.

Valanis, B. 1999. *Epidemiology in Health Care*. Stamford, CT: Appleton & Lange.

Wald, N. J., and M. R. Law. 2003. "A Strategy to Reduce Cardiovascular Disease by More than 80%." *British Medical Journal* 326 (7404): 1419.

Wilson, M. A., and T. A. Pearson. 2005. "Comprehensive Approaches to Prevention: Primary Prevention." In *Preventive Cardiology: A Practical Approach*, edited by N. D. Wong. New York: McGraw-Hill.

Yusuf, S., S. Reddy, S. Ounpuu, and S. Anand. 2001. "Global Burden of Cardiovascular Diseases: Part I: General Considerations, the Epidemiologic Transition, Risk Factors, and Impact of Urbanization." *Circulation* 104 (22): 2746–53.

HUMAN IMMUNODEFICIENCY VIRUS INFECTION

Kathleen McDavid Harrison and Steven T. Fleming

> *"By all accounts, we are dealing with the greatest health crisis in human history. By all measures, we have failed in our quest to contain and treat this scourge."* Nelson Mandela

Healthcare managers around the world are dealing with AIDS (acquired immune deficiency syndrome), which is caused by the human immunodeficiency virus (HIV). AIDS was first reported in the United States in 1981 as clusters of *Pneumocystis carini* pneumonia (now classified as *Pneumocystis jiroveci)* and Kaposi sarcoma among gay men (CDC 1981); HIV was identified as the causative agent two years later (Barré-Sinoussi et al. 1983; Gallo et al. 1984). Since that time, HIV infection has progressed to one of the most pernicious pandemics known to humankind, both in terms of human loss and costs worldwide.

In the United States and other developed countries, the burden of suffering and death, evidenced by extremely high mortality rates and short life expectancy, has been diminished by successful antiretroviral therapy, which extends life at a tremendous cost to healthcare delivery systems. Schackman and colleagues (2006) projected a 24.2 year life expectancy for persons in the United States living with HIV and estimated the discounted lifetime cost from time of infection at approximately $303,000 per person. Undiscounted costs are about twice as high, similar to the undiscounted lifetime medical costs of cardiovascular disease in women younger than 65 years. The annual medical costs of treating the approximately 1 million people in the United States living with HIV infection is about $12.5 billion.

Among adults, HIV is primarily transmitted by infected blood (e.g., sharing needles or syringes that contain contaminated blood) or during sexual intercourse with an infected partner. Perinatally transmitted HIV is the source of infection for most children currently infected in the United States (CDC 2007c). Mother-to-child transmission can occur during pregnancy, birth, or through breastfeeding (CDC n.d.).

Before 1985, when the routine HIV screening of donated blood was implemented in the United States, HIV was transmitted through the transfusion of blood or blood components or the transplantation of tissue. Currently, acquiring HIV through transfusion or transplantation is rare in Western countries (CDC 2007c).

Once in the body, HIV destroys CD4 T-lymphocytes and thus weakens the body's immune system, making infected persons vulnerable to many other infections. In the early stages of HIV infection, one may have no symptoms or only flulike symptoms. The next stage is a period of 10 to 12 years (sometimes longer or shorter) before the development of AIDS-related symptoms or advanced disease (NIAID 2007). Five-year relative survival after AIDS diagnosis in the United States is 75 percent for males and 73 percent for females (McDavid Harrison et al. 2008).

The estimates in this chapter have been adjusted for reporting delay and for cases reported without a risk factor. Also, in this chapter the term *HIV/AIDS* is used to refer to three categories of diagnoses collectively: (1) a diagnosis of HIV infection, (2) a diagnosis of HIV infection with a later diagnosis of AIDS, and (3) concurrent diagnoses of HIV infection and AIDS.

Burden of Disease

Within the past two decades, about 60 million people worldwide, an estimated two-thirds of whom live in Sub-Saharan Africa, have been infected with HIV (Joint UNAIDS 2006b). More than 20 million have died of the disease; more than 90 percent of HIV deaths have been among persons living in developing countries (Joint UNAIDS 2006a). At the end of 2003, an estimated 1,039,000 to 1,185,000 persons in the United States were living with HIV (Glynn and Rhodes 2005).

Since 1982, all 50 U.S. states, the District of Columbia, and the Commonwealth of Puerto Rico have reported AIDS cases to the Centers for Disease Control and Prevention (CDC) in a uniform format (CDC 1985, 1986). By 2002, all 50 states had HIV reporting in place: some had name-based systems; others had code-based systems (CDC does not accept coded data). Today all states but two (Vermont and Hawaii) have laws in effect that require confidential name-based HIV reporting. Given the staggered timing of the adoption of HIV reporting, the number of states that have been providing HIV data for at least four years has changed: 25 states from 1994 through 1998, 29 states in 1999, 32 states in 2000, and 33 states since 2001 (CDC 2007c).

Some states with high morbidity (e.g., California and Georgia) are not yet included in national HIV estimates because they were recently using a code-based system or their HIV surveillance system had been established recently (within less than four years). AIDS data are available for all 50 states.

Diagnoses

The name-based HIV and AIDS surveillance data collected by the states, reported without identifiers to CDC and disseminated by CDC, represent diagnosed cases. The data do not necessarily report incident infections, because some persons may have been infected in the past but have only recently been diagnosed. CDC is working with 25 areas to collect data on incident infections (CDC 2007c) by using a method for estimating HIV incidence: the serologic testing algorithm for recent HIV seroconversion (Janssen et al. 1998).

In 2005, an estimated 37,163 cases of HIV infection were diagnosed (with or without a concurrent diagnosis of AIDS, HIV/AIDS) in 33 states among persons at least 13 years old. Among males, who accounted for 74 percent of cases of HIV infection in the United States, the most prevalent HIV transmission categories for males were male-to-male sexual contact; injection drug use (IDU); male-to-male sexual contact and IDU (combination category); and high-risk heterosexual contact (heterosexual contact with someone who has, or is at high risk for, HIV infection). The most prevalent transmission categories for females were high-risk heterosexual contact and IDU (Figure 16.1).

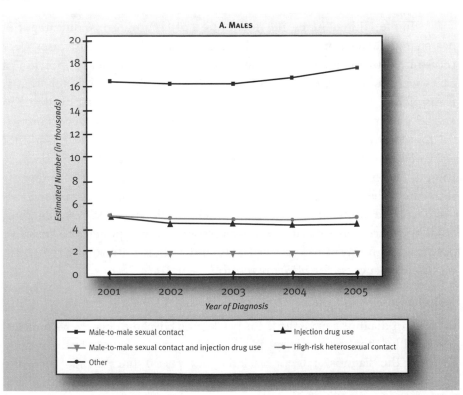

FIGURE 16.1 Estimated Numbers of HIV/AIDS Diagnoses, by Year of Diagnosis and Transmission Category—33 States with Confidential Name–Based HIV Infection Reporting, 2001–2005

(Continued)

FIGURE 16.1
(Continued)

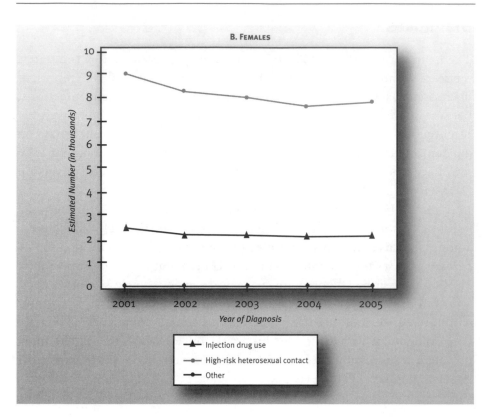

In the United States, the distribution of HIV transmission categories has changed over time. In the early years of surveillance, most cases were transmitted by male-to-male sexual contact; a much smaller proportion of cases were heterosexually transmitted. By 2005, high-risk heterosexual transmission accounted for approximately 80 percent of cases in females and 15 percent of cases in males, and male-to-male sexual contact accounted for more than 66 percent of cases in males.

Diagnosis rates by transmission category are not calculated because the population denominators for each possible combination of transmission categories are unknown. The number of perinatally transmitted cases has decreased about 95 percent (68 cases in 2005) since 1993, when antenatal and perinatal zidovudine were introduced and policies to improve prenatal testing went into effect (CDC n.d.). This noteworthy reduction represents a success for HIV prevention.

The HIV/AIDS race/ethnicity diagnosis rates decreased or remained steady during 2001–2005 (Figure 16.2). For each of the five years, the highest rates of diagnosis were those for black (not Hispanic) males and females, followed by the rates for Hispanics and American Indians/Alaska Natives. In 2005, the diagnosis rate for black females was 20 times the rate for white females, and the rate for black males was seven times the rate for white males.

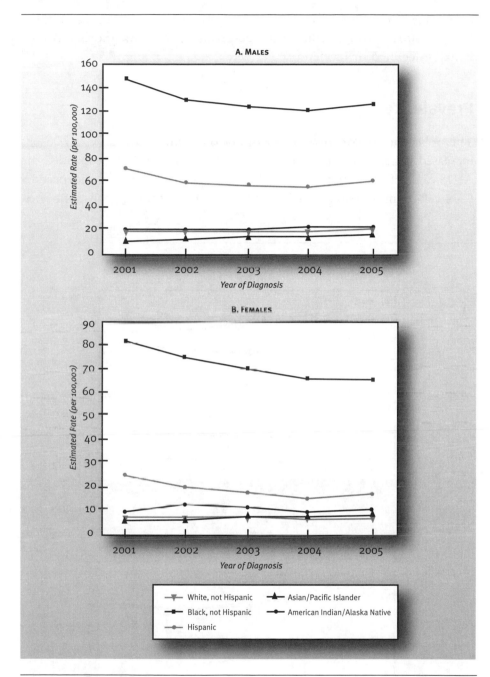

FIGURE 16.2
Estimated Annual Rates of HIV/AIDS Diagnoses, by Year of Diagnosis and Race/Ethnicity —33 States with Confidential Name–Based HIV Infection Reporting, 2001–2005

The rates of HIV/AIDS diagnosis also varied by age group. In 2005, the highest annual rate was for males 35 to 44 years of age, followed by males aged 25 to 34 and males aged 45 to 54 (Figure 16.3A). In 2005, the fourth highest rate was for males aged 13 to 24 years; however, since 2001, the diagnosis rate among males in this age group has been increasing. The highest rates of diagnosis among females in 2005 were those for females aged 35 to 44 and those aged 25 to 34, followed by females in the age groups 45 to 54 and 13 to 24 (Figure 16.3B). During 2001 through 2005, the age-group-specific diagnosis rates for females declined or leveled off.

Prevalence

The prevalence of, or the number of persons living with, HIV/AIDS has increased steadily since the early years of the epidemic. CDC expanded the AIDS case definition (effective 1993) to include HIV infection evidenced by CD4 cell counts of fewer than 200 per μL or 14 percent of total lymphocytes,

FIGURE 16.3
Estimated Annual Rates of HIV/AIDS Diagnosis, by Year of Diagnosis and Age Group—33 States with Confidential Name–Based HIV Infection Reporting, 2001–2005

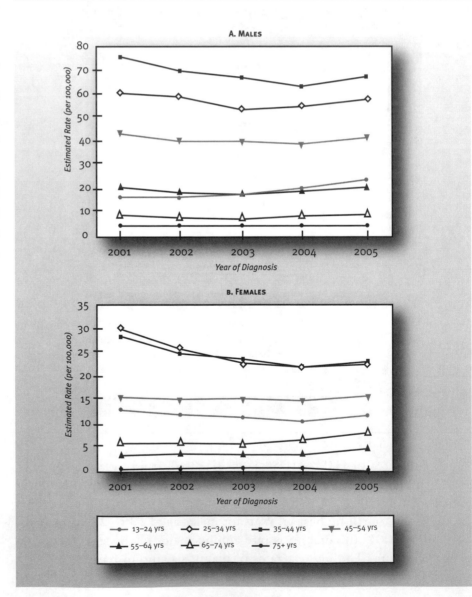

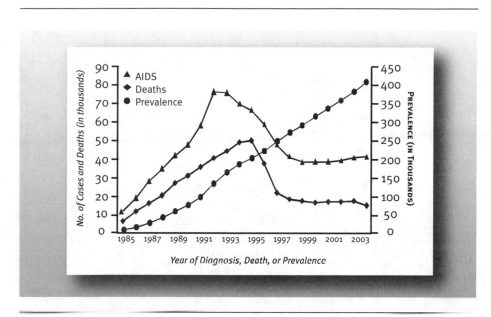

FIGURE 16.4
Estimated Numbers and Prevalence of AIDS Cases, Deaths, and Persons Living with AIDS, United States, 1985–2004

NOTE: Data adjusted for reporting delays.

pulmonary tuberculosis, severe bacterial infections, or cervical cancer. This change in definition contributed, in part, to the increased number of diagnosed cases reported in the years immediately following 1993 (CDC 1992).

By 1996, highly active antiretroviral therapy (HAART) began to be widely used. HAART is credited with increasing the survival of HIV-infected persons, thus decreasing the number of deaths of AIDS and increasing the number of prevalent AIDS cases (Figure 16.4). These data, from the national HIV/AIDS Reporting System (HARS) at CDC, are slightly different from the mortality data from the National Center for Health Statistics (NCHS), shown in Figure 16.5, because of differences in case definition criteria in HARS and the cause of death determined by the physician, the medical examiner, or the coroner. For example, a coroner could determine AIDS as the cause of death, but the deceased person may not have met the surveillance case definition for AIDS.

Another way to examine how HIV infection is distributed in the U.S. population is the geographic dispersal of cases (Figure 16.5). From this map, we can see that the rates of HIV/AIDS in 2005 tended to be higher in the Northeast, the South, California, and Nevada than in less populous states in the Midwest and Northwest.

Mortality

According to NCHS data, the median age at death due to HIV/AIDS increased from 36 years in 1988 to 45 years in 2004. People have been living longer because of the widespread use of HAART since 1996, as is clearly

FIGURE 16.5
Estimated
Rates of HIV
Infection
and AIDS in
Adults and
Adolescents
—United
States and
Dependent
Areas, 2005

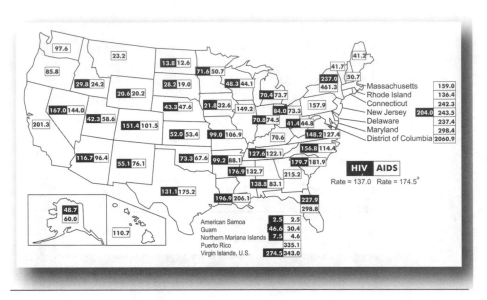

NOTE: Rates are per 100,000 population and have been adjusted for reporting delays. Rates of HIV infection include only persons living with HIV infection that has not progressed to AIDS. For some states, only the AIDS prevalence rate is displayed because CDC does not have four years of HIV data from those states.

Since 2001, the following 37 areas have had laws or regulations requiring confidential name-based HIV infection reporting: Alabama, Alaska Arizona, Arkansas, Colorado, Florida, Idaho, Indiana, Iowa, Kansas, Louisiana, Michigan, Minnesota, Mississippi, Missouri, Nebraska, Nevada, New Jersey, New Mexico, New York, North Carolina, North Dakota, Ohio, Oklahoma, South Carolina, South Dakota, Tennessee, Texas, Utah, Virginia, West Virginia, Wisconsin, Wyoming, American Samoa, Guam, the Nothern Mariana Islands, and the U.S. Virgin Islands.

[a] Includes persons whose area of residence is unknown.

SOURCE: Adapted from Centers for Disease Control and Prevention (2007c).

demonstrated in the decline in the age-adjusted rate of death due to HIV/AIDS (Figure 16.6). The age-adjusted death rate decreased 28 percent from the end of 1995 to the end of 1996 and 45 percent from the end of 1996 to the end of 1997. After 1998, the annual percentage decrease ranged from 3 percent to 5 percent. The decrease in the rate in 1996 and 1997 was largely due to improvements in antiretroviral therapy (ART). Prophylactic medications for opportunistic infections and the prevention of HIV infection may also have contributed to the decrease, but they were in use before 1995.

The leveling, or steady rate, after 1998 may reflect a lack of access to, or the effectiveness of, therapy among some persons. Possible reasons are delay in diagnosis of HIV infection until the emergence of symptoms, inadequate treatment after diagnosis, difficulty in adhering to medication regimens, and the development of viral resistance.

The age-adjusted rate of death due to HIV/AIDS varies by region of the United States. In 2004, death rates were generally higher in the Northeast, the South, and the Southwest, especially in states with large

FIGURE 16.6
Trends in
Annual Age–
Adjusted
Rate of Death
due to HIV
Disease—
United States,
1987–2004

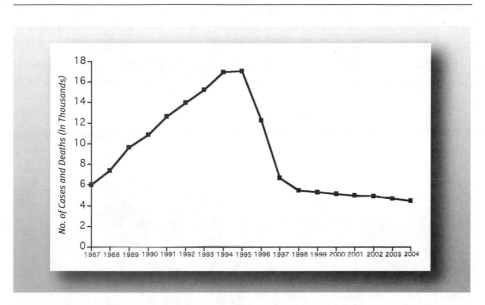

NOTE: For comparison with data for 1999 and later years, data for 1987–1989 were modified to account for ICD-10 rules instead of ICD-9 rules. Standard is age distribution of 2000 U.S. population.

SOURCE: Centers for Disease Control and Prevention (2007a, slide 4).

cities, than in states in the Midwest or the Northwest (Figure 16.7). This pattern is consistent with the pattern of prevalence rates (see Figure 16.5).

Finally, the average annual age-adjusted rate of death was higher for males than for females during 2000 through 2004, and variability by race/ethnicity was evident (Figure 16.8). The highest average annual age-adjusted death rates were those for blacks: 34 per 100,000 for males and 14 per 100,000 for females, threefold the rates for other race/ethnic categories. The next highest death rates were those for Hispanics, followed by those for American Indians/Alaska Natives.

Screening and Diagnostic Tests

Currently the protocol for HIV infection diagnosis in the United States is to use a screening test, such as an HIV-1 enzyme immunoassay (EIA), followed by a confirmatory test, to detect HIV antibodies, which signal the body's response to the infection. This two-stage screening process has very high sensitivity and specificity (both greater than 99 percent). The most common HIV tests use blood to detect HIV infection. For some tests, results take a few days, but rapid tests can produce results in 20 minutes or less. Rapid tests must be followed by confirmatory tests, which can take a few days to a few weeks.

An initial diagnosis is confirmed by Western blot or indirect immunofluorescence assay, which detects the body's serologic response to HIV.

About 4 percent to 20 percent of sera that are repeatedly reactive (or positive) by EIA are indeterminate by Western blot. One reason for indeterminate Western blot results is testing during the window period, when HIV antibodies are still forming. A few months may elapse before confirmatory tests produce positive results (i.e., until antibodies to the infection develop)

FIGURE 16.7
Age–Adjusted
Rate of Death
Due to HIV
Disease—
United States,
2004

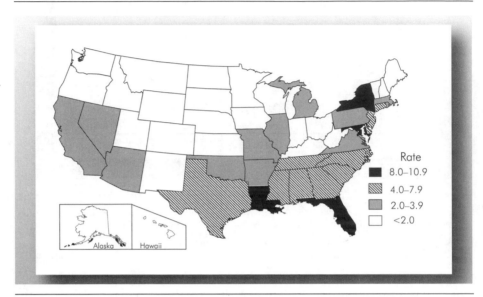

NOTE: Standard is age distribution of 2000 U.S. population. Rates are per 100,000 population.

SOURCE: Centers for Disease Control and Prevention (2007a, slide 10).

FIGURE 16.8
Age–Adjusted
Average
Annual Rate
of Death Due
to HIV
Disease, by
Sex and
Race/Ethnicity,
2000–2004

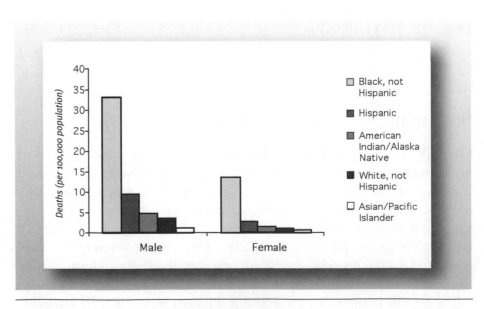

NOTE: Standard is age distribution of 2000 U.S. population.

SOURCE: Centers for Disease Control and Prevention (2007a, slide 15).

(Mylonakis et al. 2000). The Western blot has a specificity of 97.8 percent (CDC 1990); however, it has a high false-positive rate (>2 percent), rendering it of modest use as a screening test. Its use should be preceded by an EIA or a licensed rapid test (Mylonakis et al. 2000).

If confirmatory test results are positive, viral load tests, which measure the amount of HIV in the blood, should be performed. To determine whether an HIV-infected person has AIDS (advanced disease), a blood test to determine the CD4 cell count is performed. A CD4 cell count of fewer than 200 cells per μL of blood indicates advanced disease, or AIDS (CDC, in press).

Case Study 16.1. HIV-1 Enzyme Immunoassay for HIV

The HIV-1 enzyme immunoassay was developed to help diagnose HIV infection, and the recommended strategy is to use either the automated EIA or rapid testing EIA with a repeat test by automated EIA on those who test positive.

Assume that the automated EIA has a sensitivity of 99.90 percent and a specificity of 99.85 percent. Paltiel et al. (2005) conducted a cost-effectiveness study of various HIV testing strategies on three populations: (1) a high-risk population, for which the prevalence of HIV was 3 percent and the annual incidence was 1 percent; (2) the former CDC threshold population, for which prevalence was 1 percent and incidence was 0.12 percent; and (3) the U.S. general population, for which prevalence was 0.1 percent and incidence was 0.01 percent.

QUESTIONS

1. Can we say anything about the average "duration" of disease in these three populations?
2. If specimens from 1 million people in each of the three populations were subjected to the automated EIA, how many false positives and false negatives would result?
3. What is the ratio of false positives to true positives in the three populations?
4. Does the confidence that patients place in a positive EIA test result depend on the population that is tested?
5. How might we improve the confidence in a positive test result (positive predictive value) by repeat testing?

ANSWERS

1. The ratio of prevalence to incidence rates is 3 to 1 for a high-risk population, 8 to 1 for a CDC threshold population, and 10 to 1 for the U.S. general population. If we assume that HIV in these three populations is in a steady state, it appears that the duration of time "living with HIV" is longer in the general

population than for those in higher risk populations.

2. See Table 16.1 for the answers. The number of false negatives would be 30 in a high-risk population, 10 in a CDC threshold population, and 1 in the U.S. general population. The number of false positives would be 1,455 in a high-risk population, 1,485 in a CDC threshold population, and 1,498 in the U.S. general population.

3. Referring to Table 16.1, the ratio of false to true positives would be 0.05 to 1 for the high-risk population, 0.15 to 1 for the CDC threshold population, and 1.5 to 1 for the U.S. general population.

4. We can measure confidence by the positive predictive value (PPV). Referring to Table 16.1, the PPV for the high-risk population would be $[29,970/(29,970 + 1,455)] \times 100 = 95.4\%$; for the CDC threshold population, the PPV would be $[9,990/(9,990 + 1,485)] \times 100 = 87.1\%$; for the U.S. general population, the PPV would be $[999/(999 + 1,498)] \times 100 = 40\%$. Thus, members of the high-risk population who test positive can be nearly two and one-half times as confident in a positive EIA test result as can members of the U.S. general population.

5. Refer to Table 16.2 to calculate the PPV of a two-test sequence. For the high-risk population, this would be $[29,940/(29,940 + 2)] \times 100 = 100\%$; for the CDC threshold population, this would be $[9,980/(9,980 + 2)] \times 100 = 100\%$; for the U.S. general population, this would be $[998/(998 + 2)] \times 100 = 99.8\%$. Running the test a second time results in an increase in PPV from 95.4 percent to 100 percent for the high-risk population, from 87.1 percent to 100 percent for the CDC threshold population, and from 40 percent to 99.8 percent for the U.S. general population.

TABLE 16.1. RESULTS OF INITIAL ENZYME IMMUNOASSAY (EIA), BY POPULATION

	HIV+	HIV−	Total
	High-Risk Population (prevalence = 3 percent)		
EIA+	29,970	1,455	31,425
EIA−	30	968,545	968,575
Total	30,000	970,000	1,000,000
	CDC Threshold Population (prevalence = 1 percent)		
EIA+	9,990	1,485	11,475
EIA−	10	988,515	988,525
Total	10,000	990,000	1,000,000
	U.S. Population (prevalence = 0.1 percent)		
EIA+	999	1,498	2,497
EIA−	1	997,502	997,503
Total	1,000	999,000	1,000,000

TABLE 16.2. RESULTS OF REPEAT ENZYME IMMUNOASSAY (EIA), BY POPULATION

	HIV+	HIV–	Total
	High-Risk Population (prevalence = 3 percent)		
EIA+	29,940	2	29,942
EIA–	30	1,453	1,483
Total	29,970	1,455	31,425
	CDC Threshold Population (prevalence = 1 percent)		
EIA+	9,980	2	9,982
EIA–	10	1,483	1,493
Total	9,990	1,485	11,475
	U.S. Population (prevalence = 0.1 percent)		
EIA+	998	2	1,000
EIA–	1	1,496	1,497
Total	999	1,498	2,497

Prevention and Control Measures

Currently no vaccine is available to prevent HIV infection. The only way to prevent infection is to avoid behaviors (e.g., sharing needles, having unprotected sexual contact) that put one at risk for infection. The use of latex condoms has been proven effective in reducing the transmission of HIV (Carey et al. 1992; Rietmeijer et al. 1988; Van de Perre, Jacobs, and Sprecher-Goldberger 1987). Research has shown that access to sterile syringes reduces syringe sharing and prevents the spread of HIV (NIDA 2002).

In addition, cohort studies have shown that many infected persons engage less often in behaviors that help transmit infection to sex or needle-sharing partners once they are aware of their positive HIV status (Cleary et al. 1991; Coates, Morin, and McKusick 1987; Doll et al. 1990; Fox et al. 1987; Gibson et al. 1999; Rhodes and Malotte 1996; Rietmeijer et al. 1996; Van Griensven et al. 1989).

Because many people infected with HIV have no symptoms and 25 percent are unaware that they are infected (Glynn and Rhodes 2005), CDC recommends routine testing of adults and adolescents (13–64 years) in healthcare settings and annual testing of persons at high risk for HIV infection (CDC 2006). Making testing more accessible (e.g., in nonclinical settings) and focusing on areas where prevalence is high are prevention strategies that CDC adopted in 2005 (CDC 2005).

Researchers are searching for effective microbicides that can be put in creams or gels that can be applied vaginally before sexual contact, to prevent HIV transmission. The search for an effective microbicidal agent continues through several lines of research, including conducting laboratory and animal studies to evaluate the safety and the efficacy of microbicides before they are studied in humans and clinical trials to assess the safety of microbicides in humans (CDC 2007b).

As noted earlier, the prevention of mother-to-child (perinatal) transmission of HIV infection is a noteworthy success. The 95 percent reduction in perinatally transmitted infections was achieved because of the treatment of pregnant women and their infants (CDC 2007c). Therapy is effective when it is administered to the pregnant woman as early as possible during pregnancy or to the infant at the time of birth (CDC 2005).

Measures of Quality of Care

A number of measures of the quality of care of HIV-infected persons have been proposed.

For example, surveillance data have been used to examine whether AIDS was diagnosed at the same time as, or within 6 to 12 months after, an HIV diagnosis. A diagnosis within that period would mean the HIV diagnosis was late—since HIV takes a long time to develop into AIDS—and would thus be a sign that that person was missed by the healthcare system (CDC 2007c; Hall et al. 2006; McDavid, Li, and Lee 2006). As age at HIV diagnosis increases, the proportion of late diagnoses increases (CDC 2007c). In 2004, larger proportions of Asians/Pacific Islanders, Hispanics, American Indians/Alaska Natives, and blacks (40 percent to 44 percent), compared with whites (37 percent), were given a diagnosis late in the course of disease.

Other indicators of quality of care relate to whether patients receive appropriate treatment. Treatment recommendations for adults and adolescents include ART for all patients with a history of AIDS-defining illnesses or severe symptoms of HIV infection (regardless of CD4 cell count) and for asymptomatic patients with "350 CD4 cells per μL" (Panel on Antiretroviral Guidelines 2008).

Another measure of quality of care is the proportion of HIV-infected persons who are in care (defined as persons for whom a CD4 cell count is recorded in the national surveillance data set), and the percentage of those who receive ART. In 2003, a U.S. national estimate based on medical record reviews for patients aged 15 to 49 years in ten cities put the proportion of eligible persons in care who received ART at 79 percent (Teshale et al. 2005). However, that study estimated that of all persons who were living with HIV/AIDS and who were eligible for ART, only 56 percent received it (a measure of quality of, and access to, care). To go a step further, studies have found that after the introduction of HAART, or potent combinations of ART, morbidity and mortality related to HIV infection have been significantly reduced (CASCADE Collaboration 2003). Yet Teshale and colleagues (2005) found that of the 56 percent of eligible patients who received ART, just 66 percent of them received HAART.

The literature is rich with studies of the number of outpatient clinic/office visits, receipt/utilization of ART and HAART, receipt of prophylaxis against *Pneumocystis* pneumonia, access to HIV drugs, treatment volume, and type of care (case managed versus multidisciplinary) received (Fleishman et al. 2005; Goldstein et al. 2005; Handford et al. 2006; Kahn et al. 2002; Katz et al. 2001; Morin et al. 2002; Palacio et al. 2002; Rutstein et al. 2005; Shapiro et al. 1999; Teshale et al. 2005). These various measures, used to assess HIV patient morbidity and mortality outcomes, can be affected by the race/ethnicity of patient and provider, the type of health insurance, and barriers such as language and culture (Betancourt and Maina 2004).

A summary measure used to determine the net effect of a healthcare system's performance is *relative survival*. The *observed* (or *crude*) *survival proportion* (also often referred to as *survival rate*) is the estimated probability of survival to the end of a period, regardless of the cause of death or the background mortality of the population. The relative survival proportion is the ratio of the observed survival in the population of interest (HIV and AIDS patients) to the survival that would have been expected had the patients experienced only the mortality of the general population from which they were drawn (Berkson and Gage 1950; Cutler and Ederer 1958; Ederer, Axtell, and Cutler 1961). Recent five-year relative survival estimates for HIV infection indicate that older persons, blacks, injection drug users, and patients living in poor counties fared worse than their counterparts (Hall et al. 2006; McDavid et al. 2008).

Study Designs Used to Examine Risk Factors

Epidemiologic methods are designed to identify risk factors for various diseases, even when the specific etiologic agent is unknown, as it was in the early years of the AIDS epidemic.

During the early 1980s, when scientists and the medical community were just becoming widely aware of AIDS, individual case studies were conducted and reported in CDC's *Morbidity and Mortality Weekly Report*. In addition, active case surveillance by local and state health departments and CDC was conducted for Kaposi sarcoma, *Pneumocystis* pneumonia, and opportunistic infections in persons without known predisposing or underlying disease (CDC 1981).

In September 1981, a case-control study was conducted to provide information on risk factors (Dowdle 1983); later, numerous observational studies as well as longitudinal cohort studies were undertaken to better understand the risk factors and transmission of what was later defined as HIV.

Since 1985, surveillance systems have monitored virtually the same set of risk factors for HIV transmission, and today surveillance systems continue to closely monitor risk factors so as to identify potential new routes of HIV transmission.

Summary

As HAART becomes ever more widely used in the United States and other Western countries and as more effective therapies are developed, policymakers, program managers, and care providers have to deal with the reality of an increased prevalence of HIV. The improved therapies are a treatment success. However, due to this success, the burden of ensuring equity in care and recommended therapy usage becomes ever greater on a healthcare system that already faces challenges in terms of access, resources, and utilization.

Successful healthcare managers, who know that prevention is the key to reducing incidence, will have to find a way to use the resources available and optimize them for prevention services. Further, as resources become ever scarcer, healthcare managers will want to integrate, insofar as possible, prevention and care programs for tuberculosis, sexually transmitted infections, and HIV infection.

Case Study 16.2. Cost-Effectiveness of HIV Screening

Sanders and colleagues (2005) conducted a cost-effectiveness analysis of HIV screening in which they compared onetime screening or recurrent screening (every five years) and no screening. Costs and quality-adjusted life years were calculated according to two scenarios: (1) the index patient only (excluding transmission to partners) and (2) the index patient and sexual partners. They used decision-making software that provides for lifetime follow-up of a cohort of patients.

QUESTIONS

1. What kinds of costs do you think the authors included in this analysis?
2. What epidemiologic measures need to be included in the analysis?
3. What important test characteristics must be estimated?
4. Considering only the index patient, the authors reported costs of $51,517 for no screening, $51,850 for onetime screening, and $52,086 for recurrent screening. Considering the index patient and sexual partners, the authors reported costs of $52,623 for no screening, $52,816 for onetime screening,

and $53,022 for recurrent screening. What are the incremental costs of onetime screening (compared with no screening) and recurrent screening (compared with onetime screening) under both scenarios?

5. Under the index patient scenario, the authors reported life expectancies of 21.063 years for those with no screening, 21.073 for those with onetime screening, and 21.076 for those with recurrent screening. For index patients and sexual partners, the authors reported life expectancies of 21.015 years for those with no screening, 21.030 for those with onetime screening, and 21.034 for those with recurrent screening. What are the incremental life expectancies of persons with onetime screening (compared with no screening) and those with recurrent screening (compared with onetime screening) under both scenarios?

6. For the index patient scenario, quality-adjusted life years (QALYs) are reported to be 18.626 for those with no screening, 18.634 for those with onetime screening, and 18.636 for those with recurrent screening. For the index patient and sexual partners scenario, QALYs are reported to be 18.576 for those with no screening, 18.589 for those with onetime screening, and 18.592 for those with recurrent screening. Why are the QALYs lower than life expectancy estimates in question 5? Calculate the incremental QALYs under both scenarios.

7. What is the incremental cost-effectiveness ratio (ICER) under both scenarios, when both life expectancy and QALY are used as measures of effect?

8. In this scenario, which strategies would be recommended with the guideline of $50,000 per QALY (a guideline used by policy analysts for years)?

9. The authors conducted a sensitivity analysis to determine how sensitive ICERs were to changes in key variables. In this scenario, what would happen to the ICERs as the prevalence of unidentified HIV in the population decreased? What would happen to the ICERs if the incidence of HIV in the population increased?

ANSWERS

1. The authors included the costs of HIV testing, HIV counseling, antiretroviral therapy, and side effects.

2. The authors included many variables. Some of the important epidemiologic variables that need to be estimated are the prevalence of unidentified HIV infection; the annual incidence of HIV; transmission rates for men who have sex with men, and for heterosexual men and heterosexual women; and the progression rates from HIV to AIDS and from AIDS to death.

3. Test sensitivity was estimated at 60 percent for the first three months after infection and at 99.5 percent thereafter. Specificity was estimated at 99.9994 percent.

4. The incremental costs of onetime screening are $51,850 − $51,517 = $333 (index patient only) and $52,816 − $52,623 = $193 (index patient and sexual partners). The incremental costs of recurrent screening are $52,086 − $51,850 = $236 (index patient only) and $53,022 − $52,816 = $206 (index patient and sexual partners).

5. The incremental life expectancy of onetime screening is 21.073 − 21.063 = 0.01 years (index patient) and 21.030 − 21.015 = 0.015 years (index patient and sexual partners). The incremental life expectancy of recurrent screening is 21.076 − 21.073 = 0.003 years (index patient) and 21.034 − 21.030 = 0.004 years (index patient and sexual partners).

6. The QALYs are lower because they take into consideration quality of life as well as length of life. For example, the authors estimated the quality of life of one year living with AIDS to be only 0.73, compared with living in perfect health (1.0). The incremental QALYs of persons with onetime screening are 18.634 − 18.626 = 0.008 years (index patient) and 18.589 − 18.576 = 0.013 years (index patient and sexual partners). The incremental QALYs of those with recurrent screening are 18.636 − 18.634 = 0.002 years (index patient) and 18.592 − 18.589 = 0.003 years (index patient and sexual partners).

7. Table 16.3 summarizes these results. Using life expectancy, the ICERs for onetime screening would be $333/0.01 = $33,300 per year (index patient) and $193/0.015 = $12,867 per year (index patient and sexual partners). ICERs for recurrent screening would be $236/0.003 =$78,667 per year (index patient) and $206/0.004 = $51,500 per year (index patient and sexual partners). Using quality-adjusted life expectancy, the ICERs for onetime screening would be $333/0.008 = $41,625 per QALY (index patient) and $193/0.013 = $14,846 per QALY (index patient and sexual partners). ICERs for recurrent screening would be $236/0.002 =$118,000 per QALY (index patient) and $206/0.003 = $68,667 per QALY (index patient and sexual partners).

TABLE 16.3. INCREMENTAL COST-EFFECTIVENESS OF HIV TESTING

Strategy	Incremental Cost-Effectiveness ($/LY*)	Incremental Cost-Effectiveness ($/QALY**)
Index Patient		
One-time screening	33,300	41,625
Recurrent screening	78,667	118,000
Index Patient and Sexual Partners		
One-time screening	12,867	14,846
Recurrent screening	51,500	68,667

NOTE: *LY indicates life year; **QALY indicates quality-adjusted life year.

SOURCE: Adapted from Sanders et al. (2005 p. 578, Table 3).

8. In this case study, one-time screening would be recommended under both scenarios, whether one uses years or QALYs as the measure of effect. Recurrent screening may be cost-effective, particularly if a more "reasonable" guideline of $100,000 per QALY is adopted.

9. ICERs increase as the prevalence of unidentified HIV in the population decreases because the "yield" of screening is lower; that is, fewer new cases are found and treated. As the incidence of HIV in a population increases, recurrent screening becomes more cost-effective (i.e., the ICERs are lower).

References

Barré-Sinoussi, F., J. C. Chermann, F. Rey, M. T. Nugeyre, S. Chamaret, J. Gruest, C. Dauguet, C. Axler-Blin, F. Vézinet-Brun, C. Rouzioux, W. Rozenbaum, and L. Montagnier. 1983. "Isolation of a T-Lymphotropic Retrovirus from a Patient at Risk for Acquired Immune Deficiency Syndrome (AIDS)." *Science* 220 (4599): 868–71.

Berkson, J., and R. P. Gage. 1950. "Calculation of Survival Rates for Cancer." *Proceedings of Staff Meetings Mayo Clinic* 25 (11): 270–86.

Betancourt, J. R., and A. W. Maina. 2004. "The Institute of Medicine Report 'Unequal Treatment': Implications for Academic Health Centers." *Mount Sinai Journal of Medicine* 71 (5): 314–421.

Carey, R. F., W. A. Herman, S. M. Retta, J. E. Rinaldi, B. A. Herman, and T. W. Athey. 1992. "Effectiveness of Latex Condoms as a Barrier to Human Immunodeficiency Virus-Sized Particles Under Conditions of Simulated Sex." *Sexually Transmitted Diseases* 19 (4): 230–34.

CASCADE Collaboration. 2003. "Determinants of Survival Following HIV-1 Seroconversion After the Introduction of HAART." *Lancet* 362 (9392): 1267–74.

Centers for Disease Control and Prevention (CDC). 1981. "Kaposi's Sarcoma and *Pneumocystis* Pneumonia Among Homosexual Men—New York City and California." *Morbidity and Mortality Weekly Report* 30:305–8.

———. 1985. "Current Trends Update: Acquired Immunodeficiency Syndrome—United States." *Morbidity and Mortality Weekly Report* 34 (18): 245–48.

———. 1986. "Current Trends Update: Acquired Immunodeficiency Syndrome—United States." *Morbidity and Mortality Weekly Report* 35 (2): 17–21.

———. 1990. "Update: Serologic Testing for HIV-1 Antibody—United States, 1988 and 1989." *Morbidity and Mortality Weekly Report* 39 (22): 380–83.

———. 1992. "1993 Revised Classification System for HIV Infection and Expanded Surveillance Case Definition for AIDS Among Adolescents and Adults." *Morbidity and Mortality Weekly Report* 41 (RR-17): 1–19.

———. 2005. "Advancing HIV Prevention: Progress Summary, April 2003–September 2005." [Online information; retrieved 10/19/07.] www.cdc.gov/hiv/topics/prev_prog/AHP/resources/factsheets/progress _2005.htm.

———. 2006. "Revised Recommendations for HIV Testing of Adults, Adolescents, and Pregnant Women in Health-Care Settings." *Morbidity and Mortality Weekly Report* 55 (RR-14): 1–17.

———. 2007a. "HIV Mortality (Through 2004)." [Online slide set; retrieved 10/30/07.] www.cdc.gov/hiv/topics/surveillance/resources /slides/mortality/.

———. 2007b. "HIV/AIDS Among Women." [Online fact sheet; retrieved 10/19/07.] www.cdc.gov/hiv/topics/women/resources/factsheets /women.htm.

———. 2007c. *HIV/AIDS Surveillance Report, 2005,* vol. 17. rev. ed. Atlanta, GA: Centers for Disease Control and Prevention.

———. n.d. "Pregnancy and Childbirth." [Online information; retrieved 10/19/07.] www.cdc.gov/hiv/topics/perinatal/.

———. In press. "2007 Revised Surveillance Case Definitions for HIV Infection, Incorporating the HIV Classification System and the AIDS Case Definition for Adults and Adolescents, HIV Infection Among Children Aged <18 Months, and HIV Infection and AIDS Among Children ≥18 Months but <13 Years." *Morbidity and Mortality Weekly Report Recommendations and Reports.*

Cleary, P. D., N. Van Devanter, T. J. Rogers, E. Singer, R. Shipton-Levy, M. Steilen, A. Stuart, J. Avorn, and J. Pindyck. 1991. "Behavior Changes After Notification of HIV Infection." *American Journal of Public Health* 81 (12): 1586–90.

Coates, T. J., S. F. Morin, and L. McKusick. 1987. "Behavioral Consequences of AIDS Antibody Testing Among Gay Men." [Letter to the editor.] *Journal of the American Medical Association* 258 (14): 1889.

Cutler, S. J., and F. Ederer. 1958. "Maximum Utilization of the Life Table Method in Analyzing Survival." *Journal of Chronic Diseases* 8 (6): 699–712.

Doll, L. S., P. M. O'Malley, A. L. Pershing, W. W. Darrow, N. A. Hessol, and A. R. Lifson. 1990. "High-Risk Sexual Behavior and Knowledge of HIV Antibody Status in the San Francisco City Clinic Cohort." *Health Psychology* 9 (3): 253–65.

Dowdle, W. R. 1983. "The Epidemiology of AIDS." *Public Health Reports* 98 (4): 308–12.

Ederer, F., L. M. Axtell, and S. J. Cutler. 1961. "The Relative Survival: A Statistical Methodology." *National Cancer Institute Monograph* 6 (September): 101–21.

Fleishman, J. A., K. A. Gebo, E. D. Reilly, R. Conviser, W. Christopher Mathews, P. Todd Korthuis, J. Hellinger, R. Rutstein, P. Keiser, H. Rubin, R. D. Moore, for the HIV Research Network. 2005. "Hospital and Outpatient Health Services Utilization Among HIV-Infected Adults in Care 2000–2002." *Medical Care* 43 (9, Suppl. III): 40–52.

Fox, R., N. J. Odaka, R. Brookmeyer, and B. F. Polk. 1987. "Effect of HIV Antibody Disclosure on Subsequent Sexual Activity in Homosexual Men." *AIDS* 1 (4): 241–46.

Gallo, R. C., S. Z. Salahuddin, M. Popovic, G. M. Shearer, M. Kaplan, B. F. Haynes, T. J. Palker, R. Redfield, J. Oleske, B. Safai, G. White, P. Foster, and P. D. Markham. 1984. "Frequent Detection and Isolation of Cytopathic Retroviruses (HTLV-III) from Patients with AIDS and at Risk for AIDS." *Science* 224 (4648): 500–3.

Gibson, D. R., J. Lovelle-Drache, M. Young, E. S. Hudes, and J. L. Sorensen. 1999. "Effectiveness of Brief Counseling in Reducing HIV Risk Behavior in Injecting Drug Users: Final Results of Randomized Trials of Counseling With and Without HIV Testing." *AIDS and Behavior* 3 (1): 3–12.

Glynn, M., and P. Rhodes. 2005. "Estimated HIV Prevalence in the United States at the End of 2003." [Abstract T1-B1101.] Presented at the National HIV Prevention Conference, Atlanta, GA.

Goldstein, R. B., M. J. Rotheram-Borus, M. O. Johnson, L. S. Weinhardt, R. H. Remien, M. Lightfoot, S. L. Catz, C. Gore-Felton, S. Kirshenbaum, S. F. Morin, and the NIMH Healthy Living Trial Group. 2005. "Insurance Coverage, Usual Source of Care, and Receipt of Clinically Indicated Care for Comorbid Conditions Among Adults Living with Human Immunodeficiency Virus." *Medical Care* 43 (4): 401–10.

Hall, H. I., K. McDavid, Q. Ling, and A. Sloggett. 2006. "Determinants of Progression to AIDS or Death After HIV Diagnosis, United States, 1996 to 2001." *Annals of Epidemiology* 16 (11): 824–33.

Handford, C. D., A. M. Tynan, J. M. Rackal, and R. H. Glazier. 2006. "Setting and Organization of Care for Persons Living with HIV/AIDS." *Cochrane Database of Systematic Reviews* 19 (3): CD004348.

Janssen, R. S., G. A. Satten, S. L. Stramer, B. D. Rawal, T. R. O'Brien, B. J. Weiblen, F. M. Hecht, N. Jack, F. R. Cleghorn, J. O. Kahn, M. A. Chesney, and M. P. Busch. 1998. "New Testing Strategy to Detect Early HIV-1 Infection for Use in Incidence Estimates and for Clinical and Prevention Purposes." *Journal of the American Medical Association* 280 (1): 42–48.

Joint United Nations Programme on AIDS (UNAIDS). 2006a. "2006 Report on the Global AIDS Epidemic." [Online information; retrieved 10/30/07.] www.unaids.org/en/HIV_data/2006GlobalReport/default.asp.

———. 2006b. "Sub-Saharan Africa." [Online fact sheet; retrieved 10/30/07.] http://data.unaids.org/pub/EpiReport/2006/20061121_EPI_FS_SSA _en.pdf.

Kahn, J. G., X. Zhang, L. T. Cross, H. Palacio, G. S. Birkhead, and S. F. Morin. 2002. "Access to and Use of HIV Antiretroviral Therapy: Variation by Race/Ethnicity in Two Public Insurance Programs in the U.S." *Public Health Reports* 117 (3): 252–62.

Katz, M. H., W. E. Cunningham, J. A. Fleishman, R. M. Andersen, T. Kellogg, S. A. Bozzette, and M. F. Shapiro. 2001. "Effect of Case Management on Unmet Needs and Utilization of Medical Care and Medications Among HIV-Infected Persons." *Annals of Internal Medicine* 135 (8, Pt. 1): 557–65.

McDavid, K., J. Li, and L. M. Lee. 2006. "Racial and Ethnic Disparities in HIV Diagnoses for Women in the United States." *Journal of Acquired Immune Deficiency Syndromes* 42 (1): 101–7.

McDavid Harrison, K., Q. Ling, R. Song, and H. I. Hall. 2008. "Survival After HIV Diagnosis and Socioeconomic Status, United States." Manuscript submitted for publication.

Morin, S. F., S. Sengupta, M. Cozen, T. A. Richards, M. D. Shriver, H. Palacio, and J. G. Kahn. 2002. "Responding to Racial and Ethnic Disparities in Use of HIV Drugs: Analysis and State of Policies." *Public Health Reports* 117 (3): 263–72.

Mylonakis, E., M. Paliou, M. Lally, T. P. Flanigan, and J. D. Rich. 2000. "Laboratory Testing for Infection with the Human Immunodeficiency Virus: Established and Novel Approaches." *American Journal of Medicine* 109 (7): 568–76.

National Institute of Allergy and Infectious Diseases (NIAID). 2007. "HIV Infection and AIDS: An Overview." [Online fact sheet; retrieved 10/19/07.] www.niaid.nih.gov/factsheets/hivinf.htm.

National Institute on Drug Abuse (NIDA). 2002. "Principles of HIV Prevention in Drug-Using Populations: A Research-Based Guide." [Online information; retrieved 10/30/07.] www.nida.nih.gov/POHP.

Palacio, H., J. G. Kahn, T. A. Richards, and S. F. Morin. 2002. "Effect of Race and/or Ethnicity in Use of Antiretrovirals and Prophylaxis for Opportunistic Infection: A Review of the Literature." *Public Health Reports* 117 (3): 233–51.

Paltiel, A. D., M. C. Weinstein, A. D. Kimmel, G. R. Seage III, E. Losina, H. Zhang, K. A. Freedberg, and R. P. Walensky. 2005. "Expanded Screening for HIV in the United States—An Analysis of Cost-Effectiveness." *New England Journal of Medicine* 352 (6): 586–95.

Panel on Antiretroviral Guidelines for Adults and Adolescents. 2008. "Guidelines for the Use of Antiretroviral Agents in HIV-1-Infected Adults and Adolescents, October 2006." [Online information; retrieved 9/30/07.] www.aidsinfo.nih.gov/contentfiles/AdultandAdolescentGL.pdf.

Rhodes, F., and C. K. Malotte. 1996. "HIV Risk Interventions for Active

Drug Users." In *Understanding and Preventing HIV Risk Behavior: Safer Sex and Drug Use*, edited by S. Oskamp and S. C. Thompson, 207–36. Thousand Oaks, CA: Sage.

Rietmeijer, C. A. , M. S. Kane, P. S. Simons, N. H. Corby, R. J. Wolitski, D. L. Higgins, F. W. Judson, and D. L. Cohn. 1996. "Increasing the Use of Bleach and Condoms Among Injecting Drug Users in Denver: Outcomes of a Targeted, Community-Level HIV Prevention Program." *AIDS* 10 (3): 291–98.

Rietmeijer, C. A., J. W. Krebs, P. M. Feorino, and F. N. Judson. 1988. "Condoms as Physical and Chemical Barriers Against Human Immunodeficiency Virus." *Journal of the American Medical Association* 259 (12): 1851–53.

Rutstein, R. M., K. A. Gebo, G. K. Siberry, P. M. Flynn, S. A. Spector, V. L. Sharp, and J. A. Fleishman. 2005. "Hospital and Outpatient Health Services Utilization Among HIV-Infected Children in Care, 2000–2001." *Medical Care* 43 (9, Suppl. III): 31–39.

Sanders, G. D., A. M. Bayoumi, V. Sundaram, S. P. Bilir, C. P. Neukermans, C. E. Rydzak, L. R. Douglass, L. C. Lazzeroni, and D. K. Holodniym Owens. 2005. "Cost-Effectiveness of Screening for HIV in the Era of Highly Active Antiretroviral Therapy." *New England Journal of Medicine* 352 (6): 570–85.

Schackman, B. R., K. A. Gebo, R. P. Walensky, E. Losina, T. Muccio, P. E. Sax, M. C. Weinstein, G. R. Seage III, R. D. Moore, and K. A. Freedberg. 2006. "The Lifetime Cost of Current Human Immunodeficiency Virus Care in the United States." *Medical Care* 44 (11): 990–97.

Shapiro, M. F., S. C. Morton, D. F. McCaffrey, J. W. Senterfitt, J. A. Fleishman, J. F. Perlman, L. A. Athcy, J. W. Keesey, D. P. Goldman, S. H. Berry, and S. A. Bozzette. 1999. "Variations in the Care of HIV-Infected Adults in the United States: Results from the HIV Cost and Services Utilization Study." *Journal of the American Medical Association* 281 (24): 2305–15.

Teshale, E., L. Kamimoto, N. Harris, J. Li, H. Wang, and M. McKenna. 2005. "Estimated Number of HIV-Infected Persons Eligible for and Receiving HIV Antiretroviral Therapy, 2003—United States." [Abstract 167.] Presented at the Conference on Retroviruses and Opportunistic Infections, Boston.

Van de Perre P., D. Jacobs, and S. Sprecher-Goldberger. 1987. "The Latex Condom: An Efficient Barrier Against Sexual Transmission of AIDS-Related Viruses." *AIDS* 1 (1): 49–52.

Van Griensven, G. J., E. M. de Vroome, R. A. Tielman, J. Goudsmit, F. de Wolf, J. van der Noordaa, and R. A. Coutinho. 1989. "Effect of Human Immunodeficiency Virus (HIV) Antibody Knowledge on High-Risk Sexual Behavior with Steady and Nonsteady Sexual Partners Among Homosexual Men." *American Journal of Epidemiology* 129 (3): 596–603.

ALZHEIMER'S DISEASE

Suzanne L. Tyas and Iris Gutmanis

> *"From the brain and from the brain only arise our pleasures, joys, laughter, and jests as well as our sorrows, pains, griefs and tears ..."*
> Hippocrates, *The Sacred Disease*, c. 400 B.C.

The term *apocalyptic demography* reflects a doom-and-gloom perspective on the increasing number and proportion of older persons, with the resulting impact on costs for health and social services. On the positive side, the survival of more individuals to older ages reflects our success in creating a world where substantial proportions of the population are living to ages approaching the human natural life span, rather than dying prematurely from injuries or disease. The aging of our population presents both opportunities and challenges. An example of one of these challenges, Alzheimer's disease (AD), is the focus of this chapter.

It took almost all of human history to date for the world's population to reach one billion. In contrast, it is now taking only about a decade to add the next billion. In addition to these dramatic changes in the world population, there have also been changes in its structure.

The demographic transition describes an evolution from high birth and death rates and low life expectancy to low birth and death rates and high life expectancy (see McFalls 1998 for discussion of the demographic transition). Thus, the transition is from a young population (e.g., median age of 14.9 years in Uganda in 2007) to an old population (median age of 39.1 years in Canada and 36.6 years in the United States in 2007) (Central Intelligence Agency 2007). In North America, we have completed the demographic transition and thus have an increasingly older population—the apocalyptic demography mentioned earlier. All countries are experiencing this growth in older populations, although industrialized countries currently have a much greater proportion of older adults than developing countries.

Paralleling the demographic transition is the *epidemiologic transition*, which traces the long-term mortality decline in terms of changes in the cause of death. Stages in the epidemiologic transition progress from the Age of Pestilence and Famine to the Age of Receding Pandemics and then the Age of Degenerative and Man-made Diseases; a fourth stage, the Age of Delayed Degenerative Diseases and Emerging Infections, has more recently been added. A review of causes of death in North America during the 1900s shows a clear shift from mainly infectious to mainly chronic diseases, such as cancer and cardiovascular disease (see Omran 1971 for discussion of the epidemiologic transition).

The rising importance of age-related chronic diseases, such as AD, is the result of these demographic and epidemiologic transitions. This chapter will provide an overview of AD, focusing on descriptive and analytic epidemiology and the implications for health services management.

Introduction to Alzheimer's Disease

What is Alzheimer's disease?

Alzheimer's disease is a progressive, degenerative disease of the brain causing impairment in memory and other cognitive functions. These impairments are serious enough to interfere with an individual's ability to perform his or her usual daily activities. AD is the most common type of dementia, accounting for approximately two-thirds of dementia cases in North America.

Dementia is a descriptive term based on a collection of clinical symptoms of intellectual impairment. It can be caused by a variety of conditions aside from AD, including other degenerative diseases, stroke, depression, trauma, and medications (see review by Graves 2004). Some causes of dementia are reversible and treatable (e.g., dementia from medication use), and it is critical to ensure that the cause of the dementia is ascertained as quickly and accurately as possible to initiate appropriate interventions. However, it has been estimated that almost two-thirds of dementia cases in the community (that is, among people who do not live in institutions) go undiagnosed (Sternberg, Wolfson, and Baumgarten 2000).

Some of the early signs of AD (e.g., forgetfulness, lack of concentration) can be misinterpreted as part of normal aging, rather than as part of a disease process. Early warning signs may include not simply memory loss but also changes in mood, personality, and behavior; deterioration of language, judgment, and abstract thinking; disorientation; and loss of initiative. (More details are provided later in this chapter.)

The brain lesions characteristic of AD (senile plaques and neurofibrillary tangles) represent two major hypotheses as to its pathogenesis. The hypothesized mechanisms involve aggregation and deposition of beta-amyloid into senile (amyloid) plaques and hyperphosphorylation of tau protein to form fibrils (neurofibrillary tangles). Other proposed mechanisms include inflammation and oxidative stress. These pathological processes result in the death of brain cells, which alters neurochemical systems. Cholinergic deficits in AD were the first neurotransmitter changes identified in AD, with research spurred by the well-known role of cholinergic neurotransmission in memory. Although other neurotransmitter deficits have since been identified, most current pharmaceutical interventions are still based on increasing availability of acetylcholine (see review by Blennow, de Leon, and Zetterberg 2006).

The gold standard diagnostic criteria for AD rely on neuropathologic assessment of the brain after death. Neuropathologic criteria (e.g., CERAD—Mirra et al. 1991) have been developed from numbers and location of neurofibrillary tangles and senile plaques, observed by microscopic examination of brain tissue. Although these neuropathologic criteria have been useful in advancing research on AD, they are not helpful in clinical decision making in living patients. Thus, clinical criteria for the diagnosis of AD have also been developed (e.g., McKhann et al. 1984).

Different clinical criteria vary in the proportion of individuals they identify as having dementia (Erkinjuntti et al. 1997). Although AD is considered to be a diagnosis of exclusion, whereby other possible causes of dementia are ruled out, it is also a diagnosis of inclusion, with a typical pattern of progressive cognitive losses and behavioral symptoms that help differentiate it from other dementias. New technologies, such as imaging and genetic testing, in addition to new clinical tests and knowledge have improved diagnostic accuracy of AD during life to up to 90 percent in centers of AD expertise. (See later in this chapter for a more detailed discussion of diagnostic procedures for AD.)

Dementia decreases life expectancy. Age and sex are significant predictors of survival in individuals with dementia; those younger than 65 years of age, and women, live longer. Level of education, however, is not significantly associated with survival (Wolfson et al. 2001). Median survival after dementia onset is typically estimated as ranging from five to nine years. However, these estimates are based on follow-up studies that miss those with rapidly progressive disease, and thus overestimate survival (length bias). Adjusting for length bias produced estimates of 3.3 years median survival for those with dementia and 3.1 for those with probable AD (in contrast to estimates of 6.6 years for those with dementia in the same study when length bias was not considered) (Wolfson et al. 2001). In contrast, increasing ability to diagnose very early cognitive changes may extend estimates of duration if these mild cognitive impairments reflect early AD, creating a lead-time bias that may complicate estimates of treatment response with mortality outcomes. Both length and lead-time biases are discussed in Chapter 9.

Survival estimates provide information on the total duration of the disease. However, AD is usually divided into three stages: mild, moderate, and severe. Duration is typically divided fairly evenly between these stages (Gauthier 2002), with the caveat that survival duration across stages has been based on estimates of survival that were not adjusted for length or lead-time biases. Each stage has implications for care and management: those with mild AD may still be able to live independently, whereas supervision is required when an individual progresses to moderate AD. Individuals with severe AD are completely dependent on assistance from caregivers and usually are institutionalized in long-term care homes (i.e., nursing homes). (See later in this chapter for a more detailed discussion on care and management.)

Increasing interest has focused on the earliest signs of preclinical dementia symptoms. The development of pharmaceutical interventions for AD has raised interest in identifying individuals at an early stage, given the possibility that these medications may be more useful if introduced when damage in neurochemical pathways is less severe and chemical supplementation of these pathways is more likely to be effective. Strategies (e.g., imaging, neuropsychologic tests) that could be used to identify which individuals with mild cognitive impairments progress to dementia are under investigation by many research teams. One epidemiologic study addressing this topic has found that established risk factors for dementia (see below) may act by predisposing individuals to develop mild cognitive impairments; subsequent development of dementia may depend only on the passage of time and competing mortality (Tyas et al. 2007).

Risk factors for Alzheimer's disease

Age is inextricably linked to AD. The prevalence of AD is estimated to double approximately every five years after age 65 (Jorm, Korten, and Henderson 1987). Given our aging population, it is clear that the prevalence of AD will rise dramatically and present an increasing health challenge in the coming years unless effective preventive or therapeutic strategies are developed.

AD is known to have a genetic basis. Early studies recognized that a family history of dementia increased the risk of developing AD (Graves 2004). Later studies refined that association to identify specific genes associated with the disease. These genetic factors fall into two groups: genes that determine development of AD and those that merely increase the risk of developing it.

AD can be categorized into familial or sporadic subgroups. *Familial AD* is rare, with a prevalence of less than 0.1 percent (see review by Blennow, de Leon, and Zetterberg 2006). It typically develops before 65 years of age and is caused by mutations in specific genes (e.g., presenilins 1 and 2); individuals with these genetic mutations will develop AD unless they die first from another cause. In contrast, the *risk* of AD is associated with apolipoprotein E, the allele to which the genetic risk of *sporadic AD* is primarily attributed (Blennow, de Leon, and Zetterberg 2006). The E4 allele of apolipoprotein E increases the age-specific risk of AD, and affects when those individuals who are susceptible to AD will develop the disease (Meyer et al. 1998). Thus, although individuals with an E4 allele are much more likely to develop AD, some of these individuals will never develop AD despite living to a very old age.

After age and family history, a low level of formal education was the next factor consistently identified as increasing the risk of AD. It is still not clear what the mechanism might be (e.g., early-life deprivation, intellectual ability, lifelong cognitive stimulation), but studies investigating correlates of education, such as linguistic ability (Snowdon et al. 1996), have also found that lower performance on these factors was associated with a higher risk of AD later in life. A protective effect of cognitively stimulating activities in late life has also been reported (Wilson et al. 2002).

It is likely that complex gene-environment interactions are involved in the development of most cases of AD. While some risk factors, such as genetic factors, cannot be changed, many environmental risk factors for AD are modifiable. However, it is becoming increasingly clear that environmental risk factors need to be assessed in their genetic context: many risk factors have different impacts on AD depending on the apolipoprotein E allele status of the individual (Graves 2004).

As increasing numbers of AD risk factors are identified, a conceptual framework to link these predictors is needed. Graves (2004) differentiates those related to disease expression (i.e., clinical signs of AD) from those related to disease pathology (i.e., brain changes characteristic of AD). Risk factors for AD brain pathology include predominantly genetic factors. Early life conditions that maximize growth may reduce the likelihood of clinical expression of dementia. Thus, early life deprivation, associated with poverty and poor nutrition, may be reflected in reduced height and brain size, and greater risk of AD later in life. In contrast, education and linguistic ability have been suggested as protective factors, consistent with the observed neuroprotective role of cognitively stimulating activities: individuals with higher levels of education and linguistic ability are more likely to remain mentally active in later life.

In addition to mental stimulation, later-life predictors include vascular risk factors, neurotoxins, head injury, and alcohol and tobacco use (Graves 2004). The role of strokes in dementia has been recognized (i.e., vascular dementia), but the importance of the vascular system specifically in AD is becoming increasingly clear. Many risk factors for vascular diseases (e.g., hypertension, atherosclerosis, diabetes) also increase the risk of AD (Kalaria 2002). Given that vascular diseases are currently more modifiable by lifestyle and medical interventions than is AD, identification of vascular risk factors for AD may lead to new and more effective prevention and treatment strategies.

With prevalence doubling every five years after age 65 (Jorm, Korten, and Henderson 1987), even interventions that simply delay the development of AD for five years would reduce the number of AD cases by half. Epidemiologic research on modifiable risk factors, such as stroke, provides the scientific foundation on which to build such interventions.

The Magnitude of the Problem: Prevalence, Incidence, and Mortality Rates and Their Implications

Prevalence, incidence, and mortality

Twenty-four million people worldwide have dementia. With 4.6 million people developing it each year, this represents one new case of dementia every seven seconds (Ferri et al. 2005). Although prevalence is higher in developed countries, developing countries have a rate of increase in numbers of dementia cases that is three to four times higher than that of developed countries.

The majority of individuals with dementia currently live in developing countries, and this proportion is estimated to rise from 60 percent in 2001 to 71 percent by 2040. These estimates were derived by an international collaboration of experts using data based on epidemiologic studies across the world. Subtyping dementia into AD or other causes of dementia was not attempted because most of the prevalence data did not provide this level of detail.

The prevalence of dementia has been shown to vary tenfold depending on the diagnostic criteria used (Erkinjuntti et al. 1997), raising concerns about comparing estimates across studies using different criteria for dementia. However, estimates of dementia prevalence, although subject to diagnostic and other challenges, are much easier to obtain than prevalence estimates for AD or incidence rates for dementia or AD. Incidence rates for AD are the most demanding to obtain, as they require both detailed diagnostic workups to determine the subtype of dementia as well as follow-up of subjects to identify newly developed (incident) cases.

A meta-analysis of incidence studies produced age-specific estimates by geographic area (Jorm and Jolley 1998). Incidence of AD ranged from 6.1 per 1,000 person-years in 65- to 69-year-olds to 74.5 per 1,000 person-years in those 85 to 89 years of age. Rates were slightly lower in Europe, and much lower in East Asia, the other two geographic areas studied. Incidence rates were substantially lower, and less variable, when AD was restricted to cases of at least moderate severity. Another meta-analysis of incidence rates (Gao et al. 1998) reported that for every five-year increase in age, incidence rates for both dementia and AD tripled for individuals up to 65 years of age, doubled for those 65 to 74 years of age, and increased 1.5 times by approximately 85 years of age.

Although the estimates of dementia incidence are fairly consistent, rates for AD and other dementia subtypes show more variation (Canadian Study of Health and Aging Working Group 2000). It is unclear whether this variation reflects true differences in the proportion of dementia cases caused by AD or whether it is due to methodologic issues, such as differences in diagnostic criteria or imprecise estimates in studies with small samples.

Incidence rates for dementia are consistently higher in institutionalized adults than in community-dwelling adults (Bickel and Cooper 1994; Canadian Study of Health and Aging Working Group 2000; Tyas et al. 2006). For example, age- and gender-standardized incidence rates for dementia rose more than tenfold from community (15.6 per 1,000 person-years) to institutional settings (191.3 per 1,000 person-years) (Tyas et al. 2006). A national population-based study examined AD incidence rates in Canada in both the community and in long-term care homes (Canadian Study of Health and Aging Working Group 2000). For community and institutional participants combined, age-specific incidence rates, expressed per 1,000 nondemented persons per year, ranged from 7.1 (women) and 3.7 (men) for those 65 to 69 years of age, to 110.2 (women) and 99.0 (men) for those 85 years and over. Overall age-standardized rates per 1,000 nondemented persons per year were 21.8 for women, 19.1 for men, and 20.6 for both sexes combined. Incidence rates obtained from this study tended to be higher than those of other studies because of the inclusion of institutionalized subjects. In addition, the actual at-risk population (the nondemented population instead of the total population) was used as the denominator in risk calculations, again producing higher, but presumably more accurate, incidence rates.

Estimates of incidence rates were further refined by studying how attrition due to death or refusal to participate affected the underestimation of incidence rates (Tyas et al. 2006). The standardized incidence rate of 17.8 per 1,000 person-years for dementia in community and institutional subjects was significantly lower than the estimate of 25.3 per 1,000 person-years obtained after adjustment for attrition. Incidence rates did not level off at the oldest ages, consistent with other (Letenneur et al. 1994; Jorm and Jolley 1998; Andersen et al. 1999b; Hebert et al. 1995), but not all, reports (Miech et al. 2002; Andersen et al. 1999a). Rates did not differ significantly by sex in this and other studies (Letenneur et al. 1994; Aevarsson and Skoog 1996; Jorm and Jolley 1998; Andersen et al. 1999b), although such differences have been reported (Gao et al. 1998; Andersen et al. 1999a; Fratiglioni et al. 1997).

In the United States, 65,965 deaths (22.5 per 100,000 crude death rate) were attributed to AD in 2004, ranking it as the seventh leading cause of death across all ages (Miniño et al. 2007), despite known underreporting of AD on death certificates. AD ranked fifth for women (Centers for Disease Control and Prevention 2004a) and tenth for men (Centers for Disease Control and Prevention 2004b). The effect of a longer life expectancy of women is reflected in the difference between crude death rates by sex (31.5 per 100,000 for women and 13.1 per 100,000 for men) being attenuated by age-adjusted death rates (23.8 per 100,000 for women and 17.7 per 100,000 for men) (Miniño et al. 2007). Mortality from AD in the United States has rapidly increased since the 1980s, with an increase of 1.9 percent from 2003 to 2004, the most recent annual increase for which these data are available. This rise can be attributed to increased case-finding and improved diagnostic techniques and awareness; transitions in coding of cause of death (e.g., from ICD-9 to ICD-10), however, have also contributed substantially to this increase.

Management implications

As noted previously, the number of cases of dementia is expected to increase dramatically as the population ages. This growing number of people with AD will affect the healthcare system, the educational system through changes in university and college curricula, government policies, and, indeed, all of society.

Experts in dementia care have noted that management and care of persons with AD should be identified as a specialty. This specialty needs to be acknowledged across the continuum of healthcare by funders and all care providers, including those in the healthcare sector, informal caregivers, and volunteers (Alzheimer Strategy Transition Project 2007).

Individuals with AD can appear in all care settings: from the emergency room and other acute care settings, to rehabilitation and day hospitals, to palliative care, long-term care homes, and the general community. Thus, adequate numbers of care providers specifically trained in dementia care are required across the spectrum of care. For example, although 62 percent of those living in long-term care homes in Ontario have dementia, less than 10 percent of workers in these homes have received specialized dementia care training (Alzheimer Society of Ontario n.d.), demonstrating the need for additional dementia-specific education among those working in this healthcare sector.

An increase in the number of care providers who have specialized training and education can be accomplished through a number of initiatives. For example, flexible policies that promote staff education and provide incentives for additional training could be encouraged across the healthcare continuum. Specific positions or teams in various settings (e.g., the emergency room or the long-term care home) could increase the capacity of others working in the setting to deal with issues often made more complex by AD. Linking local community-based groups that focus on dementia care with funding groups (such as government agencies) would ensure that dementia-related knowledge and disease-specific strategies are incorporated into day-to-day operations as well as decision making at both personal and policy levels. The academic community could ensure that the core competencies of dementia care are included in curricula developed for and delivered to nurses, physicians, dieticians, social workers, and other care providers. Centers of care could specifically recruit peer presenters and educators to promote best dementia care and support practices.

In addition to providing dementia-specific training for those currently in the healthcare system, planners need to determine the health human resources required to deliver evidence-based care to the ever-increasing number of people with AD. Geriatrician shortages could compromise comprehensive assessment and care. For example, Canada has 0.57 geriatricians per 10,000 Canadians 65 or more years of age (Hogan et al. 2002), although a ratio of 1.25 per 10,000 has been proposed as a target (Patterson et al. 1992). Strategies that improve recruitment into geriatric medicine in Canada, such as mentorship programs (Torrible et al. 2006), need to be implemented as soon as possible.

Further, effective system-wide planning needs to start immediately in the healthcare sector. Public health has an important role in the prevention of disease and in health promotion. Initiatives that encourage healthy behaviors, such as regular physical activity in older adults, need to be further developed. Best practices and resource information can be provided to healthcare professionals and providers as well as the lay public (Centers for Disease Control and Prevention 2003). Many communities, especially suburban areas around larger cities, have grown primarily due to the influx of people born in the 1950s and 1960s (baby boomers). As these individuals and communities age, the increase in both the older population and cases of dementia will likely strain existing local healthcare resources, especially if facility development was based on past need. According to current best practices, additional day programs and other community-based programs may be needed in addition to more long-term care homes. It is estimated that more than 35 percent of all dementia care is provided by family members (Alzheimer Society of Ontario n.d.). As family structures change, more volunteer caregivers may be needed, especially if there are fewer spouses or children who are able or willing to care for the person with AD.

If those with AD and their caregivers are to live meaningful lives across the progression of the illness, planning needs to extend beyond health and social service areas. Researchers and educators will need to work collaboratively with governments, policymakers, and planners to identify enabling and supportive environments. These environments, in turn, will need to be adequately resourced and supported (Alzheimer Strategy Transition Project 2006).

Case Study 17.1. Alzheimer's Disease Incidence, Prevalence, and Mortality

As the population ages, healthcare managers are concerned about planning for the increasing number of people with AD. The need for more long-term care homes (i.e., nursing homes) has to be addressed in current and future budgets.

Planners need to know how many new cases of AD can be expected and how many cases there will be at any one time.

Table 17.1 below describes the population in Our Town. Not much happens in Our Town. In fact, on both July 1, 2005, and July 1, 2006, the total number of people living in Our Town was exactly the same, 17,000 people.

TABLE 17.1. POPULATION OF OUR TOWN, 2005–2006

Age Group (Years)	July 1, 2005		July 1, 2006
	Total Population	Existing AD Cases	New AD Cases
0–14	3,500	0	0
15–64	10,000	0	0
65–74	2,000	44	22
75–84	1,000	200	100
85+	500	170	95

QUESTIONS

1. Calculate the 2006 incidence rate for everyone 65 years of age or older.
2. Calculate the age-specific incidence rates.
3. Which age group has the highest number of new cases? Which age group has the highest incidence?
4. You have just discovered a more sensitive diagnostic tool. How would this affect your calculated incidence rate? How would this affect the calculated prevalence rate?
5. What would a plot of incidence rate by time look like after the introduction of the more sensitive diagnostic tool?
6. Management strategies for AD have changed substantially in the last ten years (e.g., new medications have increased the time spent in the early stages). If the time from diagnosis to death has doubled while incidence has remained the same, what has happened to prevalence?

ANSWERS

1. 2006 incidence
   = No. new cases/65+ population at risk
   = (22 + 100 + 95)/3,500 − (44 + 200 + 170) or 70.3 per 1,000.
2. For 65–74 year olds = 22/(2,000 − 44) or 11.2 per 1,000.
   For 75–84 year olds = 100/(1,000 − 200) or 125 per 1,000.

For 85+ years = 95/(500 – 170) or 287.9 per 1,000.
3. The highest number of new cases is among those 75–84 years of age (n = 100), whereas the highest incidence rate is among those 85 or more years of age (287.9 per 1,000).
4. The calculated incidence rate would increase. You would likely see an increased prevalence rate—if incidence increases without a change in mortality rates or disease duration, then prevalence will increase.
5. If you were graphing incidence rates by year, you would probably notice a temporary spike, which, over time, would likely fall and then plateau. This spike would reflect cases that otherwise would have been missed or diagnosed later.
6. Prevalence = incidence × average disease duration of AD. As duration increases, estimates of prevalence increase.

Cost implications

The costs of dementia are substantial. The worldwide costs of dementia care in 2005 were estimated as US$315.4 billion annually (Wimo, Winblad, and Jonsson 2007). A recent Canadian study estimated that in 2000–2001, AD and other dementias accounted for CAN$1.4 billion in combined direct and indirect costs (Canadian Institute for Health Information 2007). This same report also showed that AD and other dementias accounted for 3.5 percent of disability-adjusted life years for all illnesses in Canada. Canadian figures suggest that the annual cost of care for each person with AD varies by disease severity ($36,794 for those with severe disease, $25,724 for those with moderate disease, $16,054 for those with mild to moderate disease, and $9,451 for those with mild disease; costs are based on use of nursing home care, use of medications, use of community support services by caregivers, and unpaid caregiver time) (Hux et al. 1998).

American figures also highlight the considerable costs associated with AD. Annual inflation-adjusted estimates of the total costs associated with AD in the United States varied from $5.6 billion to $88.3 billion (Bloom, de Pouvourville, and Straus 2003). More recent information suggests that the total direct and indirect costs of Alzheimer's and other dementias (including Medicare and Medicaid costs) and the indirect cost to business of employees who are caregivers of persons with AD amount to more than $148 billion annually (Alzheimer's Association 2007a). The component of these overall costs due to institutionalization is estimated to be $100 billion annually (Leifer 2003).

In the state of New York, it is estimated that 70 percent of persons with AD reside in the community and 75 percent of their care is provided by family caregivers (University of Albany School of Public Health 2007). If unpaid caregivers were not available, the costs associated with AD would rise considerably. American estimates suggest that in 2005, 8.5 billion hours of unpaid caregiver time were provided by almost 10 million caregivers to the roughly 5 million people with AD. If these caregivers had been paid, the cost would have been approximately $83 billion (Alzheimer's Association 2007a).

As the number of individuals with AD rise, the number of healthcare interactions will increase and the associated costs will also rise. For example, in Canada, between 2000–2001 and 2004–2005, the number of individuals with AD in acute care hospitals increased by 39 percent (Canadian Institute for Health Information 2007). Further, individuals with AD represented 8.8 percent of all patient days in acute care hospitals among adult patients (those who are 19 or more years of age). Dementia is also a costly comorbidity among the hospitalized elderly. Readmission rates for those with AD were 4.3 percent within seven days and 10.9 percent within 30 days of discharge, higher than the readmission rates of 3.8 percent and 9.0 percent, respectively, for all acute adult inpatients. American studies have also demonstrated that individuals with dementia have longer hospital stays, higher costs, and a greater frequency of delirium (Lyketsos, Sheppard, and Rabins 2000).

Diagnosis and Detection

A diagnostic workup is typically initiated by individuals, family members, or close friends noticing changes in memory, difficulty in word finding, and changes in mood. Other signs of AD are listed in the box below.

CLINICAL WARNING SIGNS OF ALZHEIMER'S DISEASE

Memory loss
Difficulty performing familiar tasks
Problems with language
Disorientation to time and place
Poor or decreased judgment
Problems with abstract thinking
Misplacing things
Changes in mood or behavior
Changes in personality
Loss of initiative

SOURCE: Alzheimer's Association (2007b).

Someone with Alzheimer's Disease Symptoms	Someone with Normal Age-Related Memory Changes
Forgets entire experiences	Forgets part of an experience
Rarely remembers later	Often remembers later
Is gradually unable to follow written/spoken directions	Is usually able to follow written/spoken directions
Is gradually unable to use notes as reminders	Is usually able to use notes as reminders
Is gradually unable to care for self	Is usually able to care for self

TABLE 17.2
The Difference Between Alzheimer's Disease and Normal Age–Related Memory Changes

SOURCE: Alzheimer's Association (2007b).

Although some of these warning signs are experienced by many people as they age, changes due to aging and those due to AD differ. While there is no clear line between some of the normal changes associated with aging and the pathological changes that reflect AD, it is clear that AD is not a part of normal aging. Some of the differences between AD and normal aging are highlighted in Table 17.2.

As there are currently no universally accepted biological or radiological markers for AD, the diagnosis remains a clinical process (Robillard 2007). There are two main sets of diagnostic criteria used by the medical profession and psychologists (Yukawa, Larson, and Shadlen 2000): the *Diagnostic and Statistical Manual of Mental Disorders*, Fourth Edition, Text Revision (DSM IV-TR) (American Psychiatric Association 2000) and the National Institute of Neurological and Communicative Disorders and Stroke Alzheimer's Disease and Related Disorders Association (McKhann et al. 1984).

Although the exact criteria differ somewhat, the diagnosis of AD is a balance between excluding other health issues that lead to cognitive impairment and including criteria typical of AD (e.g., gradual onset with continuing decline). As scientific knowledge of AD grows, currently accepted criteria will evolve. Even now, some AD experts have recommended revisions to these criteria, suggesting that structural neuroimaging with magnetic resonance imaging, molecular neuroimaging with position emission tomography, and cerebrospinal fluid analysis of beta-amyloid or tau proteins provide disease biomarkers (Dubois et al. 2007).

A standard diagnostic workup for AD includes a complete medical history, a physical examination, memory tests, laboratory tests, and brain scans (Alzheimer's Disease Education and Referral Center 2007; National Institute on Aging 2007). To rule out other health issues that can present as dementia (e.g., Parkinson's disease, subdural hematoma, depression, schizophrenia), it is important to obtain a complete personal and family history from the individual, if possible, as well as information from a caregiver. A complete medication history is needed as some medications (e.g., antide-pressants, sedatives, antiarrhythmics, antihypertensives, anticholinergic agents) can produce dementia-like symptoms. The medical history should include assessment of risk factors for AD (e.g., history of head injury, fam-ily history of AD, vascular factors such as high blood pressure).

As a pattern of gradual onset with continuing decline is indicative of AD, the chronology associated with the dementia should also be doc-umented. In addition, a social/cultural history that includes information about education, socioeconomic and cultural background, and current social support networks is also needed and can be used to identify future resources and strategies.

A physical examination includes a neurological evaluation and assessments of blood pressure, vision, hearing, cardiac status, respiratory function, gait, balance, and ability to perform activities of daily living. Opinions differ as to the possible role of genetic testing in the diagnostic process. Schipper (2007) does not advise testing for the presence of the E4 allele of apolipoprotein E as a diagnostic marker for sporadic AD. In contrast, Post and colleagues (1997) have recommended genetic testing for apolipoprotein E allele status as part of the diagnostic workup for AD, although they do not advise such testing to screen asymptomatic members of the general population. Other types of genetic testing (e.g., for prese-nilins) may be appropriate in asymptomatic cases when individuals present with strong evidence of familial AD (i.e., extensive family history).

Tests of cognition and memory are also conducted (Jacova et al. 2007). Cognitive dimensions commonly examined include immediate mem-ory; short-term recall; abstract thinking; judgment; concentration; aphasia; apraxia; agnosia; and spatial, reading, writing, and mathematical ability (Holsinger et al. 2007). Common tools include the Mini-Mental State Examination (MMSE) (Folstein, Folstein, and McHugh 1975) and the Montreal Cognitive Assessment (Nasreddine et al. 2005).

Neuroimaging may be valuable in the workup for dementia. Current evidence suggests that structural neuroimaging can be useful in identify-ing concomitant cerebrovascular disease that can affect patient manage-ment (Chow 2007). A number of studies are underway to identify the role of neuroimaging in the diagnosis and monitoring of AD. Further neuropsy-chological testing may be helpful in specific cases.

Currently, there is no one single test for AD, and the diagnostic process is a lengthy one. Regular follow-up is critical after an initial assess-ment of declining mental status, both for continuous care and monitoring as well as for differentiating AD from normal aging (e.g., decline in the MMSE score of two to five points a year is common among those with untreated AD) (Han et al. 2000).

Some individuals have suggested routine screening for dementia because of the relatively high incidence of AD after the age of 85 and the availability of drug therapies that may have a beneficial effect on cognitive function. However, given concerns with diagnostic accuracy, the feasibility of screening and treatment in routine clinical practice, and the unknown potential harms of screening, the U.S. Preventive Services Task Force (n.d.) concluded that there was insufficient evidence to recommend either for or against routine screening for dementia in older adults.

Case Study 17.2. Screening for Cognitive Impairment: The Mini-Mental State Examination

Alzheimer's disease presents itself in many different ways. Multiple cognitive tests are used to help make the initial diagnosis and to monitor rates of change or decline. One of the most commonly used tests is the Mini-Mental State Examination.

The MMSE, first described by Folstein, Folstein, and McHugh in 1975, is a brief series of questions and tasks that takes about ten minutes to complete. Suppose that another test became the standard. Could the MMSE still be valuable in the diagnostic workup for AD? (See Table 17.3 below.)

TABLE 17. 3. ASSESSMENT OF ALZHEIMER'S DISEASE BY MMSE AND NEW STANDARD CRITERIA

	New Standard: AD	New Standard: No AD
MMSE score ≤23	69	74
MMSE score ≥24	11	846

QUESTIONS

1. Using the numbers in Table 17.3, calculate the prevalence of AD in this population.
2. What is the post-test likelihood of disease following a positive test?
3. What is the post-test likelihood of no disease following a negative test?
4. If you were 50 percent certain an individual had AD prior to MMSE testing and the MMSE score was 26, how confident would you be in a diagnosis of AD after administering the MMSE?
5. The MMSE is available on the Internet, so family members can coach those with AD. If there is a practice effect, would that increase the proportion of those with the disease who test negative (false negatives) or the proportion of those without the disease who test positive (false positives)?

6. What factors could increase the number of false positives? What factors could increase the number of false negatives?

7. If a newer diagnostic test for AD was developed that was more sensitive than the current test, how would results from this new test compare to those using the older, less accurate test?

8. Sensitivity of screening tests, such as the MMSE, comes at the price of specificity. Would you choose a cutoff score for the MMSE that maximized sensitivity, specificity, or both?

9. Cutoff scores for the MMSE can be stratified by age and education. What are the advantages and disadvantages of identifying cutoffs by level of education?

ANSWERS

1. 69 + 11/(69 + 11 + 74 + 846) = 80/1,000 or 8%
2. 69/(69 + 74) = 48%
3. 846/(11 + 846) = 99%
4. Assuming 1,000 people took the test, if the pretest likelihood = 50 percent, then the prevalence (a + c/a + b + c + d) = 50%; so a + c = 500 and b + d = 500. (See Table 17.4 for the distribution.)

TABLE 17.4. ASSESSMENT OF ALZHEIMER'S DISEASE BY MMSE AND NEW STANDARD CRITERIA

	New Standard: AD	New Standard: AD
MMSE score ≤23	430	40
MMSE score ≥24	70	460
Total	500	500

The post-test likelihood of disease following a negative test is 100% − (460/530 × 100%)= 13.3%. So, you have effectively ruled out AD (pre-test probability: 50%; post-test probability: 13%, a change of −37 percentage points).

5. It would increase the proportions of false negatives. Individuals who actually have AD might have improved their test performance by practicing and thus score above the MMSE cutpoint. If so, they would not be classified as having the disease according to this screening test.

6. An individual could be a false positive if he was taking medications that impaired cognitive function (e.g., anticholinergic agents), if he was feeling ill or was unable to concentrate that day (e.g., previous sleepless night or was experiencing a chest or urinary tract infection), or if the test was in English and the individual had difficulties with the English language. An

individual could be a false negative if he or she had AD with isolated frontal lobe lesions (MMSE does not test executive function) or high levels of education. Note: Because men currently in older age groups tend to have higher levels of education than women, men may be more likely to be false negatives.

7. If a new test is compared to an old (but inaccurate) test, the new test may look worse than the old test, even if it is better. If the new test is more sensitive than the standard, the additional cases identified by the new test would be considered false positives in relation to the old test. So, if an inaccurate standard of validity is used, a new test can perform no better than that standard and may look worse when it actually approximates the truth more closely. By using a poor standard, you may miss identifying a new gold standard.

8. A sensitive test should be chosen when there are important consequences for missing a disease; highly specific tests are needed when false positive results can cause harm. For AD, a false positive may be detrimental to the family and the family member. The diagnosis of AD can be frightening, and those with false positive results may suffer shame and worry. However, individuals with false negative results may not be prescribed needed medications. As there are adverse consequences to both false positives and false negatives, you would want to maximize both sensitivity and specificity in screening tests for AD.

9. A single cutpoint may miss cases among the more educated and generate false positives among those with less education. Education-specific norms may optimize performance of the MMSE as a screening tool for AD, but if there are different scores for various subgroups, clinicians may forget to adjust the score and misclassify some individuals. However, does education bias the results, or is it a risk factor? If low education is of etiological significance, scores may be overadjusted.

Management and Care

The primary care team's management of the person with AD should be client-centered and individualized, and focus on the goals set by the person with AD and his or her caregiver. Disclosure of a diagnosis of AD should include discussions regarding diagnostic certainty, treatment options, future plans, financial issues, power of attorney, wills, driving, availability of support services, and possible participation in research studies (Fisk et al. 2007). Management varies somewhat by stage and is described below for those with mild to moderate disease, those with severe disease, and those in the terminal stages of AD.

Management of mild to moderate Alzheimer's disease

Once diagnosed with AD, current best-practice evidence suggests that the primary healthcare provider should work with an interdisciplinary healthcare team, the individual, and his or her caregiver to develop and implement an ongoing treatment plan with clear, defined goals (Callahan et al. 2006). Regular monitoring of cognitive deficits and other AD-related symptoms is recommended so that response to therapies/interventions can be monitored (Hogan et al. 2007).

A number of care guidelines have been produced; recent recommendations are based on the Third Canadian Consensus Conference on the Diagnosis and Treatment of Dementia held in Montreal in March 2006. Early management of the person with AD may include referral to appropriate services (i.e., neurologists, clinical psychologists, social workers), and ongoing management of general health and existing comorbidities (Hogan et al. 2007). In addition, both individuals with AD and their caregivers may be referred to support organizations for materials on community resources, support groups, legal and financial issues, respite care, future care needs, and options.

Regarding pharmacotherapy, Hogan and colleagues (2007) advise that medications with anticholinergic effects be minimized. They also recommend that ongoing management include symptomatic treatment with cholinesterase inhibitors. Although a number of other medications, supplements, and herbal preparations have been tested as potential therapies, studies have been either inconclusive or negative and these therapies are not recommended.

Behavioral problems and mood disorders can often be managed through environmental modification, task simplification, and redirection. A number of approaches (e.g., gentle persuasion [Gentle Persuasive Approaches 2005]) have been developed to deal with aggressive behaviors. Referral to social service agencies or support organizations, such as the Alzheimer's Association's Safe Return Program (Alzheimer's Association 2006) for people who wander, may be helpful. Antidepressants should be considered in individuals with an inadequate response to nonpharmacologic interventions or those with a major affective disorder, severe dysthymia, or severe emotional lability (Hogan et al. 2007). Day programs that offer exercise and recreation may help structure both the caregiver's and the care recipient's day and improve functional performance.

As persons with AD progressively lose their ability to care for themselves, caregivers often assume increasing responsibilities. Caregivers can provide assistance with activities of daily living (i.e., eating, grooming, walking, bathing, and dressing) and help those with AD navigate the complex healthcare system. However, caring for someone with AD has attendant emotional, physical, social, and financial costs (Morris, Morris, and Britton 1998). The consequences of caring can include depression; estimates of the prevalence of depression among caregivers of people with dementia range from 28 percent to 60 percent (Redinbaugh, McCallum, and Kiecolt-Glaser 1995; Schulz et al. 1995). Other consequences for caregivers include poor physical health (Baumgarten et al. 1992) and less time for personal activities (Ory et al. 1999), highlighting the need to focus on the caregiver/care recipient dyad.

Although deteriorating memory and cognitive function increases caregiver burden, cognitive decline is often not the Alzheimer-related symptom that affects the caregiver most (Draper 2004). Changes in mood and behavioral issues often have the greatest effect on both the person with AD and his or her caregivers. Lopez and colleagues (2003) found that among those with mild AD, a high proportion exhibited mood and behavioral problems: 60 percent suffered anxiety, 55 percent had apathy, 49 percent had agitation, and 39 percent had irritability. Almost half (46 percent) of caregivers reported that their inability to deal with these behaviors was a reason for institutionalization (Buhr, Kuchibhatla, and Clipp 2006). Similarly, Thomas and colleagues (2004) found that the main problem resulting in institutionalization was dependence on the caregiver, with behavioral disorders the second most common problem.

Management of moderate to severe Alzheimer's disease

As the disease progresses, the proportion of people who exhibit agitation and aggressive behaviors tends to increase. Depression, apathy, anxiety, delusions, and hallucinations are common in severe AD (Boller et al. 2002). Ability to perform activities of daily living also declines, and individuals often lose bowel and bladder control. As a result, management goals should be reviewed and new strategies developed by the care team.

The need for assistance with daily living activities is a significant predictor of nursing home placement (hazard ratio for one or more dependencies: 1.38) (Yaffe et al. 2002). The most common reason for institutionalization identified by caregivers of individuals with dementia was the need for more skilled care (Buhr, Kuchibhatla, and Clipp 2006). Nursing home placement is best predicted by consideration of both care recipient and caregiver characteristics (Yaffe et al. 2002). Ability of the person with AD to perform daily tasks and the amount of assistance provided to the caregiver, such as overnight help, have a direct impact on the amount of care required and affect whether the person with AD is best managed at home or in an institution.

Despite few randomized controlled clinical trials on the treatment of severe AD, clinical practice guidelines for severe AD were also developed at the Third Canadian Consensus Conference on the Diagnosis and Treatment of Dementia (Herrmann, Gauthier, and Lysy 2007). It was recommended that individuals with severe AD be treated with cholinesterase inhibitors, memantine, or both. It was also recommended that treatment continue until there was no clinical improvement. Pharmacologic treatment of severe depression, psychosis, or aggression that puts the individual or others at risk of harm was also recommended. In addition, the authors noted that institutionalization is not a reason to discontinue therapy.

End of life care

Individuals with advanced dementia commonly develop difficulties eating and swallowing. Eventually, they become bedridden and dependent in all activities of daily living. At this stage, they are at high risk of dying from pneumonia or sepsis, despite antibiotic treatment (Gillick 2000), and thus management focuses on quality of life for both the person with AD and his or her family. It is recommended that palliative management of end-stage AD be similar to that of terminal cancer (Grossberg and Desai 2003).

Challenges to the Epidemiologic Study of Alzheimer's Disease

Although AD is an important public health problem and the focus of many epidemiologic studies, the disease presents substantial challenges to epidemiologic investigation. Other health conditions of older adults present many of these same challenges, while some are specific to AD.

AD is primarily a disease of old age. Thus, issues of competing comorbidities and competing mortality complicate its study. Attrition due to death is a substantial component of loss to follow-up in cohort studies of AD. Thus, although AD incidence rates are needed, they have been particularly challenging to obtain because of the need to balance the longer duration of follow-up required to accrue sufficient numbers of AD cases against the survival bias introduced by following up only on subjects who remain alive and can be assessed for incident AD. This problem is particularly acute for analysis of the oldest-old adults (i.e., those 85 years of age and older), where incidence rates often cannot be accurately calculated, particularly for men. Attrition due to death has been shown to result in significant underestimates of the incidence of AD (Tyas et al. 2006).

Other challenges are more specific to the nature of AD. As described previously in this chapter, the diagnosis of AD is an expensive and time-consuming process. It is thus not well-suited for large, epidemiologic studies, which have had to implement screening strategies to make cohort studies more feasible by restricting the number of subjects undergoing a full diagnostic workup. Death certificates remain problematic sources of AD data, with substantial underestimation of cases. Healthcare utilization data are also problematic, providing better identification of severe AD cases than milder ones (Tyas et al. 2006).

In comparison, consider other chronic conditions for which a telephone or mail survey can be used to quickly and inexpensively quantify the burden of disease. Such surveys are problematic for AD because self-reports of AD diagnosis are of questionable validity. In addition to the issue of cognitive impairment of the respondent, individuals may not be tested or told their diagnosis. The diagnosis is often expensive, complex, and not definitive, and may be associated with fear and social stigma (Fisk et al. 2007). Physicians may be hesitant to diagnose and disclose AD, especially given diagnostic challenges, as they then may need to deal with a number of challenging issues, such as driving and consent to treatment.

In addition to the resource requirements for diagnosis of AD, diagnostic accuracy remains a concern. While reliance on neuropathologic assessment is declining with improving clinical diagnostic methods, the changing diagnostic criteria hamper comparisons over time and across countries. As subtypes of dementia are refined, those cases diagnosed with AD will become more homogeneous, but substantial heterogeneity still exists. Because of its slowly progressive nature, it is difficult to determine the age at onset with precision, thus hindering investigation of risk factors. The relationship between mild cognitive impairments and preclinical AD also needs to be clarified.

Even if individuals are diagnosed with AD, impairments and disabilities associated with advancing age, such as poor vision, hearing loss, and severe arthritis, may affect performance on mental status and neuropsychological tests, leading to an increased number of false positives. False positives may also occur because of other environmental (e.g., noisy testing area) or personal (e.g., little formal education, lack of fluency in test language) factors. In addition, the likelihood of diagnosis can be affected by the individual's family members, who, for example, may coach their family member prior to testing to improve cognitive performance (Gofton and Weaver 2006).

Additional challenges relate to the cognitive impairment characteristic of AD. As new pharmacological and nonpharmacological treatments for AD are developed, care strategies need to be rigorously evaluated prior to broader implementation. Informed consent must be obtained before study participation. Although the diagnosis of AD does not in itself constitute a lack of legal capacity (Alzheimer Europe 2007), those with AD do eventually lose their capacity to consent. While laws and regulation concerning informed consent vary widely across the world, either the person participating in the study or the legal guardian must consent to study participation. Further, either the participant or the proxy must be able to withdraw the participant from the study at any time without compromise to care.

Self-reported data from cases are problematic, raising issues of data quality (e.g., bias) and influencing the selection of study designs (see

Case Study 17.3). It is also important for care and management of individuals with AD (e.g., difficulty obtaining subjective measures of pain). Proxy respondents, when available, are thus relied upon to provide much of the data, but the quality of these data then depends on many of their characteristics (e.g., relationship, status as primary caregiver). Proxy respondents may systematically report differently than the index individual, raising concerns in longitudinal studies where data may be initially self-reported and then reported by proxies as the subject's level of cognitive impairment increases (Østbye et al. 1997). This presents challenges in monitoring outcomes, such as intervention trials, when differences in outcomes may reflect different sources of data rather than actual differences in treatment response.

Case Study 17.3. Study Designs and Measures of Association (Example: Smoking and Alzheimer's Disease)

Epidemiologic studies of risk factors for AD face many challenges: the diagnosis of AD is complex and expensive, and collection of information on risk factors is hampered by the impaired cognition of cases. For example, early studies on the association between tobacco use and AD reported that smoking reduced the risk of AD; later, more methodologically sophisticated studies found that smoking increased the risk of the disease.

QUESTIONS

1. What would you want to consider in choosing an observational or experimental (e.g., randomized controlled trial) study design to examine the association of AD and smoking?
2. Calculate and interpret the odds ratio using the data below from a case control study on smoking and AD.

Number of cases with AD:	100
Number of controls without AD:	100
Number of current or former smokers among cases:	55
Number of current or former smokers among controls:	70

3. Calculate and interpret the relative risk from a cohort study on smoking and AD. This cohort study recruited 1,000 participants, 450 of whom at baseline reported smoking currently or in the past. Of these 450, 85 developed AD by the end of the study. Of the remaining 550 nonsmoking participants, 50 had developed AD.
4. Are cross-sectional or case control studies appropriate designs for examining the association between tobacco use and AD? Why or why not?

5. What might be the impact on the results of a case control study if you obtained data on smoking history from controls (cognitively intact older subjects) but used proxy respondents for cases (individuals with AD)?
6. What factors might explain the false conclusion of case control studies that smoking reduces the risk of AD?

ANSWERS

1. Experimental studies involving randomization of exposure to cigarette smoke in individuals are clearly unethical. Thus, we are restricted to observational study designs. However, we know that smokers often exhibit other risk behaviors (e.g., alcohol use), and so we need to be particularly attentive to potential confounding factors.
2. You can find this answer by setting up a 2 × 2 table, as below:

TABLE 17.5 2x2 TABLE OF ANALYSIS OF MEASURES OF ASSOCIATION

	Case	Control
Exposed	a	b
Not exposed	c	d

	Case	Control
Current or former smoker	55	70
Never smoker	45	30
	100	100

OR = ad/bc
   = (55 × 30) / (45 × 70)
   = 0.52

Cases have approximately 0.5 times the odds of smoking compared with controls (or controls have approximately twice the odds compared with cases). Smoking thus appears to be protective for AD.
3. To calculate your answer, set up a table like Table 17.6.
4. Study designs that require information from a case, such as cross-sectional or case control designs, are problematic for conditions such as AD because a case's ability to provide information is impaired. Although information from proxy respondents can be used, the quality of such information is of concern. Consider that most proxy respondents will be spouses or daughters; they will have little or no firsthand knowledge of smoking exposure of the

---

TABLE 17.6. NUMBER OF STUDY PARTICIPANTS BY AD DIAGNOSIS AND BASELINE SMOKING STATUS

Baseline Smoking Status	Developed AD	Did Not Develop AD	Total
Current or former smoker	85	365	450
Never smoker	50	500	550

RR = a/(a + b)/c/(c + d)

= (85/450) / (50/550)

= 2.08

Current or former smokers were at 2.08 times, or approximately double, the risk of developing AD compared with never smokers.

---

case in early adulthood. Thus, cohort studies, for which exposure data can be collected from participants before they develop the disease, are preferred.

5. Proxy respondents would likely underestimate the smoking history of cases due to lack of knowledge of current and, particularly, past smoking. In contrast, the smoking history of controls would be more accurately reported, creating a differential misclassification bias of exposure (Chapter 11). Thus, in the absence of any true association between smoking and AD, it would appear as if controls had more smoking exposure than cases, and that smoking was protective, or reduced the risk of AD.

6. Aside from the issue of asymmetric reporting (data from proxy respondents for cases and from self-reports for controls), confounding and survival bias can affecct the results of these studies. It is important to consider important confounders of this relationship, particularly because smoking is associated with other characteristics known to be linked to AD (e.g., education).

   In addition, we know that smoking is strongly related to mortality, and thus, heavy smokers are more likely than lighter or nonsmokers to die early. Because the risk of AD rises rapidly with increasing age, smokers will be underestimated in the older age groups who are most at risk for AD (i.e., smokers die before they develop AD). Smokers who live to an old age can be considered "hardy survivors," whose risk of all diseases may be less than the general population due to other environmental or genetic factors.

Summary

With the proportion of older adults increasing in populations across the world, age-related chronic diseases, such as AD, become more important in terms of healthcare costs and quality of life. However, the study of AD

has proven challenging. Changing diagnostic criteria and increasing awareness of the disease make the study of incidence over time difficult, and
surveys to determine disease prevalence are problematic. Identification
of risk factors is complicated by the gene-environment interactions that
contribute to the development of most cases of AD. In addition, AD is
a disease of the aged. In longitudinal studies, attrition due to death limits the accrual of sufficient numbers of AD cases to detect statistically significant risk factors and produces underestimates of incidence rates. Studies
on the management and care of those with AD are also limited, as information often needs to be collected from proxy respondents, and diagnostic tools, often not developed or tested on the very old, may not be
useful in this population.

Epidemiology has overcome considerable challenges to make substantial contributions to our understanding of AD. It is only recently that
pharmaceutical interventions have been available; we are now close to developing new therapies that go beyond temporarily augmenting neurotransmission to interventions that slow, stop, or reverse the brain damage caused
by AD. Earlier diagnosis of AD at preclinical stages will increase the effectiveness of these treatments and reduce the burden of this disease on individuals, families, and society. Given the recent increased attention to chronic
disease management generally and to AD specifically, current advances and
future research may transform the fear of an "apocalyptic demography" to
a hope for all to live longer and healthier lives.

References

Aevarsson, O., and I. Skoog. 1996. "A Population-Based Study on the
Incidence of Dementia Disorders Between 85 and 88 Years of Age."
Journal of the American Geriatrics Society 44: 1455–60.

Alzheimer Europe. 2007. "Position Paper on Research with People with
Dementia." [Online information; retrieved 7/21/07.] www.alzheimer-
europe.org/?lm2=225A8956AC31.

Alzheimer Society of Ontario. n.d. "It's Time to Act. Ontario's Dementia
Imperative." [Online article; retrieved 10/30/07.] http://
www.opga.on.ca/current-issues.asp.

Alzheimer Strategy Transition Project. 2006. *Roundtable on Future Planning
for People Affected by Alzheimer Disease and Related Dementias. An ADRD
Planning Framework*, First Edition. [Online report; retrieved 11/27/07.]
http://marep.uwaterloo.ca/other/2122ADRDPlanningFrmwrk1stEnglish
.pdf.

———. 2007. *Alzheimer's Disease and Related Dementias: Recommendations
for Prevention Care and Cure. Report 3: Health Human Resources
Strategy.* [Online report; retrieved 11/27/07.] http://
alzheimerontario.org/local/files/Web%20site/Public%20Policy/Health%

20Human%20Resource%20Strategy%20%20April%202007.pdf.

Alzheimer's Association. 2006. "Safe Return Program." [Online information; retrieved 11/26/07.] http://www.alztex.org/services/safereturn.asp.

———. 2007a. "Alzheimer's Disease Facts and Figures. [Online information; retrieved 11/27/07.] www.alz.org/national/documents/Report_2007FactsAndFigures.pdf.

———. 2007b. "Symptoms of Alzheimer's." [Online information; retrieved 10/30/07.] http://www.alz.org/alzheimers_disease_symptoms_of_alzheimers.asp.

Alzheimer's Disease Education and Referral Center. 2007. "Diagnosis." [Online information; retrieved 10/20/07.] http:// www.nia.nih.gov/Alzheimers/AlzheimersInformation/Diagnosis.

American Psychiatric Association. 2000. *Diagnostic and Statistical Manual of Mental Disorders*, 4th ed., text rev. Washington, DC: American Psychiatric Association.

Andersen, K., L. J. Launer, M. E. Dewey, L. Letenneur, A. Ott, J. R. Copeland, J. F. Dartigues, P. Kragh-Sorensen, M. Baldereschi, C. Brayne, A. Lobo, J. M. Martinez-Lage, T. Stijnen, and A. Hofman. 1999a. "Gender Differences in the Incidence of AD and Vascular Dementia: The EURODEM Studies." *Neurology* 53: 1992–97.

Andersen, K., H. Nielsen, A. Lolk, J. Andersen, I. Becker, and P. Kragh-Sørensen. 1999b. "Incidence of Very Mild to Severe Dementia and Alzheimer's Disease in Denmark: The Odense Study." *Neurology* 52: 85–90.

Baumgarten, M., R. N. Battista, C. Infante-Rivard, J. A. Hanley, R. Becker, and S. Gauthier. 1992. "The Psychological and Physical Health of Family Members Caring for an Elderly Person with Dementia." *Journal of Clinical Epidemiology* 45: 61–70.

Bickel, H., and B. Cooper. 1994. "Incidence and Relative Risk of Dementia in an Urban Elderly Population: Findings of a Prospective Field Study." *Journal of the American Geriatrics Society* 24: 179–92.

Blennow, K., M. de Leon, and H. Zetterberg. 2006. "Alzheimer's Disease." *Lancet* 368: 387–403.

Bloom, B. S., N. de Pouvourville, and W. L. Straus. 2003. "Cost of Illness of Alzheimer's Disease: How Useful Are Current Estimates?" *Gerontologist* 43: 158–64.

Boller, F., M. Verny, L. Hugonot-Diener, and J. Saxton. 2002. "Clinical Features and Assessment of Severe Dementia: A Review." *European Journal of Neurology* 9: 125–36.

Buhr, G. T., M. Kuchibhatla, and E. C. Clipp. 2006. "Caregivers' Reasons for Nursing Home Placement: Clues for Improving Discussions with Families Prior to the Transition." *Gerontologist* 46: 52–61.

Callahan, C. M., M. A. Boustani, F. W. Unverzagt, M. G. Austrom, T. M.

Damush, A. J. Perkins, B. A. Fultz, S. L. Hui, S. R. Counsell, and H. C. Hendrie. 2006. "Effectiveness of Collaborative Care for Older Adults with Alzheimer Disease in Primary Care: A Randomized Controlled Trial." *Journal of the American Medical Association* 295: 2148–57.

Canadian Institute for Health Information. 2007. *The Burden of Neurological Diseases, Disorders and Injuries in Canada*. Ottawa: Canadian Institute for Health Information.

Canadian Study of Health and Aging Working Group. 2000. "The Incidence of Dementia in Canada." *Neurology* 55: 66–73.

Centers for Disease Control and Prevention. 2003. "Public Health and Aging: Trends in Aging—United States and Worldwide." [Online article; retrieved 11/28/07.] http://www.cdc.gov/MMWR/preview/mmwrhtml/mm520 6a2.htm.

———. 2004a. "Leading Causes of Death in Females: United States, 2004." [Online information; retrieved 12/1/07.] www.cdc.gov/women/lcod.htm.

———. 2004b. "Leading Causes of Death in Males: United States, 2004." [Online information; retrieved 12/1/07.] www.cdc.gov/men/lcod.htm.

Central Intelligence Agency. 2007. "Field Listing: Median Age." *World Factbook*. [Online information; retrieved 12/5/07.] https://www.cia.gov /library/publications/the-world-factbook/fields/2177.html.

Chow, T. 2007. "Structural Neuroimaging in the Diagnosis of Dementia." *Alzheimer's & Dementia* 3: 333–35.

Draper, B. 2004. *Dealing with Dementia: A Guide to Alzheimer's Disease and Depression in Caregivers on Patients with Dementia*. Sydney: Allen and Unwin.

Dubois, B., H. H. Feldman, C. Jacova, S. T. DeKosky, P. Barberger-Gateau, J. Cummings, A. Delacourte, D. Galasko, S. Gauthier, G. Jicha, K. Meguro, J. O'Brien, F. Pasquier, P. Robert, M. Rossor, S. Salloway, Y. Stern, P. J. Visser, and P. Scheltens. 2007. "Research Criteria for the Diagnosis of Alzheimer's Disease: Revising the NINCDS-ADRDA Criteria." *Lancet Neurology* 6: 734–46.

Erkinjuntti, T., T. Østbye, R. Steenhuis, and V. Hachinski. 1997. "The Effect of Different Diagnostic Criteria on the Prevalence of Dementia." *New England Journal of Medicine* 337: 1667–74.

Ferri, C. P., M. Prince, C. Brayne, H. Brodaty, L. Fratiglioni, M. Ganguli, K. Hall, K. Hasegawa, H. Hendrie, Y. Yuang, A. Jorm, C. Mathers, P. Menezes, E. Rimmer, and M. Scazufca, for Alzheimer's Disease International. 2005. "Global Prevalence of Dementia: A Delphi Consensus Study." *Lancet* 366: 2112–17.

Fisk, J. D., B. J. Beattie, M. Donnelly, A. Byszewski, and F. J. Molnar. 2007. "Disclosure of the Diagnosis of Dementia." *Alzheimer's & Dementia* 3: 404–10.

Folstein, M. R., S. E. Folstein, and P. R. McHugh. 1975. "'Mini-Mental

State': A Practical Method for Grading the Cognitive State of Patients for the Clinician." *Journal of Psychiatric Research* 12: 189–98.

Fratiglioni, L., M. Viitanen, E. Von Strauss, V. Tontodonati, A. Herlitz, and B. Winblad. 1997. "Very Old Women at Highest Risk of Dementia and Alzheimer's Disease: Incidence Data from the Kungsholmen Project, Stockholm." *Neurology* 48: 132–38.

Gao, S., H. C. Hendrie, K. S. Hall, and S. Hui. 1998. "The Relationships Between Age, Sex, and the Incidence of Dementia and Alzheimer Disease: A Meta-Analysis." *Archives of General Psychiatry* 55: 809–15.

Gauthier, S. 2002. "Advances in the Pharmacotherapy of Alzheimer's Disease." *Canadian Medical Association Journal* 166: 616–23.

Gentle Persuasive Approaches. 2005. "Gentle Persuasive Approaches in Dementia Care." [Online information; retrieved 7/16/07.] http://marep.uwaterloo.ca/PDF/NewGPAnewsletter.pdf.

Gillick, M. R. 2000. "Sounding Board: Rethinking the Role of Tube Feeding in Patients with Advanced Dementia." *New England Journal of Medicine* 342: 206–10.

Gofton, T., and D. F. Weaver. 2006. "Challenges in the Clinical Diagnosis of Alzheimer's Disease: Influence of 'Family Coaching' on the Mini-Mental State Examination." *American Journal of Alzheimer's Disease and Other Dementias* 21: 109–12.

Graves, A. B. 2004. "Alzheimer's Disease and Vascular Dementia." In *Neuroepidemiology: From Principles to Practice*, edited by L. M. Nelson, C. M. Tanner, S. K. Van Den Eeden, and V. M. McGuire, 102–30. New York: Oxford University Press.

Grossberg, G. T., and A. K. Desai. 2003. "Management of Alzheimer's Disease." *Journals of Gerontology Series A: Biological and Medical Sciences* 58A: 331–53.

Han, L., M. Cole, F. Belavance, J. McCusker, and F. Primeau. 2000. "Tracking Cognitive Decline in Alzheimer's Disease Using the Mini-Mental State Examination: A Meta-Analysis." *International Psychogeriatrics* 12 (2): 231–47.

Hebert, L. E., P. A. Scherr, L. A. Beckett, M. S. Albert, D. M. Pilgrim, M. J. Chown, H. H. Funkenstein, and D. A. Evans. 1995. "Age-Specific Incidence of Alzheimer's Disease in a Community Population." *Journal of the American Geriatrics Society* 273: 1354–59.

Herrmann, N., S. Gauthier, and P. G. Lysy. 2007. "Clinical Practice Guidelines for Severe Alzheimer's Disease. *Alzheimer's & Dementia* 3: 385–97.

Hogan, D. B., P. Bailey, A. Carswell, B. Clarke, C. Cohen, D. Forbes, M. Man-Son-Hing, K. Lanctot, D. Morgan, and L. Thorpe. 2007. "Management of Mild to Moderate Alzheimer's Disease and Dementia." *Alzheimer's & Dementia* 3: 355–85.

Hogan, D. B., B. L. Beattie, H. Bergman, W. B. Dalziel, B. Goldlist, C.

MacKnight, F. Molnar, C. Patterson, B. Power, K. Rockwood, P. Soucie, and D. Turner. 2002. "Submission of the Canadian Geriatrics Society to the Commission on the Future of Health Care in Canada." *Geriatrics Today* 5: 7–12.

Holsinger, T., J. Deveau, M. Boustani, and J. Williams. 2007. "Does This Patient Have Dementia?" *Journal of the American Medical Association* 297: 2391–404.

Hux, M. J., B. J. O'Brien, M. Iskedjian, R. Goeree, M. Gagnon, and S. Gauthier. 1998. "Relation Between Severity of Alzheimer's Disease and Costs of Caring." *Canadian Medical Association Journal* 159: 457–65.

Jacova, C., A. Kertesz, M. Blair, J. Fisk, and H. Feldman. 2007. "Neuropsychological Testing and Assessment for Dementia." *Alzheimer's & Dementia* 3: 299–317.

Jorm, A. F., and D. Jolley. 1998. "The Incidence of Dementia: A Meta-Analysis." *Neurology* 51: 728–33.

Jorm, A. F., A. E. Korten, and A. S. Henderson. 1987. "The Prevalence of Dementia: A Quantitative Integration of the Literature." *Acta Psychiatrica Scandinavica* 76: 465–79.

Kalaria, R. N. 2002. "Similarities Between Alzheimer's Disease and Vascular Dementia." *Journal of the Neurological Sciences* 203: 29–34.

Leifer, B. P. 2003. "Early Diagnosis of Alzheimer's Disease: Clinical and Economic Benefits." *Journal of the American Geriatrics Society* 51: S281–S288.

Letenneur, L., D. Commenges, J. F. Dartigues, and P. Barberger-Gateau. 1994. "Incidence of Dementia and Alzheimer's Disease in Elderly Community Residents of South-Western France." *International Journal of Epidemiology* 23: 1256–61.

Lopez, O. L., J. T. Becker, R. A. Sweet, W. Klunk, D. I. Kaufer, J. Saxton, M. Habeych, and S. T. DeKosky. 2003. "Psychiatric Symptoms Vary with the Severity of Dementia in Probable Alzheimer's Disease." *Journal of Neuropsychiatry and Clinical Neurosciences* 15: 346–53.

Lyketsos, C. G., J.-M. E. Sheppard, and P. V. Rabins. 2000. "Dementia in Elderly Persons in a General Hospital." *American Journal of Psychiatry* 157: 704–7.

McFalls, A. J., Jr. 1998. "Population: A Lively Introduction, Third Edition." *Population Bulletin* 53 (3): 1–48.

McKhann, G., D. Drachman, M. Folstein, R. Katzman, D. Price, and E. M. Stadlan. 1984. "Clinical Diagnosis of Alzheimer's Disease: Report of the NINCDS-ADRDA Work Group Under the Auspices of the Department of Health and Human Services Task Force on Alzheimer's Disease." *Neurology* 34: 939–44.

Meyer, M. R., J. T. Tschanz, M. C. Norton, K. A. Welsh-Bohmer, D. C. Steffens, B. W. Wyse, and J. C. Breitner. 1998. "APOE Genotype Predicts When—Not Whether—One Is Predisposed to Develop

Alzheimer Disease." *Nature Genetics* 19: 321–22.

Miech, R. A., J. C. S. Breitner, P. P. Zandi, A. S. Khachaturian, J. C. Anthony, and L. Mayer for the Cache County Study Group. 2002. "Incidence of AD May Decline in the Early 90s for Men, Later for Women." *Neurology* 58: 209–18.

Miniño, A. M., M. P. Heron, S. L. Murphy, and K. D. Kochanek. 2007. "Deaths: Final Data for 2004." In *National Vital Statistics Reports,* vol. 55, no. 19. Hyattsville, MD: National Center for Health Statistics.

Mirra, S. S., A. Heyman, D. McKeel, S. M. Sumi, B. J. Crain, L. M. Brownlee, F. S. Vogel, J. P. Hughes, G. van Belle, L. Berg, and participating CERAD neuropathologists. 1991. "The Consortium to Establish a Registry for Alzheimer's Disease (CERAD). Part II. Standardization of the Neuropathologic Assessment of Alzheimer's Disease." *Neurology* 41: 479–86.

Morris, R. G., L. W. Morris, and P. G. Britton. 1998. "Factors Affecting the Emotional Well-Being of Caregivers of Dementia Sufferers." *British Journal of Psychiatry* 153: 147–56.

Nasreddine, Z. S., N. A. Phillips, V. Bédirian, S. Charbonneau, V. Whitehead, I. Collin, J. L. Cummings, and H. Chertkow. 2005. "The Montreal Cognitive Assessment (MoCA): A Brief Screening Tool for Mild Cognitive Impairment." *Journal of the American Geriatrics Society* 53: 695–99.

National Institute on Aging. 2007. "Alzheimer's Disease: Symptoms and Diagnosis." [Online information; retrieved 10/30/07.] http://nihseniorhealth.gov/alzheimersdisease/symptoms/01.html.

Omran, A. R. 1971. "The Epidemiologic Transition: A Theory of the Epidemiology of Population Change." *Milbank Memorial Fund Quarterly* 49: 509–38.

Ory, M. G., R. R. Hoffman, J. L. Yee, S. Tennstedt, and R. Schulz. 1999. "Prevealence and Impact of Caregiving: A Detailed Comparison Between Dementia and Nondementia Caregivers." *Gerontologist* 39: 177–85.

Østbye, T., S. Tyas, I. McDowell, and J. Koval. 1997. "Reported Activities of Daily Living: Agreement Between Elderly Subjects With and Without Dementia and Their Caregivers." *Age and Ageing* 26 (2): 99–106.

Patterson, C., W. B. Dalziel, B. J. Goldlist, and J. A. H. Puxty. 1992. "Geriatric Medicine in Ontario: Manpower Predictions on a Delphi Consensus Survey." *Annals of the Royal College of Physicians and Surgeons of Canada* 25: 99–102.

Post, S. G, P. J. Whitehouse, R. H. Binstock, T. D. Bird, S. K. Eckert, L. A. Farrer, L. M. Fleck, A. D. Gaines, E. T. Juengst, H. Karlinsky, S. Miles, T. H. Murray, K. A. Quaid, N. R. Relkin, A. D. Roses, P. H. St. George-Hyslop, G. A. Sachs, B. Steinbock, E. F. Truschke, and A. B. Zinn. 1997. "The Clinical Introduction of Genetic Testing for Alzheimer Disease. An Ethical Perspective." *Journal of the American*

Medical Association 277: 832–36.

Redinbaugh, E. M., R. C. McCallum, and J. K. Kiecolt-Glaser. 1995. "Recurrent Syndromal Depression in Caregivers." *Psychology & Aging* 10: 358–68.

Robillard, A. 2007. "Clinical Diagnosis of Dementia." *Alzheimer's & Dementia* 3: 292–98.

Schipper, H. M. 2007. "The Role of Biologic Markers in the Diagnosis of Alzheimer's Disease." *Alzheimer's & Dementia* 3: 325–32.

Schulz, R., A. T. O'Brien, J. Bookwala, and K. Flessiner. 1995. "Psychiatric and Physical Morbidity Effects of Dementia Caregiving: Prevalence, Correlates, and Causes." *Gerontologist* 35: 771–91.

Snowdon, D. A., S. J. Kemper, J. A. Mortimer, L. H. Greiner, D. R. Wekstein, and W. R. Markesbery. 1996. "Linguistic Ability in Early Life and Cognitive Function and Alzheimer's Disease in Late Life: Findings from the Nun Study." *Journal of the American Medical Association* 275: 528–32.

Sternberg, S. A., C. Wolfson, and M. Baumgarten. 2000. "Undetected Dementia in Community-Dwelling Older People: The Canadian Study of Health and Aging." *Journal of the American Geriatrics Society* 48: 1430–34.

Thomas, P., P. Ingrand, F. Lalloue, C. Hazif-Thomas, R. Billon, F. Viéban, and J. P. Clément. 2004. "Reasons of Informal Caregivers for Institutionalising Dementia Patients Previously Living at Home: The Pixel Study." *International Journal of Geriatric Psychiatry* 19: 127–35.

Torrible, S. J., L. L. Diachun, D. B. Rolfson, A. C. Dumbrell, and D. B. Hogan. 2006. "Improving Recruitment into Geriatric Medicine in Canada: Findings and Recommendations from the Geriatric Recruitment Issues Study." *Journal of the American Geriatrics Society* 54: 1453–62.

Tyas, S. L., J. C. Salazar, D. A. Snowdon, M. F. Desrosiers, K. P. Riley, M. S. Mendiondo, and R. J. Kryscio. 2007. "Transitions to Mild Cognitive Impairment, Dementia and Death: Findings from the Nun Study." *American Journal of Epidemiology* 165: 1231–38.

Tyas, S. L., R. B. Tate, K. Wooldrage, J. Manfreda, and L. A. Strain. 2006. "Estimating the Incidence of Dementia: The Impact of Adjusting for Subject Attrition Using Health Care Utilization Data." *Annals of Epidemiology* 16: 477–84.

University of Albany School of Public Health. 2007. "Alzheimer's Disease: A Public Health Update." [Online information; retrieved 11/29/07.] http://www.albany.edu/sph/coned/t2b2alzheimers.htm.

U.S. Preventive Services Task Force. n.d. "Recommendations and Rationale. Screening for Dementia." [Online information; retrieved 11/25/07.] http://www.ahrq.gov/clinic/3rduspstf/dementia/dementrr.htm.

Wilson, R. S., C. F. Mendes de Leon, L. L. Barnes, J. A. Schneider, J. L.

Bienias, D. A. Evans, and D. A. Bennett. 2002. "Participation in Cognitively Stimulating Activities and Risk of Incident Alzheimer Disease." *Journal of the American Medical Association* 287: 742–48.

Wimo, A., B. Winblad, and L. Jonsson. 2007. "An Estimate of the Total Worldwide Societal Costs of Dementia in 2005." *Alzheimer's & Dementia* 3: 81–91.

Wolfson, C., D. B. Wolfson, M. Asgharian, C. E. M'Lan, T. Østbye, K. Rockwood, and D. B. Hogan, for the Clinical Progression of Dementia Study Group. 2001. "A Reevaluation of the Duration of Survival After the Onset of Dementia." *New England Journal of Medicine* 344: 1111–16.

Yaffe, K., P. Fox, R. Newcomer, L. Sands, K. Lindquist, K. Dane, and K. E. Covinsky. 2002. "Patient and Caregiver Characteristics and Nursing Home Placement in Patients with Dementia." *Journal of the American Medical Association* 287: 2090–97.

Yukawa, M., E. B. Larson, and M.-F. Shadlen. 2000. "Diagnosing Dementia in Elderly Women: How to Detect and Determine Type." *Women's Health in Primary Care* 3: 245–60.

INDEX

ABOUT THE AUTHOR

STEVE FLEMING is an associate professor in the College of Public Health at the University of Kentucky, with appointments in both the departments of epidemiology and health services management. Professor Fleming has masters degrees in public administration (University of Hartford) and applied economics (University of Michigan). He also earned a Ph.D. in health services organization and policy from the University of Michigan, where he had the privilege of having Dr. Avedis Donabedian as a member of his dissertation committee. He teaches introductory and advanced epidemiology, managerial epidemiology, and cancer epidemiology. His primary research interest is in the area of cancer epidemiology, and he is particularly interested in the impact of comorbid illness on cancer diagnosis and treatment. Professor Fleming has published numerous articles in the health services research and epidemiology literature, in such journals as *Medical Care*, *Journal of Clinical Epidemiology*, *Inquiry*, *Health Care Management Review*, and *Medical Care Review*.

ABOUT THE CONTRIBUTORS

KEITH E. BOLES, PH.D, is an associate professor emeritus of health services finance in the Department of Health Management and Informatics at the University of Missouri in Columbia. He earned his doctorate in economics from the University of Arizona, and he holds a master's in economics from Florida Atlantic University. His major area of research is in risk evaluation and management in a managed care environment.

STEVEN R. BROWNING, PH.D., is an assistant professor in the Department of Epidemiology, College of Public Health, University of Kentucky. Prior to becoming a faculty member in the College of Public Health, he was a faculty member in the Colleges of Medicine and Nursing at the University of Kentucky (1994–2005). Professor Browning's research interests are in cardiovascular, environmental, and occupational epidemiology. Dr. Browning teaches graduate-level courses in advanced epidemiologic methods and cardiovascular epidemiology.

GLYN G. CALDWELL, M.D., is a part-time associate professor and vice-chairman of the Department of Epidemiology in the University of Kentucky College of Public Health. He teaches emerging and infectious disease epidemiology and the public health response to terrorism and disasters. He is currently the chairman of the faculty council of the college and a member of the University Pandemic Influenza Task Force. He serves on advisory committees for the Fatality Assessment Case Evaluation Project, the Integrated Core Injury Prevention Program, and the Kentucky Violent Death Reporting System, as well as the College Administrative Council, and Practice and Service Committee. He is a retired United States Public Health Service officer from the Centers for Disease Control and Prevention. He was the deputy director of the Arizona Department of Public Health, and the director of the Tulsa City County Health Department. He served as the state epidemiologist in both Arizona and Kentucky.

IRIS GUTMANIS, PH.D., is the director of evaluation and research, specialized geriatric services, St. Joseph's Health Centre London, Parkwood Hospital; an assistant professor in the Department of Epidemiology and Biostatistics, Schulich School of Medicine and Dentistry, University of

Western Ontario, London, Ontario; and an associate scientist, Aging, Rehabilitation and Geriatric Care Program, Lawson Health Research Institute, London, Ontario. Her current areas of research include geriatrics with a focus on measurement issues in this population, community capacity building, and knowledge exchange. Other research interests include population health surveillance, intimate partner violence, and infectious disease epidemiology. Funded through the Regional Geriatric Programs of Ontario, Dr. Gutmanis is currently working with local and provincial government agencies, as with well as researchers across Canada, on the development of senior-specific health indicators.

JOEL M. LEE, DR.P.H., holds the endowed position of University Professor of Health Services Management in the University of Kentucky College of Public Health. He has served in a variety of academic positions in the college, most recently as associate dean for academic affairs. He also has served as chair of the Department of Health Services Management and director of doctoral studies, and he has held positions in the university's undergraduate and graduate health administration programs. Dr. Lee has served on a number of association boards and advisory committees, including the Kentucky Hospital Association–affiliated Kentucky Health Care Strategy Forum, and as chair of the Association of University Programs in Health Administration, Healthcare Planning and Marketing Faculty Forum.

JOHN N. LEWIS, M.D., is the corporate medical director for Health Care Excel of Kentucky, Incorporated, where his current work is in the epidemiology of quality improvement in healthcare. He holds an MD from Johns Hopkins University and an MPH from Harvard University. He is certified by the American Board of Internal Medicine. His major areas of work have been in government public health practice and administration at the federal, state, and local levels; epidemiologic studies; and preventive medicine.

KATHLEEN MCDAVID, PH.D., has worked for more than 18 years in public health. She is currently a senior epidemiologist in the Division of HIV/AIDS Prevention in the U.S. Centers for Disease Control and Prevention, where she has worked for more than five years on surveillance issues related to women, risk-factor ascertainment and classification, socioeconomic status and relative survival, health disparities, data quality, and introduction and utilization of novel methodologies. Dr. McDavid spearheaded efforts to initiate a series of international patterns of care studies for breast, prostate, and colorectal cancers. She also served as a Peace Corps volunteer in Benin, West Africa. Dr. McDavid received her undergraduate degree from the University of Notre Dame and her master's of public health and doctorate in nutritional epidemiology from Tulane University.

KEVIN A. PEARCE, M.D., is the Michael Rankin Professor of Family and Community Medicine at the University of Kentucky (UK) College of Medicine. He is a faculty associate in the UK Center for Health Services Management and Research and holds a joint faculty appointment in the UK College of Public Health. He received his MD from the University of Florida College of Medicine and completed his residency in family practice at the Medical College of Virginia/Fairfax Hospital. He earned his MPH in epidemiology at the University of Minnesota School of Public Health. Dr. Pearce practices family medicine while pursuing his interests in medical education, practice-based research, clinical epidemiology, and evidence-based medicine.

MARY KAY RAYENS, PH.D., is an associate professor in the colleges of nursing and public health at the University of Kentucky. She earned a doctorate in statistics from the University of Kentucky. Her research interests include the design and analysis of longitudinal studies, tobacco policy research, and women's mental health.

F. DOUGLAS SCUTCHFIELD, M.D., is the Peter P. Bosomworth Professor of health services research and policy and professor of preventive medicine and environmental health at the University of Kentucky. He holds an MD from the University of Kentucky. His major areas of research are public health practice and administration, managed care, and preventive services, all areas in which he has published widely. He is editor of the *Journal of Preventive Medicine* and several textbooks on public health.

THOMAS C. TUCKER is chair of the Department of Epidemiology at the University of Kentucky College of Public Health. He is the associate director for cancer control and the senior director for cancer surveillance at the University of Kentucky Markey Cancer Center. Professor Tucker is a past president of the North American Association of Central Cancer Registries. He teaches courses in epidemiology, and he has published extensively in the cancer surveillance literature. His major research interests include cancer epidemiology, social factors associated with differing patterns of cancer care, and geographic variations in the burden of cancer.

SUZANNE L. TYAS, PH.D., is an associate professor in the Department of Health Studies and Gerontology and in the Department of Psychology at the University of Waterloo in Canada. She holds a Ph.D. in epidemiology and biostatistics and teaches courses in epidemiologic methods and the epidemiology of aging. Her research interests encompass Alzheimer's disease, cognitive reserve, and healthy aging. Dr. Tyas has been published in major scientific journals and has presented her research at scientific conferences throughout North America, Europe, and Asia.